Pathophysiology of pregnancy complications

W0043214

L.L.H. Peeters
P.W. de Leeuw
E.D. Post Uiterweer

Pathophysiology of pregnancy complications

Roadmap to early prediction and prevention

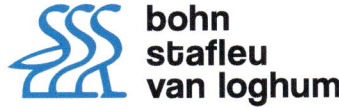

Houten 2021

L.L.H. Peeters
Utrecht, The Netherlands

E.D. Post Uiterweer
Gynecology & Obstetrics
University Medical Center Utrecht
Utrecht, The Netherlands

P.W. de Leeuw
Internal Medicine
Maastricht University Medical Center
Maastricht, The Netherlands

ISBN 978-90-368-2570-2   ISBN 978-90-368-2571-9   (eBook)
https://doi.org/10.1007/978-90-368-2571-9

NUR 876
Cover design: Studio Bassa, Culemborg
Full service vendor: Scientific Publishing Services (P), Ltd., Chennai, India

Bohn Stafleu van Loghum
Walmolen 1
Postbus 246
3990 GA Houten

www.bsl.nl

Preface Louis Peeters, MD, PhD

Pregnancy induces adaptations in maternal physiology to create the proper conditions for organogenesis and growth of the conceptus within the uterus. These adaptations ensure that the conceptus (1) has an adequate supply of O_2 and nutrients, (2) has the ability to discard metabolic waste products and (3) experiences the best possible protection against external stressors. The placenta orchestrates these adaptations in maternal physiology, with the changes in the cardiovascular function, volume regulation, metabolism and immune function having a large impact on the course of pregnancy and its outcome. Occasionally, these adaptations lead to complaints, like e.g. fatigue, nausea, heartburn, constipation and shortness of breath. Only in a small number of cases such nuisances represent early signs of a developing pregnancy complication.

This book aims to use current insights into the physiologic adaptations to pregnancy as a reference for early detection of pathophysiologic events that may complicate pregnancy. This information is expected to (1) ameliorate counseling of women that experience new-onset symptoms in the course of their pregnancy, (2) facilitate early identification of a developing relevant complication, and (3) increase self-confidence in pregnant women by explaining context and relevance of specific complaints and how these can be distinguished from early signs of a relevant pregnancy complication.

The *first chapter* elaborates on the normal physiologic adaptation to pregnancy. The *second chapter* describes the pathophysiology of common pregnancy complications in healthy women. The *third chapter* discusses the impact on pregnancy of a preexisting condition that undermines the functional reserve capacity of the maternal cardiovascular-, renal-, metabolic- and/or immune systems. The *fourth chapter* describes the effect on pregnancy of a preexistent condition that affects the functional reserve capacity of other organ systems. The *fifth and last chapter* elaborates on how our current insight in pregnancy (patho)physiology can be used to prevent, or at least early detect common pregnancy complications.

Foreword by Eric Steegers, MD, PhD

Providing good clinical care to pregnant women is totally dependent on a thorough understanding of the physiological changes in normal pregnancy and resulting from this of the pathophysiology of pregnancy complications. Only then new preventive and therapeutic modalities can be developed for obstetrical syndromes and gestational diseases like preeclampsia and placenta related fetal growth restriction. New insights in gestational physiology should not only have a direct hearing on clinical practice but also on related research as this is key to the correct interpretation of results of studies in pregnancy.

Up to the fifties in the last century, however, 'maternal physiology in pregnancy' was a much neglected research area with hardly any knowledge of the profound gestational physiological changes. In daily practice, pregnancy was often regarded by obstetricians as a pathologic medical state with life-threatening complications.

The Physiology of Human Pregnancy, a classic book by Frank Hytten and Isabella Leitch, was published in 1964. It systematically explained for the first time that there is no system in the body that does not show major physiological changes during pregnancy. The same holds true for the additional changes during labour and the subsequent puerperium during which short period most of the gestational changes are strikingly being reversed to a seemingly normal non-pregnant state. The book, and its successors, acted as a huge stimulus for the study of 'maternal physiology in pregnancy'. It also marked the beginning of the understanding of the fetal a maternal consequences of pathophysiological maternal adaptation to pregnancy which had been virtually nonexistent.

Although gestational physiological changes during pregnancy are generally beneficial to the mother and fetal growth and development in particular, they may also pose considerable risks in chronic conditions like maternal congenital heart defects. Maternal adaptive changes may often only mimic abnormality, but at the same time can result in overt clinical pathology in some patients. Risks can only be properly recognized and managed with a basic understanding of physiological and pathophysiological processes involved.

Many standard textbooks on Reproduction and Obstetrics, however, provide only limited information on physiology and pathophysiology. Louis Peeters (an obstetrician), Peter de Leeuw (an internist) and Emiel Post Uiterweer (a resident in Obstetrics and Gynaecology) have put together this textbook entitled *Pathophysiology in pregnancy* providing a unique and admirable overview of the physiology of pregnancy and the pathophysiology of common pregnancy complications. The book is abundantly and attractively illustrated. It is clearly written with reference to daily clinical practice, guiding us to improved early prediction and prevention in particular. Feedback on preliminary drafts of the text and figures was provided by a panel of experts.

Its strong conceptual framework will help in bridging the domains of clinical medicine and science. Patient care can only improve by the continuous vice versa interactions between fundamental, translational and clinical science on the one hand and daily clinical practice on the other. Although this book is not primarily focused on the management of pregnancy complications, I am convinced that it will really benefit clinical obstetric practice. It will prove popular both with scientific and clinical obstetric and midwifery junior and senior staff training and working in the field of reproduction and obstetrics. This also includes other physicians caring for pregnant women such as those working in the multidisciplinary field of *Obstetric Medicine* like internists, cardiologists and anesthesiologists. The composition of this editorial team fully matches the intellectual challenges to compile such a book, bringing in their individual extensive knowledge and creativity.

Human reproduction and obstetrics nowadays are at the center of the life course approach in medicine. This book makes a great contribution to the wellbeing and health of women during pregnancy, and in doing so to women's health in later life, as well as to that of their children before and after birth. I expect that this textbook will again result in a further upsurge of interest in the further study of 'maternal physiology in pregnancy' as did Hytten and Leitch's book in 1964.

Eric Steegers, MD, PhD
Department of Obstetrics and Gynaecology, Medical Chair of the Sophia Children's Hospital, Erasmus MC, Rotterdam, The Netherlands

Foreword by Basky Thilaganathan MD, PhD, FRCOG

It is a great honour to write the foreword for this book by Louis Peeters. I have known Louis for many years as an obstetrician who has dedicated his scientific career to the study of maternal physiology in both normal and pathological pregnancy. He is acknowledged as the pioneer in the field of maternal hemodynamic maladaptation in preeclampsia and modern approaches to the safer cardiovascular management of this condition. Louis Peeters started his specialist medical career in 1974 with a fellowship at the University of Colorado, Denver and has since worked in Nijmegen, Erasmus University of Rotterdam, MUMC Maastricht and UMC Utrecht. He retired from active clinical duty in 2013, but has continued to work in education and research in an academic career spanning nearly 50 years during which he has published over 150 scientific articles and numerous book chapters.

The belief that abnormal placentation causes preeclampsia and fetal growth restriction has been championed for several decades – to the extent that they are collectively referred to as "placental syndromes". However, consistent and emerging evidence suggests otherwise, especially for late-onset disorders which constitute the majority of cases. The inconsistencies with the placental origins' hypothesis have been attributed to disease heterogeneity or explained as the maternal form of the disorders. These are neither adequate nor actual explanations of causality. In the fabulously illustrated book on maternal pregnancy physiology, not only does Louis update our knowledge in this field to a better understanding of the profound physiological changes, but also explains how limits of maternal adaptation play a role in the pathophysiology of pregnancy disorders. Forming a better understanding of maternal physiology of placental syndromes is critical for the development of accurate diagnostic aids, improved screening, better triage by disease severity and offering targeted preventative and therapeutic measures. This book provides a state-of-the-art narrative to inform students of physiology, clinicians and researchers interested in this field.

Basky Thilaganathan MD PhD FRCOG
Director, Fetal Medicine Unit, St Georges University Hospitals NHS Foundation Trust, London UK.
E: basky.thilaganathan@nhs.net | T: +44 (0) 20 8725 0072

Clinical Director, Tommy's National Centre for Maternity Improvement, Royal College of Obstetrics and Gynaecology, London UK.
E: bthilaganathan@rcog.org.uk | T: +44 (0) 20 7772 6217 | W: ► www.rcog.org.uk

Acknowledgments

The first author (LP) prepared the first version of the text. The second author (PdL) assisted in revising and upgrading the final version of the sections involving chronic medical disorders. The third author (EPU) upgraded and supervised the preparation of the many illustrations in the book that were carried out by a professional design office.

The following colleagues contributed to the quality of the book by **upgrading text/content**: *Hans Duvekot* (Obstetrician and MFM specialist, Erasmus Medical Center, Erasmus University, Rotterdam, the Netherlands) organized and interviewed eight former patients, who had experienced a common pregnancy complication. This has resulted in eight video's, illustrating the emotions and experiences of the patients, during and after their complicated pregnancies. These video's are available online and can be accessed using a personalized code. *Gerrit Schreij* (Internal Medicine Specialist, specializing in infectious diseases, University of Maastricht, The Netherlands) assisted in preparing certain sections of the text in ▶ chaps. 3 and 4. *Bert Kaufmann* (pharmacist, Tweestedenziekenhuis, Tilburg, The Netherlands) provided valuable input in preparing the final section of ▶ chap. 4, that describes the effect of pregnancy on pharmacokinetics. *Régina Steegers-Theunissen* (Professor in Periconception Epidemiology, Erasmus University, Rotterdam, The Netherlands) gave valuable suggestions to upgrade and optimize ▶ chap. 5.

Completion of this book in its current form would not have been possible without the assistance of the following **fact checkers**, who critically reviewed the revised manuscript: *Larry Burd*, Professor in Maternal Fetal Medicine (MFM), University of Illinois, Chicago, USA; *Eric Steegers*, Professor in Obstetrics/MFM, Erasmus University in Rotterdam, the Netherlands, and *Marc Spaanderman*, Professor in Obstetrics/MFM, University of Maastricht, the Netherlands.

Finally, *Saul Gallagher* (English reader) carefully checked the manuscript for misspellings and grammatical flaws in the English language and optimized the final version of the text.

Supplementary online materials

You have unlimited access to the online version of this book including comprehensive abstracts of the five chapters and eight online interviews with former patients with either a history of a major pregnancy complication or who were at increased risk during their pregnancy because of some preexistent medical condition requiring specialized pregnancy care.

The interviews

The interviews (on video) with former patients were organized by **Hans Duvekot MD, PhD**, obstetrician at the Erasmus Medical Center in Rotterdam. The interviews (in Dutch, subtitled in English) were recorded in the BSL studio in Utrecht, the Netherlands. The topics being addressed during these interviews consisted of each patient's personal experiences related to the clinical impact of the pregnancy complication and to the concomitant communication with care providers involved in the clinical management. Pregnancy complications that were addressed were (1) (pre-) eclampsia, (2) Acute Fatty Liver of Pregnancy, (3) severe fetal growth restriction caused by placental insufficiency, (4) severe preterm birth (birth < 30 weeks), (5) gestational diabetes, (6) severe hemorrhage during childbirth due to placenta percreta, resulting in shock and ischemic CVA (7) pregnancy in a woman with trauma-induced paraplegia and (8) pregnancy in a woman with a chronic neurologic muscular disorder (Limb Gridle Dystrophy II).

To obtain access to the interviews on Mijn BSL use the activation code you can find in the back matter of the book.

Contents

Curriculum vitae of the authors

Louis Peeters
performed his PhD studies in Fetal and Maternal Medicine in Denver, Colorado, USA (1974–1976, resulting in the 'cum laude' defense of his PhD-thesis in 1978). He did his Residency training in Obstetrics and Gynecology at the University of Nijmegen (1976–1981) and started his professional career in 1981 as a post-doctoral fellow at the Erasmus University in Rotterdam, Department of Obstetrics, exploring the basic principles of the maternal adaptation to pregnancy. In 1987, he continued his career as an Associate Professor in Obstetrics at the Maastricht University Medical Center, Department of Obstetrics & Gynecology, where he combined a clinical appointment (high-risk Obstetrics) with an appointment in research (exploring the mechanisms of normal and defective maternal adaptation to pregnancy). Until his retirement in 2013, he had his own research group and accommodated/supervised many PhD projects resulting in the publication of a wide range of scientific articles, reviews and contributions to textbooks. The final two years of his professional career, he performed his clinical duties, teaching and research, both at the University Medical Centers of Maastricht and Utrecht.

Peter de Leeuw
was trained in Internal Medicine at the Zuiderziekenhuis in Rotterdam. He defended his PhD thesis at the Erasmus University in Rotterdam in 1978. Afterwards, he worked as a post-doctoral fellow at the Peter Bent Brigham Hospital and Harvard University in Boston. Upon his return to Rotterdam, he became head of the Hypertension Unit at the Zuiderziekenhuis in Rotterdam until his appointment as a Professor at the University of Maastricht. His research mainly focused on pathophysiological mechanisms in hypertension with special emphasis on the regulation of renal blood flow and renin secretion. In later years, fibromuscular dysplasia became an important part of his research work. He supervised many PhD students of whom several in collaboration with Louis Peeters. He published many scientific papers and prepared various contributions to textbooks. He has served on the Board of the International Society of Hypertension and was Editor-in-Chief of three Medical Journals.

Emiel Post Uiterweer
graduated from Medical School at Maastricht University in 2010. Afterwards, he did his PhD studies at the University of Utrecht and the University of Florida (Gainesville), exploring the maternal (uterine) immunovascular adaptations to pregnancy. After his PhD thesis defense in 2014, he worked as a post-doctoral fellow in Reproductive Immunology at the New York University. During this fellowship, he studied the immunologic events at the fetal-maternal interface, a project that was awarded a Rubicon grant by the Netherlands Organization for Scientific Research (NWO). After his return to the Netherlands in 2015, he started his residency training in Obstetrics and Gynecology at the University Medical Center of Utrecht and combined his clinical work with ongoing participation in research in the physiology and pathophysiology of human pregnancy. Throughout his still early career, he has designed medical artwork and logos for scientific publications, medical trials and conferences. He has served on the Board of the Society for Reproductive Investigation.

Hans Duvekot

performed his residency in Obstetrics and Gynecology at the Maastricht University Medical Center, Department of Obstetrics and Gynecology between 1988 and 1992. He defended his PhD thesis on the subject of early changes in maternal hemodynamics and volume homeostasis at the University of Maastricht. From 1992 until 2003, he started his professional career as a gynecologist in a secondary care hospital in Rotterdam. In 2003, he continued his career as an Assistant Professor in the Obstetrics at the Erasmus University Medical Center, Department of Obstetrics and Gynecology, in Rotterdam, where he combined his clinical appointment (high-risk Obstetrics) with research in clinical Obstetrics, with main focus being hypertensive disease in pregnancy and postpartum hemorrhage. He supervised many PhD students. Until 2020, he published over 200 scientific papers and contributed to various book chapters. Besides his regular work specified above, he performs several additional positions. He is chairman of the Dutch Gynecologic and Obstetric Guidelines Committee and is a member of the Dutch medical disciplinary committee.

Maternal adaptation to pregnancy

Abstract

The first chapter of this book describes the most important maternal adaptations to pregnancy. In the following three chapters, that information is used as a reference for the pathophysiology of common pregnancy disorders, that may develop in seemingly healthy women (▶ chap. 2), in women with a pre-existent chronic disorder that predisposes to these pregnancy complications (▶ chap. 3) and in women with a preexistent chronic disorder that does not directly predispose to these pregnancy complications (▶ chap. 4). Finally, ▶ chapter 5 discusses how the information on pathophysiology of pregnancy complications can be translated into strategies that enable early detection and/or prevention of these complications.

© Bohn Stafleu van Loghum is een imprint van Springer Media B.V., onderdeel van Springer Nature 2021
L. L. H. Peeters et al., *Pathophysiology of pregnancy complications*,
https://doi.org/10.1007/978-90-368-2571-9_1

1

Highlights

1. Development of immunotolerance towards the embryo is a key objective during implantation;
2. The formation of circulatory and metabolic buffers are key adaptations in early pregnancy. They enable the mother to meet the higher fetal demands in advanced pregnancy. These buffers are created by instituting a high-flow/low-resistance circulation and transient anabolism in the first half of pregnancy.
3. In the second half of pregnancy, these buffers are utilized by (a) redirecting the redundant shunt flow generated by the hyperdynamic circulation, to the uterus, and (b) mobilizing nutrients from the expanded energy stores to be preferentially supplied to the fetus by creating a state of normoglycemic insulin resistance;
4. Labor is triggered by the combination of (a) a fall in the progesterone/estradiol ratio, that results from fetal maturation, and (b) a rise in inflammatory mediators in the cervix and uterus, that accompany both the aging of the placenta and membranes and the concomitant increasing myometrial stretch associated with the expanding intra-uterine content.

1.1 Pregnancy-induced changes in the maternal genital tract

The maternal adaptation to pregnancy begins about three days after fertilization with the arrival of the fertilized ovum in the uterine cavity. Uterine remodeling is probably one of the first structural changes, that results in the creation of a safe, stable and easy distensible environment perfectly fit for the unborn child to grow, mature and thrive during pregnancy. The pregnant uterus accommodates the growth of the fetus, the placenta and the amniotic fluid to their maximum volume of about 3500 grams, 600 grams and 400 mL, resp. It follows that in the course of pregnancy, the capacity of the uterine cavity is to expand gradually to almost 5 L. This expansion is paralleled by myometrial growth from 60 to about 1200 grams. Most of the uterus consists of smooth muscle tissue with some connective tissue, a vascular bed and a nervous supply. In the first half of pregnancy, uterine growth mostly results from myometrial hyperplasia. Afterwards, the uterus primarily grows by hypertrophy with the expanding uterine content increasingly imposing mechanical stretch upon the uterine wall. Myometrial growth is more rapid in the uterine fundus than in its corpus, which alters the uterine shape with advanced pregnancy. This explains the more caudal position of the round ligaments at term. Accommodation of the fetal head in the pelvic inlet in the third trimester implies that more stretch will be exerted upon the anterior- than on the posterior side of the lower uterine segment.

After the first trimester of pregnancy, the uterus exhibits sporadic, irregular, painless, tonic, so-called 'Braxton-Hicks' contractions. Unlike true labor, the duration, frequency and intensity of these contractions do not increase with advancing pregnancy. From time to time they also fade and may even disappear altogether, only to re-occur again days or weeks later. Towards term, these contractions tend to increase in frequency and intensity, though, without causing changes in cervical consistency and dilation. During active labor the uterine contractions evolve to a phasic, peristalsis-like pattern resembling that observed in the intestinal and urinary tracts (Young 2015). The myometrium contains so-called 'Cajal-cells' (Hutchings et al. 2009), that have pacemaker properties and can form an integrated unit of muscle cells and bundles resembling that in the GI tract. It is conceivable that these cells propagate peristalsis-like labor contractions, most likely starting in the fundus, pulling the fundus towards the birth canal like a squeezebox. A comprehensive description of normal labor is beyond the scope of this book but has been provided in various reviews on this topic (Liao et al. 2005; Kamel 2010; Hanson and VandeVusse 2014).

The cervix forms a safe barrier preventing ascending infections and – in pregnancy – protecting the conceptus against premature expulsion. The cervix is also capable of dilating during labor to enable childbirth. The importance of the cervical barrier function to avoid colonization is indirectly supported by the observation that preterm labor is often preceded by ascending infections from the vagina (Romero et al. 2014). The cervix consists of extracellular matrix (80 % collagen) along with smooth muscle tissue (15 %), most abundant in its upper half, where it encircles the endocervical canal like a sphincter (Vink et al. 2016). The cervical canal is about 4 cm long and connects the vagina with the uterine cavity. Its lining consists of cylindrical epithelium that produces bacteriostatic mucus. Prior to labor, the consistency of the cervix is firm, to soften up during the first stage of labor, due to collagen fragmentation followed by its dissolution, resembling an inflammatory response. The mechanism of the first two stages of labor has been described in detail in two excellent and comprehensive reports (Li et al. 2010; Cahill et al. 2013).

During pregnancy the external cervix becomes hyperemic causing a blueish/purple discoloring, as can be noted by speculum exam. In the past, this phenomenon, the so-called 'Chadwick's sign', served as an early sign of pregnancy. The hyperemia leads to more transudation and with it, more discharge. Even though pregnancy does not alter the vaginal bacterial flora appreciably, enhanced transudation raises the pH in the vagina and with it, reduces the vaginal protection against infections. This may explain the higher prevalence of vaginal candidiasis during pregnancy. Also, the fallopian tubes are more hyperemic and swollen during pregnancy, but without appreciable functional impact.

In a normal menstrual cycle, the follicle stimulating hormone (FSH) and luteinizing hormone (LH) from the pituitary gland regulate the maturation of the dominant ovum, enabling it to ovulate by day 14 of the menstrual cycle. After ovulation, the remnant of the ovulated follicle transforms into the corpus luteum (CL) and gradually develops into the primarily production source of progesterone and various other substances involved in the endometrial transformation from the proliferative into the secretory phase (Conrad et al. 2019). In the absence of conception, the natural lifespan of the CL is 10–12 days.

1.2 Local adjustments to secure implantation and early placentation

After conception, the fertilized ovum is picked up by the fallopian tube, while still covered by a zona pellucida shell. This cover protects the fertilized ovum against possible hostile influences, partly related to the immunologically different intra-fallopian environment. The fertilized ovum undergoes various mitotic divisions during its circa three-days lasting journey to the uterus, where it 'hatches', indicating that it loses its zona-pellucida cover (◘ fig. 1.1).

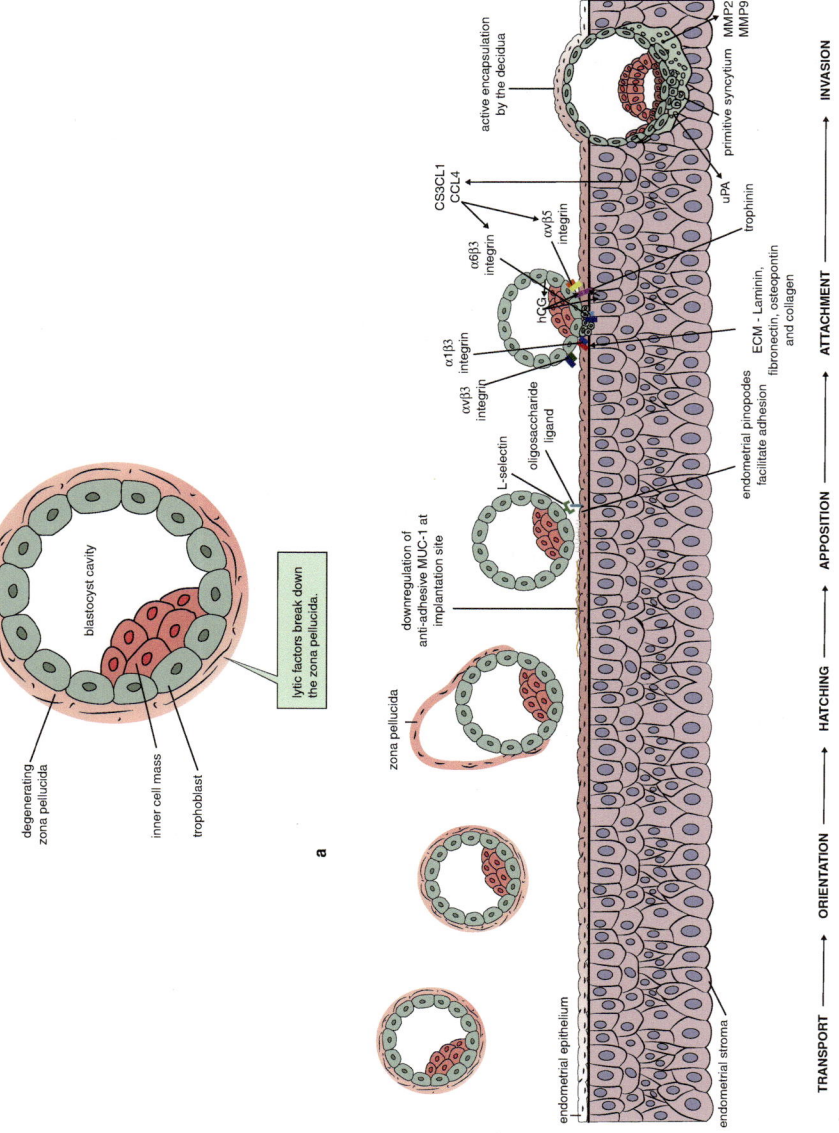

Figure 1.1 (a) Embryo (blastula) at arrival in the uterine cavity, with trophectoderm lining (green cells) and inner cell mass or embryoblast (red cells). (b) Sequence of events regulated through crosstalk between embryo and decidua by locally released chemokines, cytokines and hCG. These events evolve in a progesterone-dominated steroid environment, and eventually result in embryo implantation (*adopted from* Weimar et al, 2013)

Presumably, hatching shortly after blastocyst's arrival in the uterine cavity is important for two reasons. Firstly, the uptake of O_2 and nutrients from its surroundings by diffusion across the zona pellucida may no longer be sufficient to sustain growth and development of the blastula. Secondly, the blastula has differentiated into an inner cell mass (embryoblast), a cavity and an outer lining of trophectoderm capable of interacting with the endometrium. This interaction synchronizes their mutual development and promotes the selection of a suitable implantation site. The concomitant endometrial development consists of 'decidualization', which refers to the preparation of a receptive state for embryo implantation. Decidualization is a process, controlled by progesterone, cAMP and various transcription factors. It includes changes in the phenotype of the endometrial stromal cells (Okada et al. 2018; Liu et al. 2020) with influx of a wide range of immune cells (Solano 2019). Decidualization transforms the endometrium into an immunotolerant state, which is crucial for embryo implantation. The initial steps of this process also occur in an ovulatory cycle without conception, but the 'finishing touch' requires crosstalk between preimplantation embryo and endometrium as shown in ◘ fig. 1.1 (Gellersen et al. 2007, 2014; Craciunas et al. 2019). During decidualization, natural killer (NK) cells accumulate around the decidual spiral arteries, where they interact with decidual stromal cells, which then induce their differentiation into uterine NK (uNK) cells with a typical immunotolerant, growth-promoting and anti-killing phenotype, pivotal during embryo implantation (◘ fig. 1.2).

From an immunological point of view, the decidualized endometrium in reproduction has unique properties, because of its ability to harbor highly specialized, active leukocyte populations, such as uNK cells, that have properties found nowhere else other than in the pregnant uterus. In addition, the decidua is restrictive with respect to the

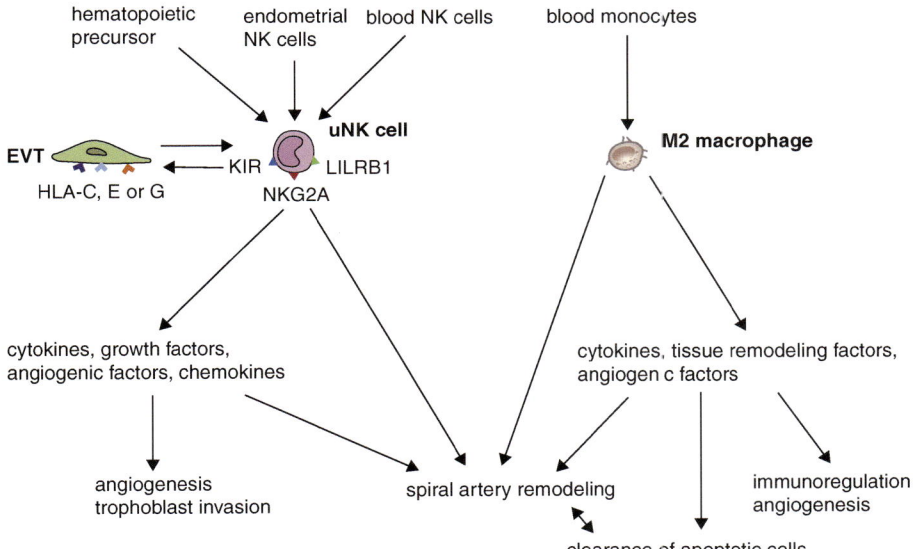

◘ **Figure 1.2** Diagram illustrating how invading extravillous trophoblasts (EVT) cells activate uterine NK (uNK) cells to become instrumental in spiral artery (SA) remodeling. uNK cell activation coincides with M2 macrophages recruitment, that are involved in both spiral artery remodeling and the removal of the tissue debris generated during SA remodeling (*adopted from* Faas et al. 2017)

1

entrance and accumulation of other immune cell types (Erlebacher 2013). It appears that the maternal immune tolerance is entirely restricted to the decidua at the fetal-maternal (F-M) interface (Deryabin et al. 2019) with no concomitant functional changes of the maternal innate immune system elsewhere in the body or of the adaptive immune system. It is a unique process only observed in mammalian pregnancy and has negligible impact on the maternal immune response to exogenous pathogens as recently reviewed (Racicot et al. 2014; Bonney 2016).

During implantation and early placentation, uNKs play a key role by their interaction with invading extravillous trophoblast cells (EVTs) (Moffett et al. 2014; Tessier et al. 2015), which enables EVTs to remodel the uterine spiral arteries (■ fig. 1.3) (Tessier et al. 2015; Ander et al.2019; Harris et al. 2011, 2019).

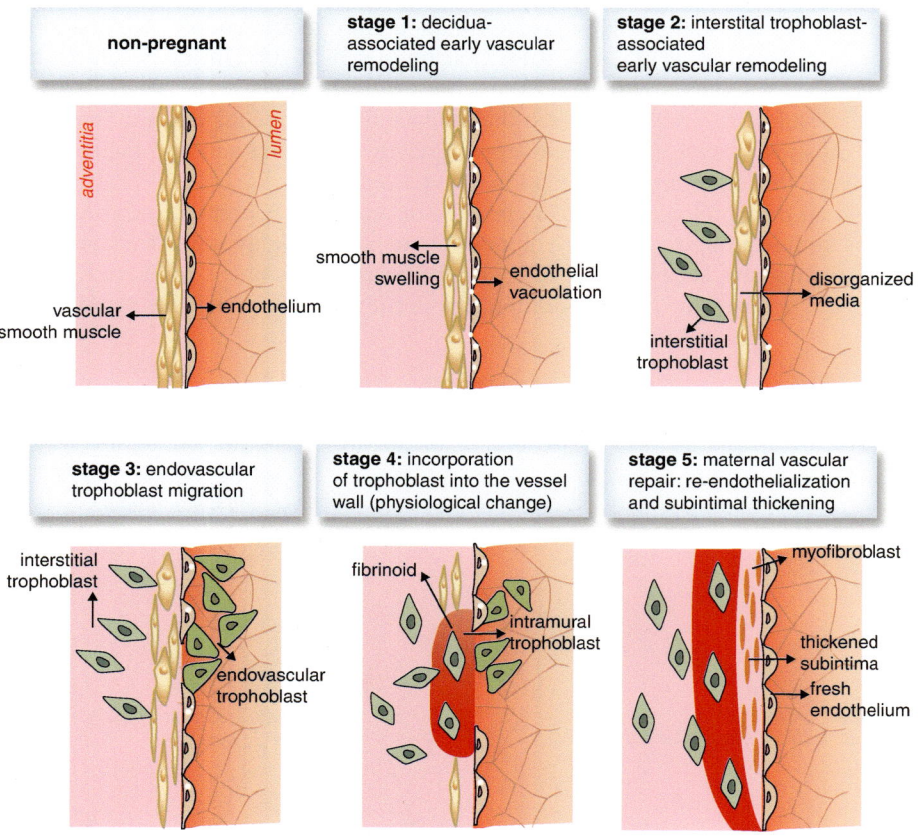

■ **Figure 1.3**   Presumed steps in spiral artery (SA) remodeling. Spiral artery structure in the non-pregnant state; Decidual natural killer (uNK) cells trigger both vacuolization of endothelial cells and swelling of vascular smooth muscle cells (VSMCs) (**stage 1**); Invading interstitial extravillous trophoblast cells (EVTs) cause disorganization of VSMCs (**stage 2**); Endovascular EVTs also invade the SA along the endothelial lining, thus becoming involved in SA remodeling (**stage 3**); Fibrinoid replaces the VSMC layer, EVT cells are embedded intramurally within this layer (**stage 4**); Reendothelialization, occasionally accompanied by the appearance of subintimal cushions containing α-actin immunopositive myofibroblasts (**stage 5**).

Shortly after implantation, the amount of human chorionic gonadotrophin (hCG), released by trophoblast cells, that reaches the maternal blood stream (by diffusion) increases rapidly and with it, the likelihood of emerging systemic effects, most importantly, the rescue of CL function to prolong its lifespan by about five weeks. This effect allows the primitive placenta to reach sufficient capacity to take over the steroid production. This transition – the 'luteo-placental shift' – occurs at about 8 weeks amenorrhea.

About 70 % of the decidual leukocytes are uNK cells, with the remainder consisting of macrophages ($\pm$ 20 %), T-regulatory cells ($\pm$ 10 %) and dendritic cells (DCs, $\pm$ 1 %) (Erlebacher 2013). The role of decidual macrophages has only been partly elucidated. These cells not only contribute to spiral artery remodeling. They are also involved in the removal of apoptotic debris accumulated locally during spiral artery remodeling. At term, the macrophages may also contribute to the initiation of labor by activating inflammatory pathways. The role of the sparsely present DCs is still unclear. It is conceivable that their low density in the decidua minimizes their normal role of providing immune surveillance, and that the few DCs that are present, are just remnants of the endometrium from the time of implantation, when they surveyed the uterine mucosa for pathogens.

The depth of spiral artery remodeling is closely regulated as indicated by its sharp cut-off in the myometrial portion of the spiral artery, proximal to the decidual-myometrial junction and just distal of the arteriovenous (a-v) shunts, that are located at a level that corresponds with the outer one-third portion of the myometrium (■ fig. 1.4).

Spiral artery remodeling is accompanied by the formation of plugs in the arterial outlets made up of accumulated debris consisting of apoptotic cells andEVTs. These plugs (■ figs. 1.4 and 1.5) hinder the blood flow in the spiral arteries causing most of the blood stream to be redirected to the myometrial a-v shunts. Between 10- and 12-weeks pregnancy these plugs gradually dislodge, presumably due to pressure building up proximal

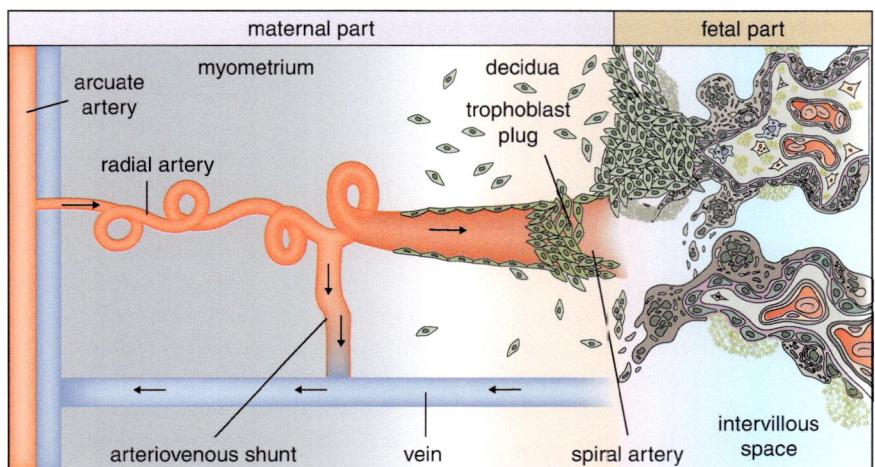

■ **Figure 1.4** Arteriovenous shunts prevent the upstream extravillous trophoblast invasion into the spiral arteries to infiltrate into the inner two-thirds of the myometrium proximal to the decidual-myometrial junction. The resulting stasis downstream to the shunts creates favorable conditions in the spiral artery outlets for the formation of trophoblast plugs, thus preventing maternal blood to reach the intervillous space until around 10-12 weeks pregnancy.

1

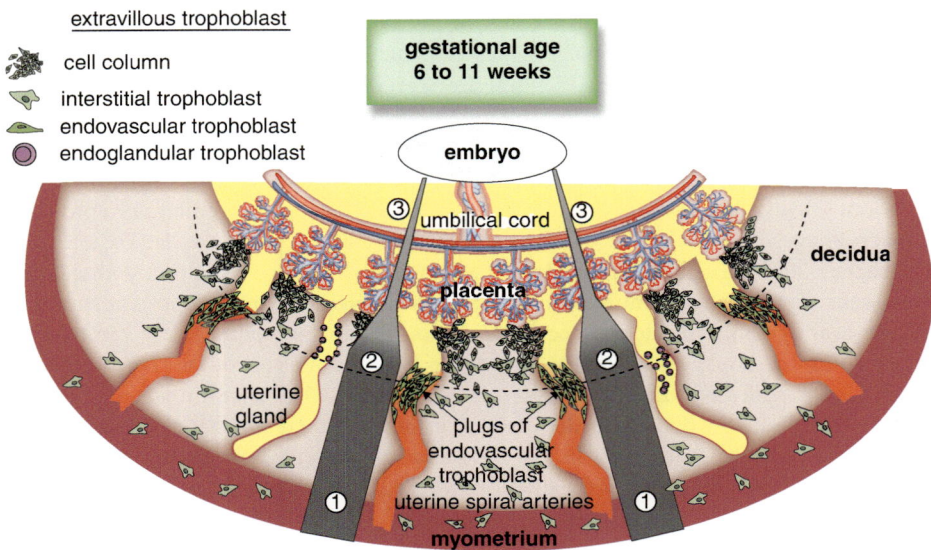

① stable oxygen from myometrium to decidua
② steep oxygen gradient from endovascular plugs to placenta
③ moderate oxygen gradient from placenta to embryo

▫ Figure 1.5 Schematic illustration of the invasion and differentiation of extravillous trophoblast cells (EVTs) into the decidua between ± 6 and around 11-weeks amenorrhea and how this process is regulated by the O_2 gradient [2]. Trophoblastic cell columns underneath the villi adhere the placenta to the decidua. They form the source of EVTs. Invasive interstitial EVTs leave the cell columns to invade and differentiate, partly into uterine glands and partly into the spiral arteries. The latter cells cluster with locally generated cell debris into plugs that prevent maternal blood of reaching the intervillous space (adapted from Huppertz et al. 2014)

to the plugs in conjunction with the rapidly increasing uterine blood flow, that gradually exceeds the draining capacity of the myometrial a-v shunts. These plugs differ from blood clots by being created differently, and without a key role for (sticky) fibrin formation. The latter may also explain their different behavior within a blood vessel (Weiss et al. 2016; James et al. 2018), e.g. indicated by their loose attachment to the vessel wall and their ability to allow plasma to seep through to the intervillous space.

The absence of maternal blood flow in the intervillous space, caused by the partial obstruction of the spiral arteries (until 10–12 weeks) creates an O_2 gradient perpendicular to the implantation site. This gradient is pivotal in regulating EVT proliferation, migration, invasion and differentiation, as these processes utilize the hypoxia-inducible-factor-1 (HIF-1) signalling pathway (Caniggia et al. 2002). These events evolve in a delicate, low-O_2 environment and in a pre-arranged order, indicating their vulnerability to disruption. For instance, disrupted EVT-related actions increase the risk of premature plug dislodgement, and with it, loss of the O_2 gradient. Such an event would be an extra setback of – in that case – the already compromised EVT actions and associated spiral artery remodeling (James et al. 2018). Premature unplugging also abolishes the early defence against excessive oxidative stress at the fetal-maternal interface (Burton et al. 2010).

Impaired spiral artery remodeling not only reduces the eventual placental blood flow capacity. It also raises the risk of mechanical damage of villous trophoblast later in pregnancy, as (partial) absence of trumpet-shaped remodeling spiral-artery outlets changes the blood flow properties within the intervillous space with a higher fraction of flow being turbulent, entering the intervillous space at a higher pressure and shear rate. These effects increase the risk of mechanical damage of free-floating villi (Roth et al. 2017). It follows, that EVT invasion is a tightly regulated process resulting in both the secure placental anchorage to the uterine wall and the stable placental access to maternal O_2 and nutrients (Von Rango et al. 2008).

The trophoblastic plugs in the spiral-artery outlets dislodge between 10 and 12 weeks. Until then, the nutrient and O_2 supply to the embryo is regulated by so-called 'histotrophic nutrition' as shown in ◘ fig. 1.6 (Burton et al. 2001). This unique form of nutrition consists of diffusion from the intervillous space to the vitelline microcirculation and occurs without direct transfer of O_2 and nutrients from the maternal blood. The fluid in the intervillous space consists of endometrial glandular secrete supplemented with maternal plasma seeping through the spiral-artery plugs.

Presumably, the contact of the embryo with maternal blood is postponed for two reasons. Firstly, to protect the vulnerable embryo against potentially toxic external influences, such as oxidative stress caused by free oxygen radicals. Secondly, the oxidative metabolism of the embryo is probably low, as the functional role of the immature embryonic tissues is still limited with most metabolic activity consisting of tissue growth and differentiation, an activity requiring only small amounts of ATP. In the first trimester of pregnancy, an important part of the embryonic metabolic functions that would require ATP, such as preserving body temperature and regulating the uptake and removal of nutrients, O_2 and waste products, are executed by the placenta and the mother.

1.3 Systemic adaptations in support of implantation and early placentation

1.3.1 Creating a progesterone-dominated endocrine environment

A progesterone-dominated endocrine environment generated by the CL, together with rapidly rising peripheral hCG levels produced by the trophoblast, are key for normal early placental development. Low levels of progesterone and/or hCG in the peri-implantation period predispose to implantation failure as progesterone is essential for the postovulatory transformation of the endometrium from the proliferative to the secretory phase, which is essential to enable decidualization. Progesterone also promotes myometrial quiescence, raises uterine blood flow and modulates the local immune function towards adopting an embryo-friendly profile (Druckmann and Druckmann 2005). Luteal insufficiency predisposes to implantation failure and/or spontaneous miscarriage. Besides preserving CL function, hCG is also involved in regulating implantation by promoting endometrial angiogenesis and enhancing trophoblast differentiation (Licht et al. 2007). After the 8th pregnancy week, the CL regresses, conveying most of its endocrine functions to the primitive placenta.

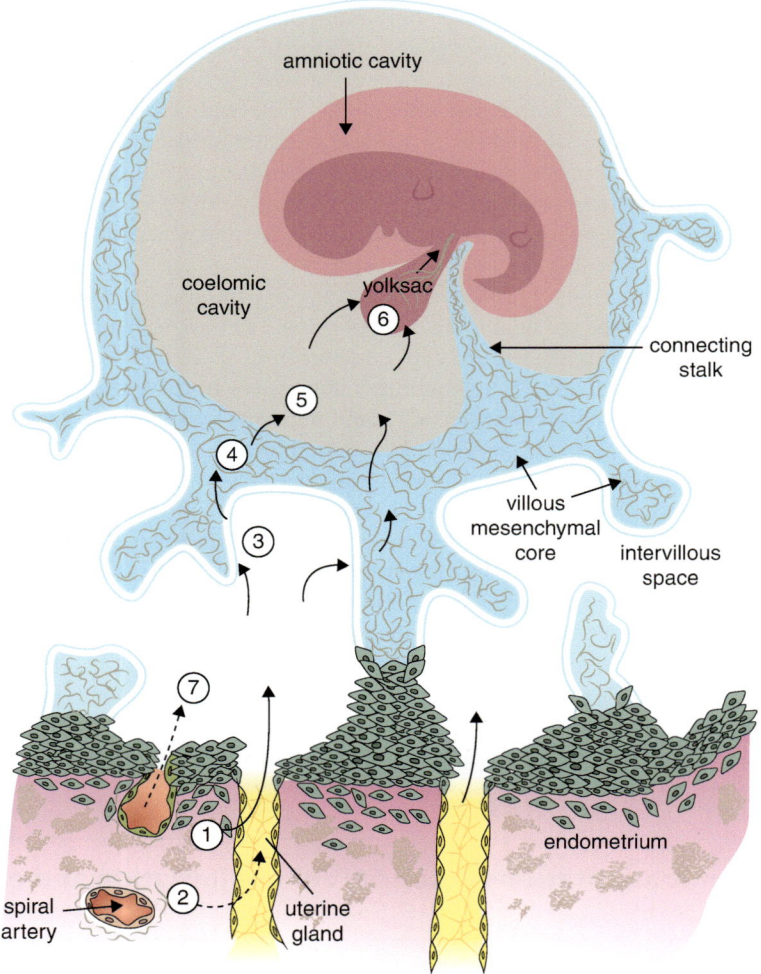

◘ Figure 1.6 Cartoon illustrating the histiotrophic nutrition of the human embryo. Secretions from the uterine glands into the intervillous space (arrows, 1, 2). This fluid is taken up and utilized by trophoblast, partially passed on to the villous mesenchymal core and diffused along stromal channels into the coelomic fluid (3, 4, 5). From here, this fluid may be absorbed by the epithelia of the yolk sac (6) and passed on to the embryo using the vitelline circulation. Presumably, the uterine secretions are supplemented by maternal serum transudate from the spiral arteries (7)

1.3.2 Mobilizing the functional reserves of the maternal cardiovascular system, kidneys and metabolism

Already by 5th pregnancy week, the trophoblast releases factors that induce systemic vasorelaxation, requiring a compensatory 30–40 % rise in cardiac output (CO) to prevent systemic blood pressure to fall. Insufficient cardiovascular reserves, but also insufficient renal and metabolic reserves, will trigger a stress response resulting in a rise in cardiovascular sympathetic tone and the adrenal release of catecholamines. This response induces the redistribution of CO in favor of heart and brain and at the expense of the so-called 'nonvital' organs, which also includes the uterus. Therefore, this stress response leads to a rise in uterine vascular resistance and with it, hampers early placental development. The functional reserve capacity of affected organ systems is often reduced in women with preexistent cardiovascular, renal and metabolic disorders. Obviously, this will also affect these women's capacity to adapt to pregnancy. These disorders are often associated with a higher risk of defective early placental development, as has been elaborated in ▶ chap. 3.

1.3.3 Utilizing the maternal ability to remove syncytiotrophoblast microvesicles (STBMs)

Subnormal maternal capacity to remove STBMs may trigger the development of late-onset PE in a healthy pregnant woman (Redman et al. 2012), particularly in women with a relatively large placenta, such as in multiple pregnancy, severe anemia, or when living at high altitude. In (advanced) normal pregnancy, the placenta sheds large amounts of STBMs (◘ fig. 1.7) into the maternal systemic circulation, usually without noticeable adverse effect on maternal health and wellbeing, because of their rapid clearance by the lungs (Redman et al. 2012). Yet, there are certain conditions in which these STBMs have developed toxic properties (◘ fig. 1.8) that may jeopardize maternal health. For instance, it is conceivable that unfavorable external factors may trigger a maternal stress response, as detailed earlier. This response reduces placental perfusion, and with it, increases oxidative stress in the intervillous space causing excessive placental release of these toxic STBMs thus inducing late-onset PS (detailed in ▶ chap. 2).

1.4 Role of the endocrine system during pregnancy

Maternal adaptation to pregnancy consists of (1) the timely preparation of endometrial receptivity to enable embryo implantation, (2) responding to hCG to preserve CL function long enough to support the early stages of placental development, (3) being able to respond to triggers from the conceptus, to adapt her organism in such a way that it favors fetal growth and development (Tan et al. 2013), and (4) preparing the pregnant woman for labor, lactation and motherhood (Feldt-Rasmussen et al. 2011).

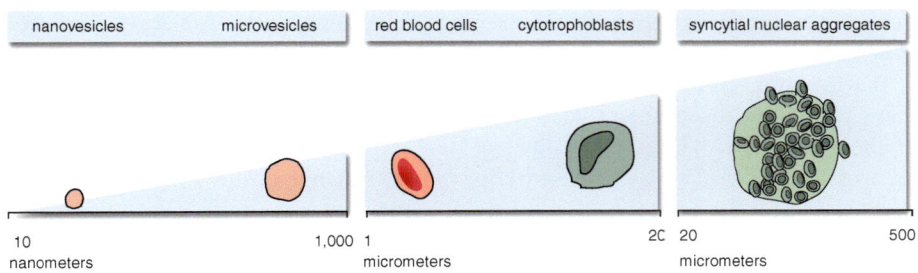

◘ **Figure 1.7**   This illustration shows the relative size of the components included in the trophoblast debris. A red blood cell has been added to serve as a reference for size (adapted from Chamley et al. 2014)

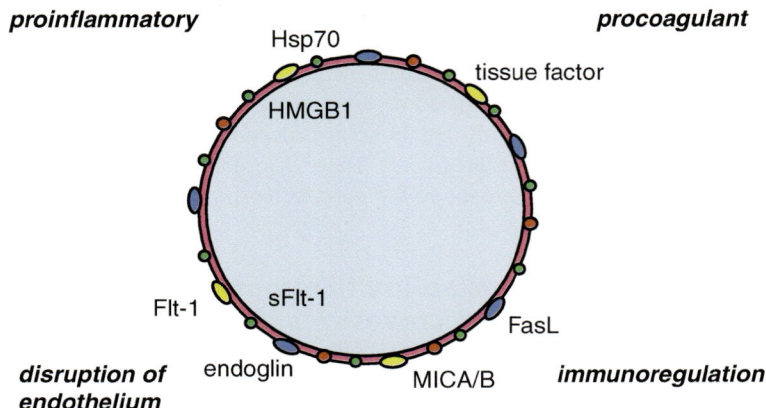

Figure 1.8 Functional activities of syncytiotrophoblast microvesicles (STBMs) and relevant molecular cargo they carry. STBMs may have pro-inflammatory properties by expressing 'danger molecules' (Hsp70, HMGB1) and displaying procoagulant activity (tissue factor). They may also carry the anti-angiogenic factors, sFlt-1 and endoglin, thus capable of inducing endothelial dysfunction. Expression of MICA/B and FasL is consistent with their immunoregulatory effects, reflected in suppression of NK and T cell responses (*cartoon based on a report* by Redman et al. 2012)

The embryonic endocrine system is the earliest system that develops in prenatal life. Obviously, early in pregnancy, this system relies almost entirely on precursors secreted by either the trophoblast or the mother. Towards the end of pregnancy, the infant's endocrine system is mature enough to cope with independent extra-uterine life.

The earliest-detectable pregnancy hormone in the maternal blood is hCG, almost entirely produced by the syncytiotrophoblasts (STBs), that develops from CTBs shortly after embryo implantation. Already by circa 2 days post-implantation, β-hCG is detectable in the maternal serum (Fournier et al. 2015). It has a wide range of effects. Initially, it is locally involved in the regulation of CTB invasion and syncytialization, SA remodeling and immunotolerance (Costa 2016; Theofanakis et al. 2017). The more distant effects of β-hCG, such as the rescue and maintenance of the steroid production by the CL, only develop at about 4 days post-implantation, presumably since these effects are only triggered, when the serum β-hCG level exceeds a particular threshold. hCG has also thyrotrophic effects as discussed in ▶ chap. 3, in the subsection on thyroid disorders. For a detailed description of the local regulation of implantation, the interested reader is referred to a number of comprehensive reviews elaborating on this subject (Sharma et al. 2016; Aplin et al. 2017; Kong et al. 2019).

The invading CTBs together with the STBs form the so-called 'primitive placenta' (characterized by absent intervillous flow), a structure that gradually develops into the definite placenta (with intervillous flow) by 10–12 weeks. The definite placenta has a fetal and a maternal circulation enabling bidirectional exchange of nutrients, O_2 and waste products (▶ fig. 1.9).

The definite placenta also plays a key role in orchestrating the maternal adaptations, by regulating it's owns functions using autocrine, paracrine and endocrine mechanisms, as well as by orchestrating the adaptive changes in the mother to achieve favorable conditions for the fetus to grow and mature in line with its genetic potential. Finally, near term, the placenta responds to signals generated by fetal maturation and placental aging,

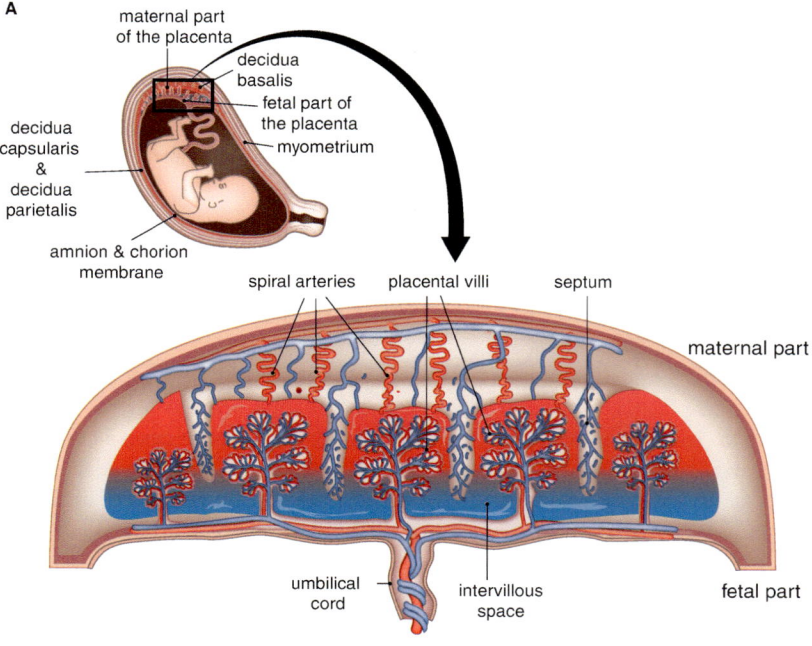

A

maternal part
of the placenta

decidua
basalis

fetal part of
the placenta

myometrium

decidua
capsularis
&
decidua
parietalis

amnion & chorion
membrane

spiral arteries   placental villi   septum

maternal part

umbilical
cord

intervillous
space

fetal part

B

maternal part

fetal part

myometrium

decidua

intervillous space

syncytial knot

maternal
spiral artery

extravillous
invading
smooth   trophoblast
muscle

maternal blood flow

villous
trophoblast

cytotro-
phoblasts

vascular
endothelium

endovascular
trophoblasts

vein

intervillous space

🔲 **Figure 1.9   A**: Mature placenta with both fetal and maternal vascular beds, enabling bidirectional exchange. **B**: Close-up of a remodeled spiral artery: 1. Anchoring villus; 2. Trumpet-shaped spiral artery; 3. Endothelial cells replaced by endovascular trophoblast cells; 4/5. High volume, low velocity intervillous flow; 6/7. Free-floating placental villus; 8. Venous inlet, with micro-vesicles shed by the adjacent placental villus; 9. Shedding of trophoblast material into the inter-villous space

1

that act in concert, to trigger the onset of labor. These diverse and complex placental functions have been reviewed recently (Fowden et al. 2015; Costa 2016).

With so many functions, it is not surprising that the placenta has a high metabolic rate, as also reflected in its utilization of a large fraction of uteroplacental O_2 and glucose uptake. The pregnancy-induced adaptations in the most important maternal organ systems and how they are induced, are discussed in the sections below. The placental role in creating the proper conditions for fetal growth and maturation has been reviewed recently (Larqué et al. 2013; Murthi 2014; Nelson 2015).

1.5   The maternal cardiovascular function in pregnancy

Pregnancy induces a high-flow and low-resistance circulation, accompanied by renal hyperfiltration and plasma volume expansion. These adaptations develop in response to primary systemic vascular relaxation, that activates – and in some cases also resets – a number of cardiovascular and volume regulatory systems. The exact purpose of the initial systemic vasorelaxation is unclear. However, it is conceivable that the creation of a volume-expanded, 'hyperdynamic' maternal circulation with a properly remodeled heart already in early pregnancy, can be considered as the timely creation of an extra cardiovascular buffer in a period of pregnancy, when metabolic demands are only modestly raised. This reserve is then available to be utilized in the second half of pregnancy to facilitate the then exponentially rising uteroplacental blood flow. Indirect support for the importance of these adaptations comes from pregnancies complicated by a placental syndrome. A typical feature of these pregnancies is the abnormal early-pregnancy hemodynamic adaptation (Spaanderman et al. 2001).

1.5.1   Pregnancy-specific changes in cardiovascular function and volume homeostasis

The pregnancy-induced systemic vascular relaxation (Schrier et al. 1994) develops about six days after implantation and includes an extra rise on top of the normal luteal vasodilation. This event appears to be linked to the time of implantation and coincides with a rapid decline in plasma osmolality (◘ fig. 1.10) and various changes in the local immune function and endocrine environment (Tkachenko et al. 2014; Conrad 2011). Important in this response is (1) its timing, (2) its abruptness and (3) the systemic character of its effect. This combination of features supports the view that, about 6 days after embryo implantation, a bidirectional interaction between CL and the implanting embryo results in (1) hCG-mediated preservation of the CL function, and (2) the onset of luteal relaxin release. Relaxin induces – possibly in concert with some concomitantly released other vasodilator – such a strong systemic arterial relaxation that both cardiac pre- and afterload are challenged, and with it, cardiac output and blood pressure (Schrier et al. 2010; Conrad and Shroff, 2011; Leo et al. 2017).

To prevent this strong arterial relaxation disrupting the cardiovascular functional integrity, the fall in cardiac afterload activates both the carotid body and aortic baroreceptors (◘ fig. 1.11). These receptors perceive increased stretch resulting from smooth muscle relaxation in the arterial bed inducing both short- and long-term responses

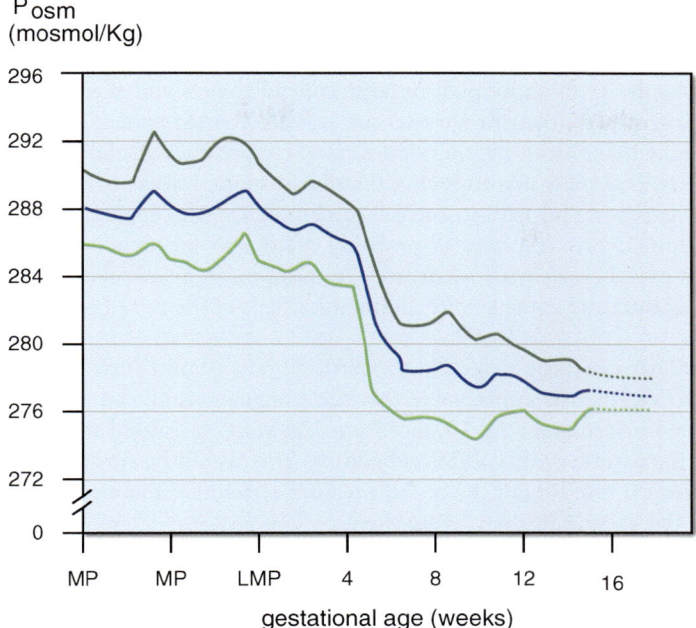

Figure 1.10 Mean osmolality ($P_{osmol} \pm 1$ SD) measured weekly from pre-conception until 16 weeks pregnancy in nine healthy women with normal pregnancy outcomes. MP and LMP indicate menstrual and last menstrual periods, respectively (*based on data reported by* Davison et al. 1981)

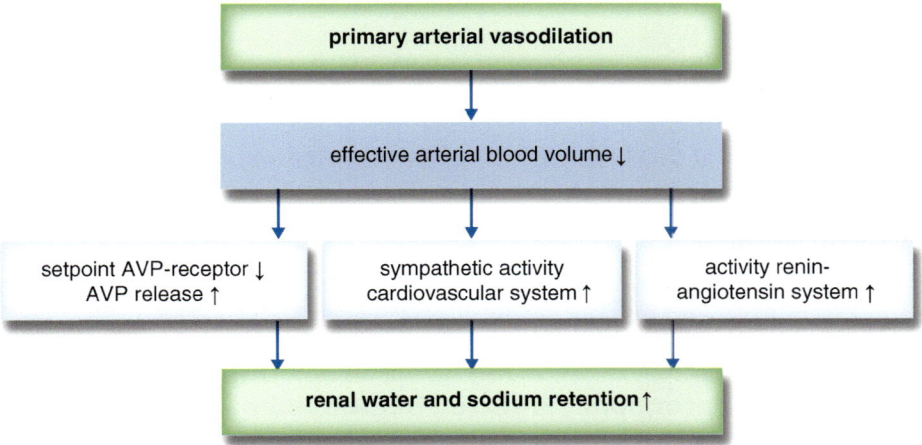

Figure 1.11 Responses of the volume regulatory systems to the initial systemic arterial relaxation in pregnancy. In this figure, the higher activity of the arterial baroreceptors enhances the release of arginine vasopressin (AVP). Besides, the higher activity of the carotid baroreceptors increases the cardiovascular sympathetic activity

(Tkachenko et al. 2014). The *short-term response* is to preserve blood pressure, and the myocardial and cerebral blood flows by increasing cardiovascular sympathetic tone (Reyes et al. 2018). The latter leads to selective vasoconstriction in so-called 'non-vital' organs, such as the intra-abdominal organs, skeletal tissues and skin, and a rise in the activity of the renin-angiotensin-aldosterone system (RAAS), which accelerates sodium retention. Meanwhile, the *long-term response* is to restore the vascular filling state by further raising RAAS activity and inducing the non-osmotic release of vasopressin, resulting in water retention and with it, the fall in osmolality. The apparent absence of renal vasoconstriction in this response is probably related to the concomitant presence of relaxin in the peripheral blood, a hormone with strong renovascular dilator properties (Conrad 2011) and thus, capable of revoking the effects of the raised cardiovascular sympathetic tone.

The central baroreceptor located in the carotid body is embedded in vascular smooth muscle tissue (VSM). It is conceivable that the pregnancy-induced decline in diastolic and systolic blood pressures by 10 and 5 mmHg, resp., is caused by the concomitant relaxation of the carotid body's VSM embedding. This would be consistent with the idea that the downward resetting of the blood pressure setpoint is merely a side-effect of the lower tone of the VSM at this particular site.

The responses elaborated above have the following functional effects:

1. The higher cardiovascular sympathetic tone leads to CO redistribution in favor of the heart and brain and is a short-term response. It limits the fall in cardiac afterload and also bridges the period needed to restore the reduced vascular filling state and associated reduced cardiac preload. Therefore, the initially induced increase in cardiovascular sympathetic activity can be expected to decline gradually in concert with the normalization of cardiac preload.
2. Inherent to the high-output and low-resistance circulation is a higher wall shear stress in the arterial bed, which causes extra mechanical strain exerted upon the endothelium and with it, increases the endothelial release of nitric oxide and prostacyclin. These vasorelaxants raise the compliance of the entire vascular bed, though, with most functional impact on the arterial bed.
3. The high-output and low-resistance circulation develops without concomitant rise in basal metabolic rate (Spaanderman et al. 2000). Therefore, the generated extra systemic flow is directed towards a-v shunts to protect the systemic capillary beds against excessive flow.
4. The extra shunt flow created in early pregnancy, is mobilized in the second half of pregnancy to support the then rapidly increasing uteroplacental blood flow.

1.5.2 Impact of pregnancy-induced hemodynamic changes on cardiac structure

Pregnancy induces (physiological) *eccentric* myocardial hypertrophy resembling the one that develops in response to endurance sport (◘ fig. 1.12) (Chung et al. 2014; Melchiorre et al. 2012).

Both left-ventricular end-diastolic diameter and wall thickness increase by about 15 %. The increased wall thickness not only lowers wall stress, but also maintains myocardial

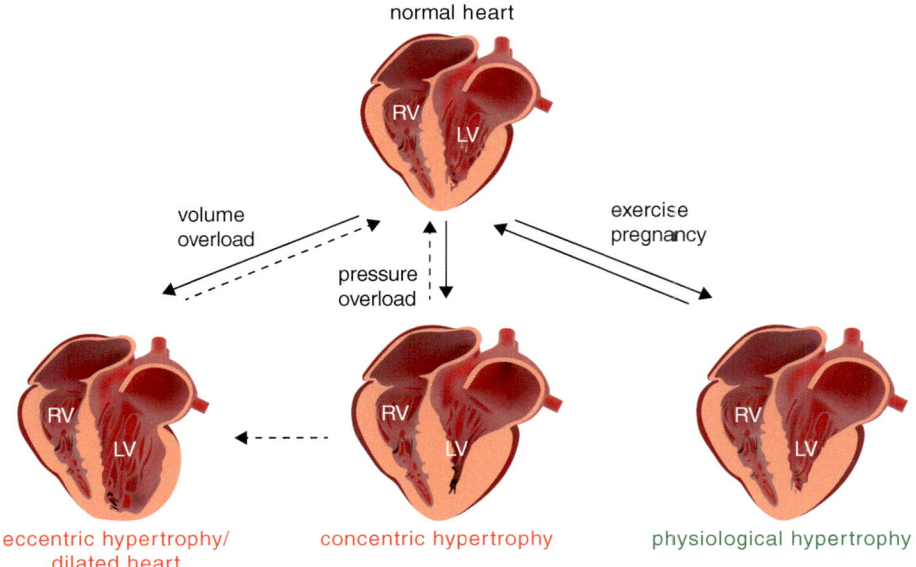

Figure 1.12 Cardiac remodeling in normal human pregnancy differs from that developing in response to volume- or pressure-load. Note rise in left ventricular dimensions and wall thickness. Most of the pregnancy-induced structural changes caused by cardiac remodeling reverse postpartum, which is not the case in both other (pathologic) forms of cardiac remodeling (*based on a report from* Chung et al. 2014)

oxygenation during a prolonged state of elevated cardiac preload and reduced cardiac afterload (Melchiorre et al. 2012). The following stimuli induce pregnancy-related cardiac remodeling:

1. Increased cardiac workload caused by the higher heart rate and higher stroke volume.
2. Higher right ventricular preload caused by the expanded total blood volume.
3. The pregnancy-induced endocrine environment.

By mid-pregnancy, cardiac workload defined as the triple product of heart rate (↑20 %), stroke volume (↑20 %) and systolic blood pressure (↓5 %) (Melchiorre et al. 2012), has increased to a level that is about one-third above pre-pregnancy levels. Cardiac remodeling involves an increase in left-ventricular mass by about 20 %, which reverts back almost completely within 6 months postpartum without any functional aftereffect (Savu et al. 2012; Melchiorre et al. 2016).

During pregnancy, cardiac efficiency (cardiac work per unit O_2 uptake) improves, mostly because of the higher preload, and – to a lesser extend – the lower afterload. The higher preload raises cardiac filling enabling a higher stroke volume to be generated by the so-called 'Frank-Starling mechanism'. However, it is conceivable that this adaptation has limited reserve capacity, particularly in late pregnancy, when the heart is likely to operate close to the flat portion of the Starling curve. This would imply that an extra rise in preload generates little, if any, extra stroke volume (Marques et al. 2015). Conversely, the high incidence of pregnancy complications in women, who fail to adequately raise their plasma volume in early pregnancy emphasizes the importance of instituting a hyperdynamic circulation in early pregnancy for the pregnancy course afterwards (Aardenburg et al. 2003). To meet the rising demands for systemic blood flow in advanced pregnancy, these women lack this CO buffer and thus, are obliged to respond with an extra rise in heart rate (Savu et al. 2012), which requires a rise in cardiovascular sympathetic tone. This 'plan-B' compensation has limited yield, when cardiac preload is already subnormal (Spaanderman et al. 2001). Another drawback of this alternative compensation is that a higher cardiovascular sympathetic tone raises the vascular resistance in the uterus.

In the second half of pregnancy, the heart adopts a more horizontal position within the thorax associated with the upward movement of the diaphragm caused by the rapidly growing uterus. As a consequence, the electrocardiogram (ECG) shows a more leftwards deviation of the QRS axis and flatter T-waves, often accompanied by abnormal T-waves (Sunitha et al. 2014). Also, the higher cardiac output without wider aortic annulus often produces a (physiologic) ejection murmur.

1.5.3 Pregnancy-induced changes in cardiac output, arterial pressure and the arterial bed

In the first two trimesters of pregnancy, resting CO and total blood volume increase to a plateau of about 40 % above the pre-pregnant level (Tan et al. 2013). Until the 8th week, the rise in CO primarily results from a rise in stroke volume (■ fig. 1.13). The additional rise in CO with advancing pregnancy is to be achieved by an increase in heart rate. In the third trimester, stroke volume falls slightly, partly due to the higher intra-abdominal pressure, which increasingly hinders lower body venous drainage. In this period, a fall in CO is prevented by a rise in heart rate. It follows that at term, heart rate and stroke volume have increased by about 20 % relative to pre-pregnant values (Sanghavi et al. 2014).

At 6-weeks amenorrhea, mean arterial pressure has already fallen by 3–5 mmHg relative to pre-pregnancy with an additional fall of about 2 mmHg in the remainder of the first trimester (Nama et al. 2011). Between the 12th and the 28th week, the mean arterial pressure increases again, though, only by 2 mmHg. This rise in blood pressure becomes slightly steeper towards the end of pregnancy, as indicated by an additional 6 mmHg

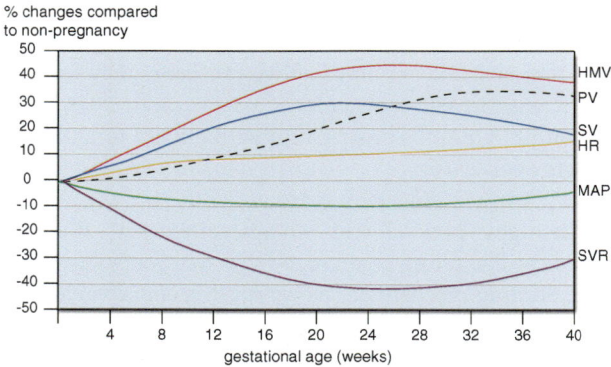

■ Figure 1.13 Relative change in various hemodynamic parameters over the course of pregnancy. *Abbreviations:* HMV: cardiac output; PV: plasma volume; SV: stroke volume; HR: heart rate; MAP: mean arterial pressure; SVR: systemic vascular resistance

◻ **Table 1.1** Pregnancy-induced circulatory and volume changes. Values are means, retrieved from various sources (Robson et al. (1989), Clark et al. (1989), Duvekot et al. (1993), Duvekot and Peeters (1994), Halligan et al. (1993)). Changes are statistically significant (except for that in α-natriuretic peptide)

pregnancy-induced changes in cardiovascular and volume parameters	pre-pregnant state	24–28 weeks amenorrhea
cardiac output (L/min)	4.5	6.0 (↑33 %)
heart rate (beats/min)	70	85 (↑21 %)
stroke volume (mL)	65	72 (↑11 %)
plasma volume (mL)	2500	3800 (↑52 %)
erythrocyte volume (mL)	1500	1800 (↑20 %)
active plasma renin concentration (pg/dl)	16	41 (↑156 %)
systolic blood pressure (mmHg)	110	105 (↓5 %)
diastolic blood pressure (mmHg)	80	70 (↓12 %)
colloid-osmotic pressure (mmHg)	21	18 (↓14 %)
total peripheral vascular resistance (dyne·s/ cm^6)	1600	1000 (↓37 %)
pulmonary vascular resistance (dyne·s/cm^6)	119	78 (↓35 %)
α-atrial natriuretic peptide (pmol/dl)	54	30 (↓44 %)
osmolality (mOsm/dl)	288	277 (↓4 %)

rise to reach a term blood pressure comparable to the pre-pregnant one. This pattern indicates that already by 12 weeks pregnancy, the nadir in arterial blood pressure may have been reached, as opposed to the classical view that this lowest blood pressure is not reached before midpregnancy. ◻ Table 1.1 lists a number of pregnancy-induced changes in circulatory and volume parameters.

1.5.4 **Pregnancy-induced changes in the systemic microcirculation**

Hemodilution along with a higher cardiovascular compliance alters the transcapillary fluid balance in the systemic microcirculation (◻ fig. 1.14). Hemodilution reduces the plasma oncotic pressure, and with it, enhances interstitial fluid accumulation. This effect explains why orthostatic edema tends to develop, particularly in advanced pregnancy. Whether the higher vascular compliance also alters the hydrostatic pressure in the arterioles at the level of the precapillary sphincters, is unknown. Theoretically, a higher arteriolar compliance would imply that a larger fraction of the kinetic energy generated by the heart during systole is stored in the arteriolar wall to be released again as extra volume flow during diastole. At the level of the precapillary sphincters this extra volume flow is most likely preferentially directed to a-v shunts to protect the downstream capillary bed.

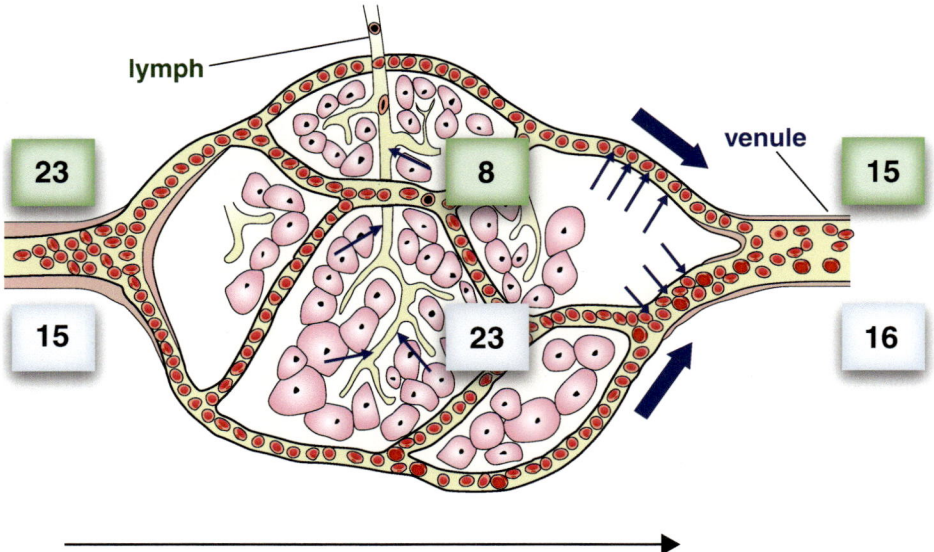

Figure 1.14 Driving forces for transcapillary fluid exchange based on the Starling principle. Hydrostatic (mmHg, green boxes) and oncotic pressures (mmHg, grey boxes) at the precapillary sphincter, in the capillary bed and at the venular outflow site, respectively. Pressure gradients enable serum to leave and re-enter the vascular bed during blood passage across the capillary bed

1.5.5 Pregnancy-induced changes in the venous bed

About 70 % of the total blood volume resides in the venous bed. Veins are 30× more compliant than arteries, particularly in the splanchnic bed. Therefore, physiologic changes in venous filling have a negligible effect on venous pressure. The venous system returns the blood from the peripheral tissues to the heart and, of importance, the splanchnic bed serves as the most important back-up reservoir to preserve venous return. The venous bed consists of 2 imaginary components, the 'unstressed-' and 'stressed volumes'. The unstressed volume represents two-thirds of the venous compartment and is defined as the volume that can be contained at zero transmural pressure, which refers to the pressure gradient across the venous wall. Meanwhile, the stressed volume refers to the one-third of the total venous blood volume, needed to raise the transmural pressure to the mean circulatory filling pressure (MCFP) of about 7 mmHg (Pang 2001). The stressed volume determines venous return and thus cardiac preload (Berlin et al. 2014). A fall in CO activates the central baroreceptors in the carotid body and with it, leads to constriction of the most compliant part of the venous compartment, the splanchnic bed, particularly the hepatic sinusoidal microcirculation (Gelman 2008). This induces an immediate shift of unstressed to stressed volume to preserve cardiac preload.

Pregnancy induces venous relaxation and with it, a relatively underfilled venous bed, leading to RAAS activation as discussed earlier in this chapter. Pregnancy also raises the responsiveness of the respiratory center to the CO_2 dissolved in the circulating blood. Hence, the (respiratory) tidal volume rises and with it, amplifies the average negative intrathoracic pressure and the pressure gradient between central veins and the right atrium. These effects boost both cardiac preload and venous return (Cong et al. 2015).

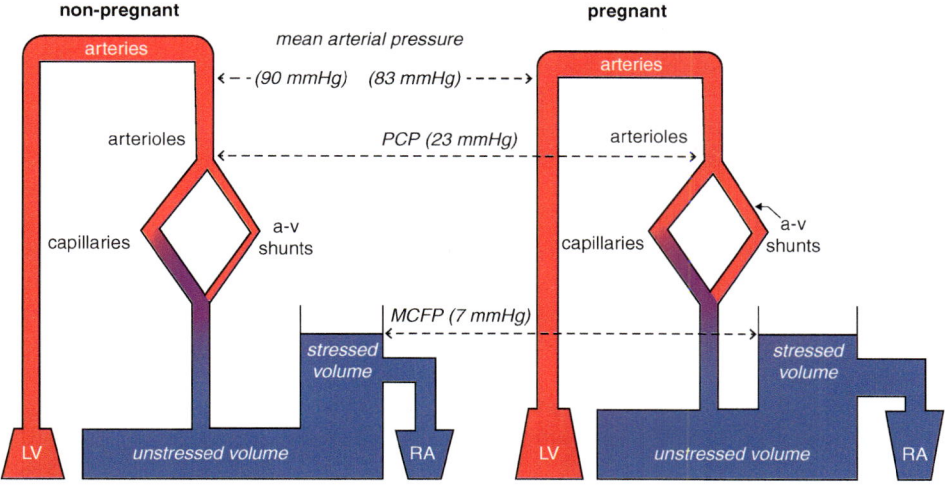

■ **Figure 1.15** Pregnancy-induced change in cardiovascular function, with emphasis on the venous compartment. The venous compartment becomes larger, but preserves relative distribution between stressed & unstressed volumes. Excess cardiac output is directed towards a-v shunts in order to protect the systemic microcirculation from excessive flow. *Abbreviations*: PCP, precapillary hydrostatic pressure; a-v shunts, arteriovenous shunts; MCFP, mean circulatory filling pressure

■ Figure 1.15 shows how pregnancy-induced volume expansion accumulates in the venous bed, proportionally distributed between stressed and unstressed volumes. The extra stressed volume enables CO to be maintained at approx. 40 % above the pre-pregnant level for an extended period of time with limited extra sympathetic activity.

From the 10th week of pregnancy onwards, venous pressure in the iliac veins that drain the blood from the lower body increases gradually from 10 to 25 mmH$_2$O, due to gravity and partial venous obstruction by the growing uterus. With advancing pregnancy, this effect increasingly raises the venular pressure in the microcirculation of lower body tissues. Besides, the pregnancy-induced hemodilution leads to an about 15 % fall in plasma colloid-osmotic pressure. Both effects may hinder reabsorption of interstitial fluid in the microcirculation indicating that orthostatic edema in advanced pregnancy is to be considered a normal physiologic phenomenon.

1.5.6 Pregnancy-related changes in regional blood flows

During pregnancy, CO not only increases, but is also redistributed. Shortly after embryo implantation, the blood flow to mammary glands, kidneys and skin increases. The rise in mammary flow is probably induced by accelerated mammary growth and higher metabolic rate. Meanwhile, the marked increase in renal perfusion is probably an effect induced by the raised circulating relaxin levels (Conrad 2011). Finally, the higher skin flow is likely to result from increased arteriovenous shunting combined with raised tissue perfusion to radiate the extra heat generated by the higher basal metabolic rate (Forsum et al. 2007).

1

1.6 Impact of pregnancy on the maternal metabolism

The maternal metabolism is anabolic until around the 24th week of pregnancy, as reflected in accelerated glycogen and fat accretion. During this period, the endocrine environment induces hyperphagia, which not only boosts glycogen accretion, but also *de novo* lipogenesis, as indicated by raised intracellular glycerol utilization and with it, increased formation of triglycerides (Zeng et al. 2017). After the 24th weeks of pregnancy, a transient 'low-threshold' insulin resistance (IR) develops acting within the normoglycemic range. It serves to redirect the available glucose away from the insulin-dependent maternal organs, such as skeletal tissues, skin and liver (Schwartsburd 2016). Hormones involved in inducing this IR are placental growth factor (PlGF), cortisol, progesterone, and the cytokine TNFα (Vejrazkova et al. 2014). This physiologic form of IR is particularly beneficial for insulin-independent organs, such as the brain and in pregnancy, the uterus. The transplacental glucose uptake is determined by the gradient between the uterine- and umbilical arterial blood glucose levels. Glucose is the most important metabolic substrate to fuel the fetal oxidative metabolism and its tissue growth (Hadden et al. 2009). To prevent circulating maternal glucose levels from falling in between meals and overnight, this low-threshold IR forces insulin-sensitive tissues to switch to alternative energy sources (fatty acids, amino-acids and glycerol) to fuel their oxidative metabolism. These substrates are readily available, as this particular IR is also responsible for the breakdown of glycogen, protein and fat in the normal glucose range. The low-threshold IR requires at least a twice as high concomitant insulin release capacity compared to non-pregnancy to enable postprandial storage of glucose and fat, and with it, also avoiding excessive postprandial hyperglycemia. ◘ Figure 1.16 illustrates that the low-threshold IR both preserves maternal circulating glucose levels and raises non-glucose substrates levels in-between meals.

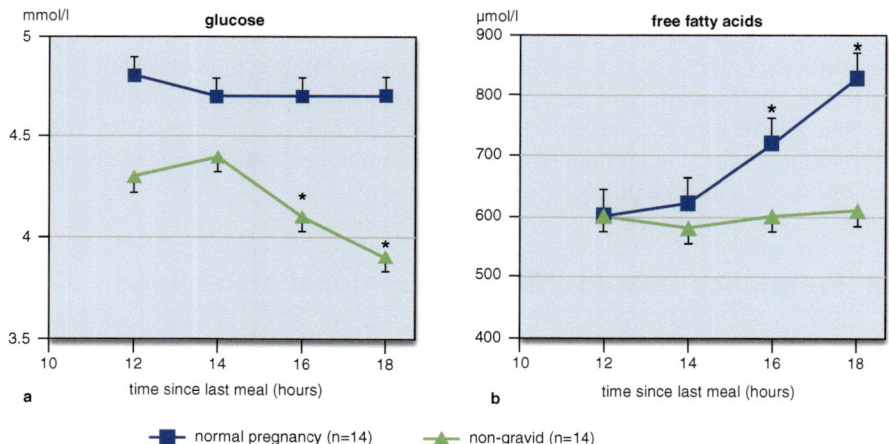

◘ **Figure 1.16**   Post-prandial changes in plasma levels of glucose (**a**) and free fatty acids (FFAs) (**b**) in 14 non-gravid and 14 late-pregnant women. In the postprandial hours, pregnant women differ from non-gravid controls by preserved glucose levels along with rising levels of FFAs. The latter effect is also paralleled by rising amino acids and ketoacids (not shown). The beneficial effects of this adaptation for the fetus has been detailed in the text (*data from* Hadden et al. 2009)

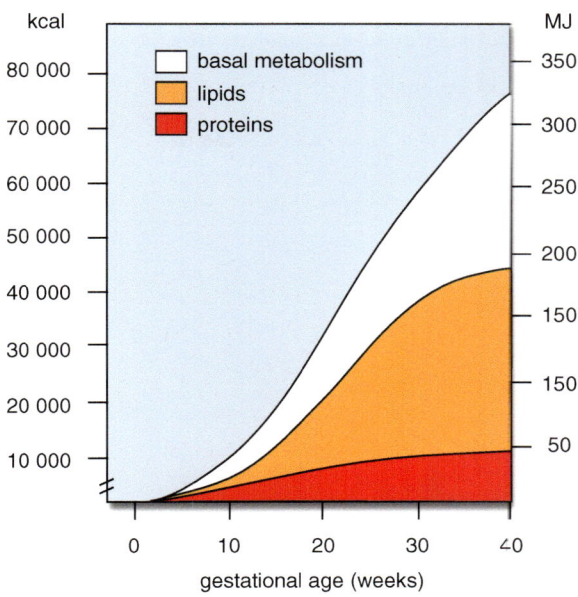

Figure 1.17   Distribution of extra caloric uptake with advancing pregnancy. In the second half of pregnancy, ca. two-thirds of the extra caloric uptake is transferred to the fetus to fuel its growth and metabolism, with only one-third of this extra caloric uptake being utilized to fuel the raising maternal basal metabolic rate

Particularly fetal growth benefits from the combination of maintained glucose levels and rising levels of non-carbohydrate substrates, such as FFAs, amino acids and ketoacids, which are preferentially directed to the conceptus in-between meals (and overnight). These substrates are essential for fetal tissue accretion, particularly in the second half of pregnancy (▶ fig. 1.17). The latter is reflected in the rise in total fetal fat mass from only 2 % of fetal body weight at 28 weeks to 16 % at term (Battaglia et al. 1988; Zeng et al. 2017).

The maternal basal metabolic rate in pregnancy increases by about 400 kcal or 16 % (Battaglia et al. 1981), mostly because of an extra rise in oxidative metabolism in the last trimester of pregnancy as illustrated in ▶ fig. 1.17, when not only fetal growth, but also its oxidative metabolism as a fraction of the maternal oxidative metabolism, is at its highest level (▶ tab. 1.2). Finally, ▶ fig. 1.18 summarizes the most important pregnancy-induced metabolic changes.

1.7 Pulmonary adaptation

The endocrine environment, volume homeostasis and cardiovascular function, and – in the last trimester – also the increasing intra-abdominal pressure modulate the respiratory function. The changes in volume homeostasis may lead to some mucosal swelling of the naso- and oropharynx causing breathing discomfort due to increased airflow resistance. In severe cases, this is reflected in symptoms such as snoring, mouth breathing and sleep disturbances. Up to 75 % of pregnant women complain about shortness of breath,

1

■ **Table 1.2**   Maternal O_2 consumption during human pregnancy

O_2 uptake (mL/min)	non-pregnant	10 wks	20 wks	30 wks	40 wks
total	250	260	270	280	290
myocardium	20	25	27	27	27
respiratory muscles	7	8	9	10	12
kidneys	18	25	25	25	25
myometrium	0.3	ca. 0.5	1	2	4
placenta	–	< 0.5	1	2	4
fetus	–	< 0.5	1	8	18

Data shown were determined using information provided in reports by Battaglia FC et al. 1978, 1981, Butte 2000 and Lotgering et al. 1991.

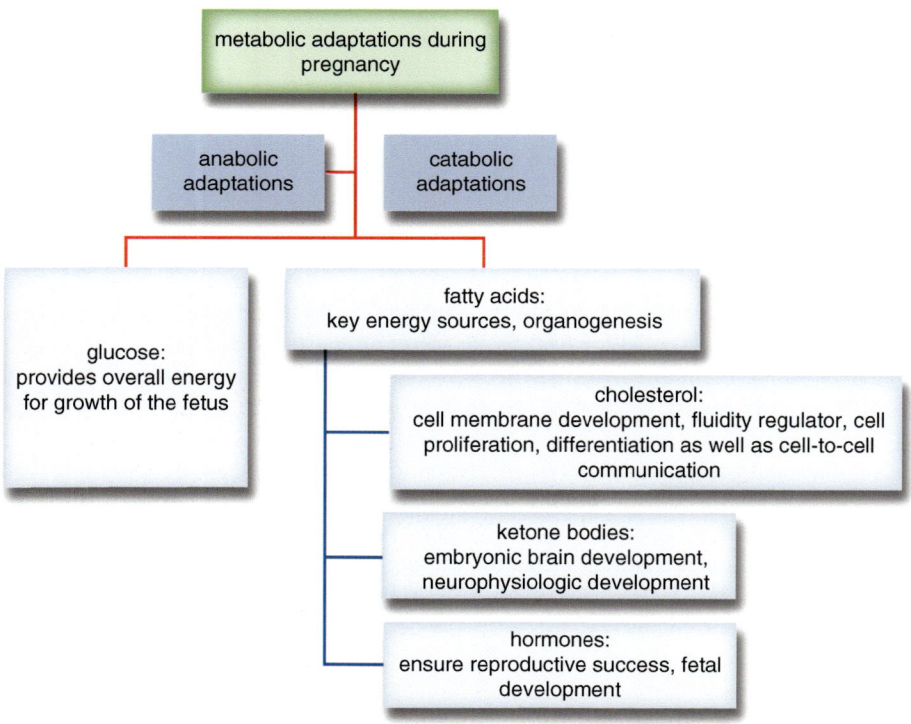

■ **Figure 1.18**   Metabolic adaptation to pregnancy. Anabolism in the 1st half of pregnancy primarily serves to enlarge *maternal* energy stores. The low-threshold insulin resistance afterwards not only preserves fetal glucose availability between meals and overnight, but also the steady uterine supply of non-carbohydrate substrates needed to secure ongoing fetal growth.

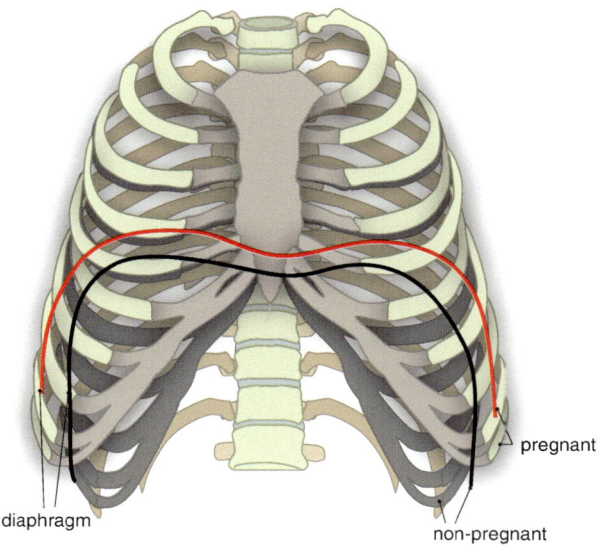

pregnant

diaphragm

non-pregnant

■ Figure 1.19 The shape of the thorax before – (black line, dark-grey ribs) and during pregnancy (red line, yellow ribs). During pregnancy, the diaphragm is pushed upwards, increasing both the cross section and subcostal angle (from 70° to 100°)

presumably related to the 40 % higher respiratory minute ventilation and more airflow resistance in the upper respiratory tract (Jensen et al. 2008). This breathing discomfort often begins in midpregnancy to ease again in the last trimester. Usually, this discomfort does not interfere with normal daily activities.

In early pregnancy, structural changes in the thorax lead to expansion of the lower surface area of the rib cage, reflected in an almost 50 % rise in the subcostal angle, a 4-cm elevation of the diaphragm with a 2-cm compensatory wider chest diameter (■ fig. 1.19) (Bobrowski 2010). With advancing pregnancy, the functional effects of these changes in thoracic shape are increasingly influenced by the growing uterus pushing the woman's center of gravity upwards and with it, reducing her stability in the upright position. This will unconsciously urge her to adopt a more upright posture. Both effects together raise her respiratory efficiency, thus reducing the extra metabolic demands to maintain the approx. 40 % higher tidal volume throughout pregnancy.

The higher respiratory minute volume results from a higher tidal volume triggered by progesterone, that increases the sensitivity to PCO_2 of the respiratory center in the medulla (Bobrowski 2010). The resulting hyperventilation lowers maternal circulating PCO_2 and with it, increases the transplacental PCO_2 gradient. This effect facilitates both the transplacental CO_2 clearance (Meschia 2011) and the alveolar O_2 uptake, favorable effects considering the also 20 % higher O_2 demands of the maternal oxidative metabolism in pregnancy.

The pregnancy-induced anatomic changes reduce the functional residual capacity, expiratory reserve volume and residual volume by about 20 % and raise the inspiratory capacity by 5–10 % (■ fig. 1.20). ■ Table 1.3 lists the effects of the pregnancy-induced changes in lung function on maternal blood gases.

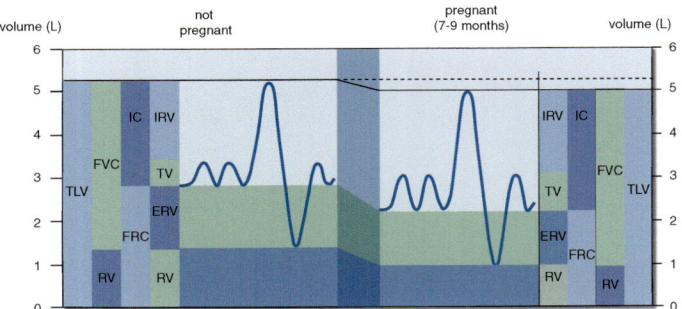

● **Figure 1.20**   Pregnancy-induced changes in lung volumes. *Abbreviations*: TLC: Total lung capacity; FVC: Forced vital capacity; IC: Inspiratory capacity; FRC: Functional reserve capacity IRV: Inspiratory reserve capacity; TV: Tidal volume; ERV: Expiratory reserve capacity; RV: residual volume. The most relevant changes are the rises in IC and VT and decreases in FRC and its subcomponents ERV and RV

● **Table 1.3**   Changes in pH, arterial blood gases and HCO₃ level in human pregnancy. (*Data adopted from* Hegewald et al. 2011)

arterial blood gas measurement	nonpregnant state	first trimester	third trimester
pH	7.40	7.42–7.46	7.43
P_aO_2 (mmHg)	93	105–106	101–106
P_aCO_2 (mmHg)	37	28–29	26–30
Serum HCO_3 (mEq/L)	23	18	17

1.8   Adaption of the digestive tract, liver and pancreas to pregnancy

Pregnancy alters both eating habits and digestion, resulting in maternal anabolism and reflected in (maternal) weight gain and a number of related common annoyances as specified below.

1.8.1   Pregnancy-induced changes in the functioning of the gastrointestinal (GI) tract

Placental steroids not only inhibit GI motility and peristalsis. They also relax the lower esophageal sphincter (LES) and pylorus (Body et al. 2016). These effects often lead to GI discomfort, which may vary in the course of pregnancy. In the first trimester, altered taste sensation influences eating patterns and may contribute to the development of morning sickness. This annoyance seems to occur more often, when elevated steroids levels are paralleled by markedly raised circulating levels of human chorionic gonadotropin (hCG). The mechanism that causes nausea and *vomiting* in pregnancy is not fully understood (London et al. 2017). Moreover, not only the combination of elevated circulating levels of hCG and steroids, but also emotional factors are involved. Interestingly, women who are expecting a female infant experience the pathological form of vomiting and nausea more often (hyperemesis gravidarum, discussed in ▶ chap. 2) than their counterparts, who are expecting a male infant (Veenendaal et al. 2011). Meanwhile, these GI-tract annoyances are often the earliest signs of pregnancy and also the most common complaints in early pregnancy, sometimes even lasting until term. In late pregnancy, the mechanical impact of the enlarged uterus pushing the stomach upwards may be an additional instigator of nausea, vomiting and gastroesophageal reflux.

Constipation has a prevalence of up to 40 % in pregnancy (Shin et al. 2015), and is one of the most common complaints that may last throughout pregnancy, but is most pronounced in the 1st and 2nd trimester. It is probably related to the pregnancy-induced endocrine changes, such as the progesterone-induced slower peristalsis and prolongation of bowel transit time. This complaint may benefit from more fibre and fluid intake, and more physical activity (Body et al. 2016). Constipation may lead to mechanical damage of the pelvic floor in general and of the anal canal in particular. In up to 25 % of pregnant women, *hemorrhoids* may develop, caused by increased local venous pressure and as a complication of constipation (Shin et al. 2015). Hemorrhoids are varicose rectal veins covered with mucosa located at or near the end of the anal canal. They may cause symptoms, such as itching, bleeding, prolapse and infection. Their pathogenesis involves a degeneration of anchoring supportive tissue of the anal cushions that tend to descent with venous distention and engorgement plus stasis owing to lack of support (Avsar et al. 2010). Conservative management may often suffice to obtain acceptable relief. Postpartum, symptoms usually diminish gradually over a period of months.

1.8.2 Pregnancy-induced change in liver function

The placenta is key in securing both a balanced supply of nutrients and oxygen to the pregnant uterus and removal of its metabolic waste products. These functions differ in various stages of pregnancy. In the first half of pregnancy, raised circulating levels of growth factors, progesterone and prolactin induce maternal anabolism leading to enhanced fat and glycogen accretion. During the 2nd half of pregnancy, these energy reserves are mobilized again, with glucose preferentially being taken up by the pregnant uterus at the cost of insulin-dependent maternal tissues, as detailed previously (Lacroix et al. 2013).

Liver tests are abnormal in about 10 % of pregnant women despite a seemingly normal liver function. It is conceivable that raised metabolic demands in late pregnancy in some of these women exceed the hepatic metabolic and excretory capacity. This may result in impaired clearance of some compounds, that subsequently may be excreted into the bile. With pregnancy advancing into the 2nd half, serum levels of cholesterol and triglycerides increase markedly, paralleled by the accumulation of cholesterol and triglycerides in the liver. This effect is partly due to the progressive rise in placental output of steroids with advancing pregnancy. It is plausible that an enlarged gallbladder filled with bile, that is supersaturated with cholesterol, in combination with the reduced mobility of the biliary ductal system, is responsible for the about 10-fold higher risk of gallstone formation in pregnant and puerperal women, compared to age-matched nulliparous controls (De Bari et al. 2014).

1

1.8.3 Pregnancy-induced changes in pancreas function

Most of the exocrine pancreas consists of acinar cells (80 %) that closely interact with the 5 % ductal cells to produce the pancreatic secretions. The latter consist of various digestive enzymes dissolved in an isotonic fluid. There is no evidence in support of a pregnancy-induced change in pancreatic exocrine function (Ramin et al. 2001). On the other hand, in early pregnancy, both number and size of the insulin-producing ß-cells in the pancreatic islets of Langerhans increase, presumably triggered by placental lactogen, and in anticipation of the transient low-threshold IR, that develops in the second half of pregnancy (Baeyens et al. 2016). Postpartum, the enlarged pool of ß-cells shrinks again in response to the lower metabolic load exerted upon the mother. The endocrine, exo-crine and ductal systems of the pancreas interact with one another thus optimizing their individual functional performances (Bertelli et al. 2005; Lammert et al. 2019). How this plays out in human pregnancy is not yet fully elucidated.

1.9 Adaptation of kidneys and urinary tract

1.9.1 Pregnancy-induced changes in renal function

The about 40 % rise in cardiac output during pregnancy is paralleled by an even larger rise in renal plasma flow (RPF) and thus also, renal blood flow (RBF) (Odutayo et al. 2012). The strong renal vasodilation probably develops in response to the rapidly ris-ing peripheral levels of relaxin, released by the CL shortly after ovulation (Conrad et al. 2014, 2011). The renal vasodilation induced by relaxin is enhanced by the concomitantly markedly elevated circulating levels of progesterone, as detailed elsewhere (Carvalho et al. 2012; Lumbers et al. 2014).

A disadvantage of the higher RBF and with it, higher glomerular filtration rate (GFR) is the associated marked increase in filtered sodium load, an effect that, on the one hand, is boosted by the higher circulating levels of α-ANP in pregnancy, but on the other hand, attenuated by the coinciding lower peritubular filtration pressure. Never-theless, the most important renal effect of progesterone in pregnancy is not enhancing vasodilation, but rather limiting sodium loss by protecting the formation of aldosterone, as sodium conservation is pivotal for normal pregnancy course and outcome (Lumbers et al. 2014). Actually, sodium conservation, such as normally develops in response to the raised plasma levels of aldosterone and deoxycorticosterone, does prevail in preg-nancy, as reflected in the about 1,000 mEq of sodium sparing, required to meet the extra sodium demands needed by the fetus to grow, mature and thrive (summarized in ◘ tab. 1.4).

In the first half of pregnancy, the GFR increases rapidly to a plateau of over 60 % above the pre-pregnant level, coinciding with the rise in ERPF (◘ fig. 1.21). This level is maintained until term and normalizes again within 6 weeks postpartum (Odutayo et al. 2012). Most of the increase in GFR seems to be triggered by the rise in ERPF, proba-bly with some contribution of the fall in plasma oncotic pressure. It is unlikely that the marked changes in renal hemodynamics are associated with a rise in the intra-glomer-ular pressure, as indicated by the postpartum absence of glomerular damage after an uncomplicated pregnancy. While the GFR remains high throughout pregnancy, the RBF decreases gradually in the last trimester (◘ fig. 1.21). Presumably, this decline relates to

▣ **Table 1.4** Regulation of Na$^+$ and K$^+$ homeostasis in pregnancy (*adopted from* Odutayo et al. 2012)

physiologic change	effect during pregnancy	change during pregnancy
glomerular filtration rate	natriuretic	↑ from early pregnancy until delivery
atrial natriuretic peptide	natriuretic	↑ at 12 weeks; until > 36 weeks
progesterone	natriuretic/antikaliuretic	↑ from ovulation until ca. 36 weeks
aldosterone	*antinatriuretic/kaliuretic*	↑ from 6 weeks until delivery
deoxycorticosterone	*antinatriuretic*	↑ in 1st trimester, peaks in 3rd trimester
Na$^+$/K$^+$ transporters	*antinatriuretic*	↑ in pregnancy

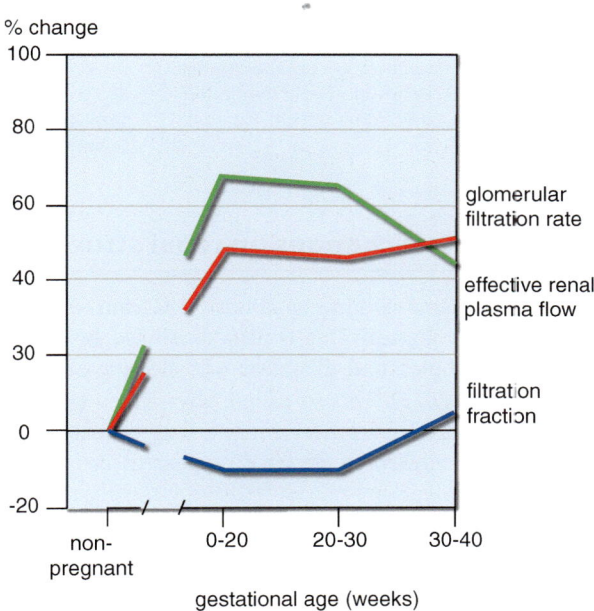

▣ **Figure 1.21** Relative rise during pregnancy in glomerular filtration rate (GFR, red line), effective renal plasma flow (ERPF, green line), along with a small decline in filtration fraction (GFR/ERPF, blue line), measured by inulin & para-aminohippurate clearance, respectively.

the progressively increasing claim of the growing conceptus on the finite maternal circulatory and metabolic reserves, as suggested by the concomitant rise in the sympathetic contribution to the autonomic control of the circulation (Reyes et al. 2018).

The elevated GFR not only raises the filtered load of sodium, but also that of readily filtered substances, such as uric acid, glucose, amino acids and some smaller proteins such as albumin. Nevertheless, this effect only rarely causes certain compounds to surpass their maximum reabsorption capacity in the proximal tubules. Plasma osmolality falls by circa 10 mOsmol/L in pregnancy, probably resulting from a lower threshold of the osmoreceptor for thirst, presumably in concert with the non-osmotic release of antidiuretic hormone (ADH or vasopressin) (Lindheimer et al. 1989).

1

■ **Table 1.5** Pregnancy-induced changes in renal structure and function (Jeyabalan and Lain 2007)

change	functional effect	clinical relevance
renal enlargement	radiographic ± 1 cm elongation; no functional effect;	no clinical relevance, postpartum no loss of renal parenchyma during renal shrinkage;
dilation renal pelvis and urinary tract (R > L)	no functional effect, but change may mimic hydronephrosis;	not to be confused with obstructive uropathie;
renal vasodilation	GFR & ERPF increase by 40–60 %;	lower serum creatinine & urea levels; no clinical relevance;
shift in acid-base balance;	renal HCO_3 threshold ↓; progesterone-induced hyperventilation	± 5 µml/L and ± 10 mmHg lower serum bicarbonate and PCO_2 levels, respectively;
renal water handling	lower setpoint of the osmoreceptor (located in hypothalamic supra-optical nucleus)	serum osmolality falls by ± 10mOsmol/L; higher ADH turnover, occasionally causing (transient) diabetes insipidus

1.9.2 Impact of functional changes on renal structure

Pregnancy leads to a rise in renal volume by about 30 %, caused by expansion of both the vascular and interstitial volumes. This is also paralleled by an approximate 30 % elongation of the proximal tubules, and dilatation of collecting ducts, calices, renal pelvis and ureters (Cheung et al. 2013). This so-called 'physiologic hydronephrosis of pregnancy' is partly induced by pregnancy hormones, partly by external pressure exerted by the enlarged uterus. Normally, these effects disappear in the first week postpartum (■ tab. 1.5).

1.9.3 Volume homeostasis

Volume homeostasis is determined by the balance between volume dissipation and volume retention. During pregnancy, the intravascular compartment expands by about 1400 mL, divided over circa 1100 mL extra plasma volume (De Haas et al. 2017) and circa 300 mL extra red blood cells (RBC) mass, as shown in ■ fig. 1.22.

Plasma volume expansion during pregnancy develops in response to elevated levels of aldosterone and ADH, which raise sodium and water retention, and thus also hemodilution. The early-pregnancy fall in effective arterial blood volume activates RAAS and accelerates ADH release as detailed earlier in this chapter. The balance between volume retention and dissipation in pregnancy is delicate. Disturbance of this balance diminishes the cardiovascular reserve capacity and with it, the capacity to adapt to the initial fall in systemic vascular resistance. An inadequate volume response to the initial fall in arterial filling state triggers a so-called 'fight or flight' back-up consisting of a larger sympathetic contribution to the autonomic cardiovascular control. This 'plan-B' response will rescue cardiovascular function, though, at the expense of the uteroplacental blood supply.

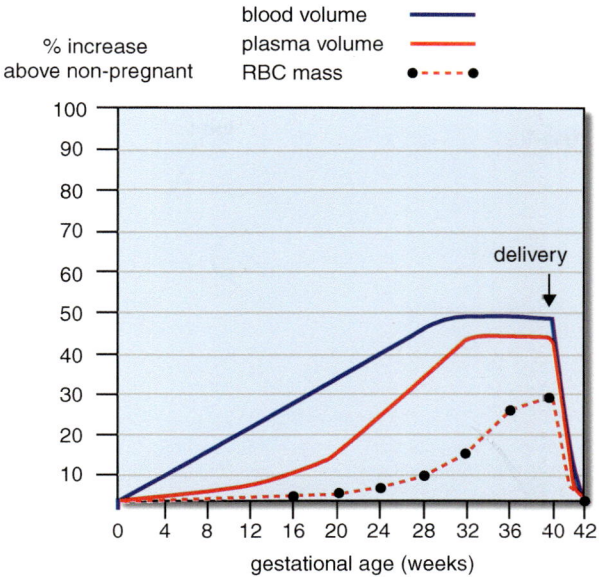

% increase
above non-pregnant

blood volume ──────
plasma volume ──────
RBC mass ●----●

delivery

gestational age (weeks)

■ Figure 1.22 The pregnancy-induced increases in plasma volume, red blood cell (RBC) mass, and the resulting expansion of total blood volume, presented as a function of gestational age

1.10 Impact of pregnancy on the hematologic function

Pregnancy alters the composition of circulating blood cells, firstly because of the physiologic hemodilution that coincides with the institution of the high-flow and low-resistance circulation, and secondly, because of the growth-promoting endocrine environment that induces an increase in total red blood cell (RBC) volume (■ fig. 1.22). The larger rise in plasma volume (+40 %) than in RBC volume (−25 %) leads to a fall in Hct during pregnancy, which reaches a nadir of about 10 % below pre-pregnant values by 30 weeks. The rise in RBC volume limits the pregnancy-induced decline in Hct. The physiologic dilutional anemia of pregnancy together with iron deficiency are the two most common causes of anemia in pregnancy and are discussed in more detail in ► chap. 2.

Pregnancy induces a state of hypercoagulability, reflected in higher circulating levels of fibrinogen and the clotting factors I, V, VII, VIII, IX and X, along with lower levels of prothrombin, free protein S and clotting factor XI (■ tab. 1.6). An additional factor that enhances the hypercoagulability is the reduced fibrinolytic activity associated with the elevated circulating levels of placenta-derived plasminogen activator inhibitor type-2 (PAI-2). The hypercoagulability of pregnancy is reflected in a fall in the 'International Normalized Ratio' (INR) to below 0.9 (Hellgren 2003).

It is unclear, whether the hypercoagulability in pregnancy is functionally relevant. It is plausible that it is a side-effect of some of the many verifiably beneficial adaptive changes. The hypercoagulability is unlikely to protect against excessive intrapartum hemorrhage caused by the tear-off of up to 120 remodeled decidual spiral arteries from the placental bed at the time of placental detachment. These transformed arteries are structurally unable to constrict and with it, occlude in response to injury.

1

◻ **Table 1.6**   Hemostatic changes during pregnancy (*adopted from* Brenner 2004)

factors affecting hemostasis	increased	decreased	no change
systemic changes			
– procoagulant factors	I, V, VII, VIII, IX, X	XI	
– anticoagulant factors	Soluble TM	Protein-S	Protein-C
– adhesive proteins	vWF		
– fibrinolytic proteins	PAI-1, PAI-2	t-PA	TAFI
– microparticles and antiphospholipid antibodies	MP		APLA
local placental changes	TF	TFPI	

Abbreviations: TM, thrombomodulin; vWF, von Willebrand factor; PAI, plasminogen activator inhibitor; t-PA, plasminogen activator; TAFI, thrombin-activatable fibrinolysis inhibitor; MP, microparticles; APLA, antiphospholipid antibodies; TF, tissue factor; TFPI, tissue factor pathway inhibitor

The hypercoagulability in this condition may help to limit bleeding, however, *only* after the real cause of bleeding has been eliminated by inducing myometrial constriction e.g. by administrating a uterotonic agent, such as ergotamine (Lockwood 2006). Yet, the pregnancy-induced hypercoagulability is associated with a clear disadvantage as it predisposes a pregnant woman to thromboembolism, particularly postpartum, when the resolving adaptive changes of pregnancy may transiently even enhance the hypercoagulability (Bates 2011). Therefore, it is important to emphasize that some typical pregnancy-induced maternal effects (nausea, constipation, melasma, orthostatic edema and probably also hypercoagulability) are mere side-effects or 'collateral damage' accompanying the really relevant and beneficial adaptive changes.

Already in the first trimester of pregnancy, the circulating white blood cells count has risen by ± 40 % above pre-pregnant levels with only a small additional increase during the remainder of pregnancy (Kühnert et al. 1998). The leucocytosis appears to be 'spillover' from the activated innate immune system at the F-M interface, that leads to a mild systemic inflammatory state (Garlanda et al. 2008).

1.11 Impact of altered body shape in pregnancy on posture, balance and gait

In the second half of pregnancy, maternal body shape changes rapidly giving rise to an upwards and posterior shift of the woman's center of gravity. This leads to a more pronounced lumbar lordosis to balance the asymmetric distribution of the extra body weight, mostly accumulated in the woman's abdomen and breasts (Cakmak et al. 2016). These changes are paralleled by a rise in the joints' laxity (Schauberger et al. 1996) and altered proprioception in the woman's musculoskeletal structures. In response to all these changes, pregnant women will intuitively alter their posture, balance and gait. It follows that with advancing pregnancy, they will lower their walking speed and adjust their spatiotemporal gait pattern. This includes a shorter step length and longer duration of both their stance and double-support phases (Blaszczyk et al. 2016). These changes improve dynamic stability and thus, reduce the risk of falling. On the other hand, these adjustments may also increase lower back pain, pain and discomfort in the hip abductors and extensors, and pain in the ankle plantar flexor muscles, probably due to musculo-skeletal overuse injuries (Foti et al. 2000). These potential adverse effects raise the question, whether physical activity or moderate exercise during pregnancy is beneficial or unsafe. Many studies have provided convincing evidence for moderate exercise to be safe for both mother and fetus and should be recommended to all pregnant women in the absence of absolute contraindications (Nascimento et al. 2012). During exercise, women should monitor themselves, maintain hydration, prevent exposure to heat and humidity, and avoid hypoglycemia. Warning signs of a potential problem include regular painful contractions, vaginal bleeding, dyspnea on exertion, dizziness, headache, chest – or calf pain. If these symptoms develop, they should discontinue exercising immediately and consult their physician. Overexertion and strenuous aerobic exercise ought to be discouraged as these could compromise fetal well-being due to redirecting blood supply at the cost of the uteroplacental unit. Exercise during pregnancy improves control of weight gain, gestational diabetes, and may also prevent urinary incontinence and low back pain (Shiri et al. 2018). Regular exercise does not harm or impose risks to the fetus and may even have a positive effect on fetal growth and adaptation. Therefore, low-risk pregnant women should be encouraged to participate on a weekly base, in aerobic and strength training at moderate intensity sessions.

1.12 Impact of pregnancy on the maternal skin

Endocrine, metabolic and immunologic changes in pregnancy have an effect on the skin, reflected in alterations in pigmentation, blood vessels, nevi, connective tissue, glands, hair, nails, and mucous membranes. Even though these skin changes are benign, they may cause significant cosmetic distress (Geraghty et al. 2011). The most common skin effect of pregnancy is hyperpigmentation as indicated by a prevalence of up to 90 %, most pronounced in women of darker skin. The mechanism responsible for *pregnancy-induced hyperpigmentation* is not completely understood, as elevated levels of estrogen, progesterone, β-endorphin in early pregnancy, and α- and β-melanocyte-stimulating hormone (MSH) in more advanced pregnancy are all melanogenic and may be involved (Tyler 2015). The hyperpigmentation is unevenly distributed, concentrated in already darker areas of the skin, such as the areolae, nipples, genitalia, but also the axillae, inner thighs and peri-umbilical skin with darkening of the adjacent linea alba ('linea nigra'). Up to 75 % of the women with pregnancy-induced hyperpigmentation may also develop circumscribed areas of hypermelanosis affecting face, neck and forearms, also called 'melasma', or 'mask of pregnancy' (◘ fig. 1.23). Sun exposure enhances its development, indicating that exacerbation of hyperpigmentation by exposure to sunlight can be controlled by sunscreens. In general, hyperpigmentation regresses postpartum, but persists in 10 % of the cases, to recur again in a future pregnancy.

Many women notice the development of *thicker scalp hair* during pregnancy, an effect related to prolongation of the anagen or 'growing phase' of hair follicles, resulting in a larger fraction of hair follicles residing in this stage. This effect reverses in the first five months postpartum, when these hair follicles enter the telogen ('resting') phase, resulting in increased hair loss.

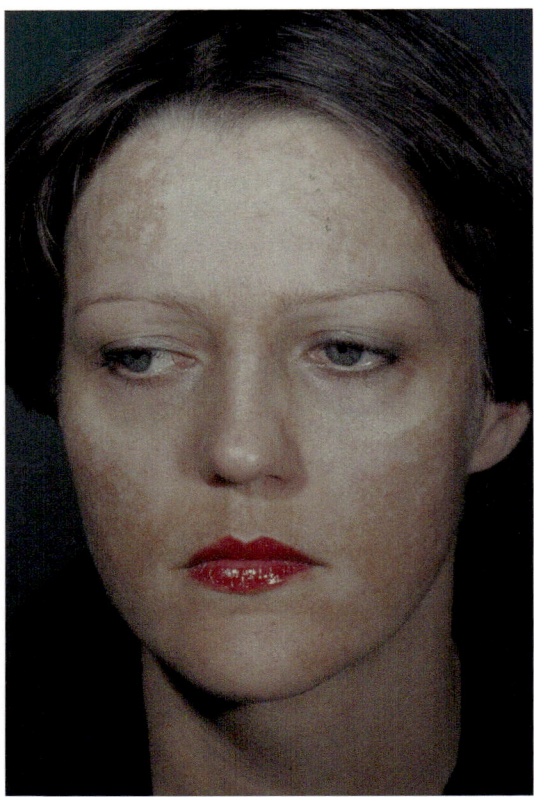

◘ Figure 1.23   Melasma in a late-pregnant woman, characterized by dark-brown patchy hyperpigmented skin spots on the cheeks

Striae gravidarum are another common skin effect of pregnancy, often developing by the end of the second trimester, particularly in Caucasian women (Panicker et al. 2017). Their development is caused by physical factors (such as stretch by abdominal distension) combined with hormonal changes (corticosteroids, relaxin, estrogens), which lead to thinning of elastic fibres and fibrillin microfibrils in the dermis and a change in the fibre orientation. Linear violaceous bands emerge on the abdomen and occasionally also on the thighs, arms, breasts, axillae and buttocks, gradually evolving into pale, skin-colored atrophic bands at term. Other factors involved in the development of striae gravidarum are maternal weight gain and genetic predisposition. The efficacy of preventive measures, such as massage with oil or water and creams, still awaits scientific confirmation.

Less common pregnancy-induced skin changes have been described in two recent reviews on this topic (Tyler et al. 2015; Panicker et al. 2017).

1.13 Impact of pregnancy on brain functioning and upcoming motherhood

During pregnancy, a wide range of circulating neurochemicals (neuropeptides and neurotransmitters) act in concert with various hormones (e.g. steroids, prolactin, oxytocin) to modulate not only maternal physiology, but also socio-psychologic functions, such as caregiving behavior, cognition, emotions and mood (Galea et al. 2013; Brunton 2019). Studies in nonhuman primates indicate that high circulating estrogen levels during pregnancy raise the maternal motivation and responsiveness to infant stimuli (Saltzman et al. 2011). Studies in transgenic rodents provide evidence for maternal nurturing responses being modulated by the inhibitory neurotransmitter γ-aminobutyric acid (GABA) and the neuropeptide oxytocin (Lonstein et al. 2014). Yet, it is questionable whether these findings in animal studies can be extrapolated to humans, because of the huge cognitive, social and communicative differences between animals and humans. This aspect challenges any comparison of psycho-emotional or behavioral endpoints. Therefore, better understanding of the complex mechanisms that control these cognitive and emotional effects in human remains elusive for the time-being. Actually, in human these effects depend on a pregnant woman's physical/mental wellbeing and personal background, which is the outcome of interactions between intrinsic (emotional stability, maternal affect and stress systems, and intelligence) and extrinsic factors (early adverse experiences, current observed mothering behavior, level of education, cultural/family context and socioeconomic situation), as recently reviewed (Stolzenberg et al. 2016; Moses-Kolka et al. 2014).

1.14 Mechanism regulating onset of (normal) parturition at term

The fetus requires time to reach sufficient maturity in order to survive in an aerobic environment. In humans, this period lasts from the first day of the last menstrual period until the 37th pregnancy week. During this period, the uterus must be hospitable to pregnancy by promoting uterine quiescence. Hence, the uterus is kept in a relaxed state, grows in concert with its contents, and keeps its cervix rigid and closed. Also, the decidua is kept in an immunologically dormant state to prevent rejection of the allogeneic fetal tissues. Progesterone promotes all these effects in pregnancy by blocking gap-junction formation, and by inhibiting the production and release of uterotonic prostaglandins and oxytocin. It also has potent anti-inflammatory properties and, last but not least, anti-progestins have been shown to induce cervical ripening.

Parturition refers to the physiologic chain of events that enables the safe, reliable and timely uterine expulsion of fetus and placenta. Labor is a physiologic event at term, defined by regular, painful and coordinated uterine contractions leading to progressive cervical effacement and dilatation from 4 cm to full dilatation. Labor develops after a quiescent period of irregular myometrial contractions without cervical changes, known as Braxton-Hicks contractions and detailed in ▶ sect. 1.1 of this chapter (Liao et al. 2005). Towards term, the number of progesterone receptors in the uterus and cervix fall, in spite of no consistent decline in circulating progesterone levels. Yet, the changes at the tissue level are expected to reduce the functional effect of progesterone on the myometrium and cervix. The decline in progesterone receptors coincides with a rise in

1

the circulating levels of estradiol and estriol. Estrogen opposes the actions of progesterone as reflected in a rise in uterine oxytocin receptors and in prostaglandin production, leading to an increase in myometrial contractility. Prostaglandins also promote cervical ripening.

Although our insight in normal parturition is still incomplete, experimental evidence supports fetal control over the onset of labor. As a matter of fact, the latter coincides with the fetal hypothalamic-pituitary-adrenal axis reaching a critical level of maturation (Liao et al. 2005), reflected in the fetal adrenals having reached the capacity to produce and release cortisol. This hormone enhances fetal lung maturation by raising the release of surfactant components (Mendelson et al. 2017) and by promoting the biosynthesis of estrogen, which is key in inducing both cervical ripening and inflammatory gene expression. Estrogen also prevents progesterone from binding to its receptor, which is another mechanism that supports a role of inflammation during the process of parturition (Keelan 2018). This mechanism for labor onset has been extensively studied in sheep (Challis et al. 2000), which only partly resembles that in humans. Mechanically, the difference relates to the birth canal in the human being curved with the fetal head being large relative to the diameter of the birth canal. These features cause more mechanical resistance that needs to be overcome during fetal expulsion, requiring more forceful, coordinated and peristaltic uterine contractions.

Human labor involves a series of coordinated processes (see ◘ fig. 1.24) including (1) a switch from progesterone to estrogen dominance, (2) actions triggered by (placental) corticotropin releasing hormone (CRH) that increase shortly before labor, and (3) the concomitant increase in oxytocin sensitivity, gap junction formation and activity of prostaglandins (Vannuccini et al. 2016). These actions are further amplified by concomitant effects related to aging of the fetal membranes, circadian endocrine clocks, inflammatory and mechanical factors (Menon et al. 2016).

In normal pregnancy, inflammatory responses could be involved in maternal self-preservation, provoked by specific external threats with labor being an intended direct consequence. Actually, emptying an infected body cavity that jeopardizes maternal health not only serves the woman's self-preservation. It also protects her future reproductive capacity. It is plausible that this defence mechanism is also key in the onset of normal human labor. However, such a mechanism requires finetuning of both its time-regulation (term pregnancy) and its effects being limited to the target site (birth canal), thus avoiding the amplification to a systemic inflammatory response.

Interestingly, the conceptus self is responsible for the late-pregnant change in the (1) mix of placental steroid output and CRH production, (2) maturity-related fetal cortisol output and (3) aging of the fetal membranes. This aspect can be expected to further finetune their composite impact on the timing of labor onset. The processes regulating human parturition, have been elaborated in various recent reviews on this topic (Li et al. 2010; Hanson et al. 2014; Ravanos et al. 2015; Norwitz et al. 2015; Vannuccini et al. 2016; Mendelson et al.; 2017; Menon et al.; 2016 *and* 2017; Keelan 2018).

Both pregnancy length and fetal maturity at term vary widely among viviparous species and are not related to size at birth. Nevertheless, all viviparous species studied so far, have in common that the near-term uterus undergoes a pre-labor process of activation (phase 1), that precedes the phase of stimulation (phase 2, or active labor) (◘ fig. 1.25) (Vannuccini et al. 2016). Uterotropins like estrogens induce phase 1 by activating select

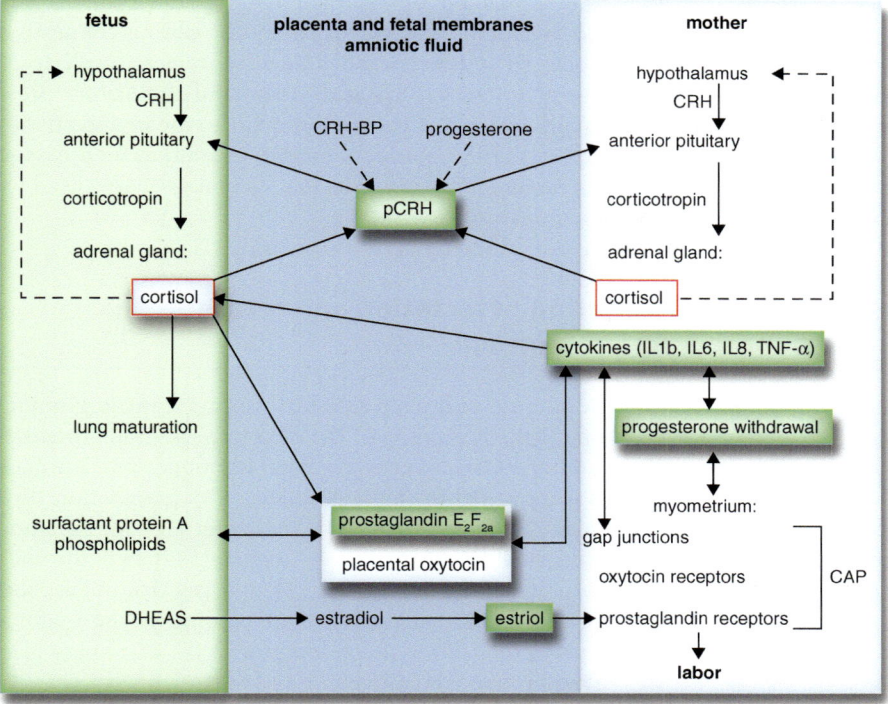

Figure 1.24 Interactions between fetal, placental and maternal factors prior to normal labor onset. *Abbreviations*: CRH: corticotropin releasing hormone, CRH-BP: CRH-binding protein, pCRH: placental CRH, DHEAS: dehydroepiandrosterone sulfate, CAP: contraction activating proteins.

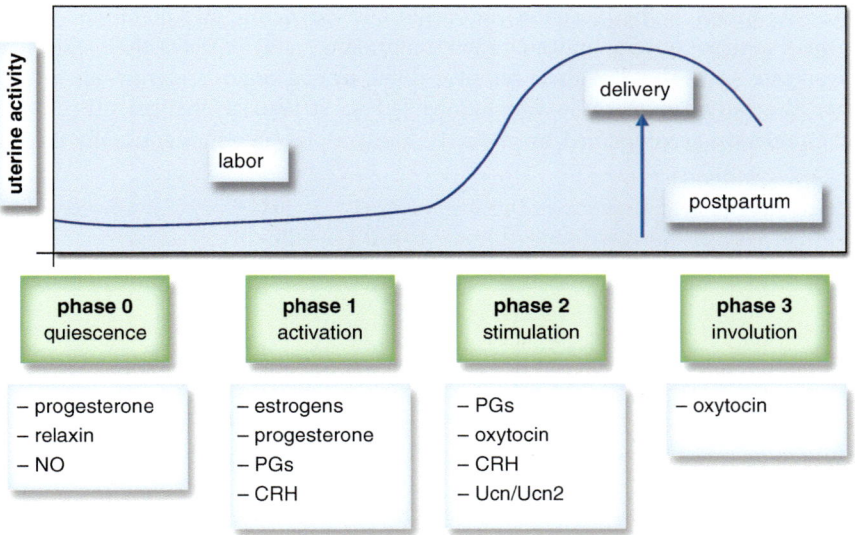

Figure 1.25 Phases of human parturition. *Abbreviations*: NO: nitric oxide, CRH: corticotropin releasing hormone, PGs: prostaglandins, Ucn: urocortin (*adopted from* Vannuccini et al. 2016)

ion-channels, by increasing the expression of contraction-associated proteins (such as myometrial receptors for prostaglandins and oxytocin) and by raising connexin-43, a key component of gap junctions. These effects enable the advancement to phase 2 by raising the uterine receptivity to uterotonics, such as oxytocin and stimulatory prostaglandins (PGE_2 and $PGF_{2\alpha}$). Finally, phase 3 of parturition refers to the period after placental expulsion and consists of events that promote uterine involution with oxytocin playing a central role. Unique in *human* labor is a fetus that combines a large head with various organ systems still being immature.

1.15 Puerperium, initiation of lactation and return to nonpregnant physiology

Placental detachment from the uterine wall after childbirth forms a turning point in the maternal physiology and marks the beginning of the next stage in motherhood, the puerperium. The abrupt interruption of the input of placental hormones into the maternal blood stream impacts the maternal physiology as follows. (1) termination of the endocrine support of the pregnancy-induced changes in the maternal body (2) almost complete cessation of the uteroplacental blood supply that utilized 15–20 % of the maternal cardiac output, (3) discontinuation of the maintenance of an organ that utilizes about 15 % of total maternal O_2 and metabolic demands, and (4) ending of the inhibiting effects of placental steroids on prolactin's affinity to its receptor in the mammary gland, thus preparing the next step in motherhood, breastfeeding and nurturing.

Most of the physical health issues caused by pregnancy and delivery (perineal pain after vaginal birth or abdominal pain after cesarean birth, but also constipation, bowel/urinary incontinence, back pain, hemorrhoids) fade in over 90 % of women within 2 weeks postpartum (◘ tab. 1.7), although mental issues – if present (e.g. depressive symptoms) – tend to persist for much longer (Chang et al. 2015).

The withdrawal of the placental endocrine, hemodynamic and metabolic functions from the maternal system indicates their redundancy and initiates their elimination. However, rate and extend of their removal differ among organ systems, depending on whether the duration of these adaptations led to structural changes. The hyperdynamic circulation accompanied by about 1.5 L extra plasma volume, usually returns to

◘ **Table 1.7**   Postpartum persistence of pregnancy- or childbirth-induced physical complaints reported by mothers over a period of 8 weeks (Cooklin et al. 2015)

general self-rated health	week 1 (n=212)	week 2 (n=210)	week 3 (n=210)	week 4 (n=210)	week 8 (n=222)
good/excellent	88 %	92 %	92 %	94 %	91 %
fair/poor	12 %	8 %	8 %	6 %	9 %

the prepregnant level within two weeks along with the 'normalization' of the maternal metabolism and peripheral vascular resistance. Obviously, it should be kept in mind that the postpartum maternal metabolism differs from that prevailing before pregnancy, as in this period the uterus gradually evolves to its nonpregnant form, shape and function, whilst metabolic demands also increase due to breastfeeding. With cardiovascular function almost normalized, the now redundant extracellular fluid accumulated during pregnancy in the intravascular compartment (about 1.5 L) and in the interstitial space (about 4 L) is to be dissipated, resulting in a negative fluid balance for about 10 days. This process of regaining the nonpregnant volume state is accompanied by a transient rise in plasma volume, preload and CO, along with a transient rise in α-ANP, indicative of the concomitant accelerated natriuresis. Since the pregnancy-induced change in renal function – hyperfiltration and altered tubular function – developed without structural renal changes, it is not surprising that renal function returns to the pre-pregnant state within 6–8 weeks (Odutayo et al. 2012). In contrast, the cardiovascular adaptation to pregnancy includes eccentric myocardial hypertrophy that requires 6 to 12 months to fully resolve (Savu et al. 2012; Melchiorre et al. 2016). Most of the pregnancy-induced changes in respiratory function relate to the progesterone-induced rise in sensitivity for PCO_2 of the respiratory center in the medulla oblongata, leading to a rise in tidal volume. It also follows that this effect can be expected to resolve shortly postpartum. The same applies to the adaptive changes in the maternal immune, hematologic and hemostatic functions. These are all induced by placental hormones without concomitant structural changes in the organs involved. Therefore, these changes can be expected to resolve shortly postpartum. Maternal weight loss between ten days postpartum and the subsequent six months ranges from 0.5–0.9 kg per month with some variation related to breastfeeding (Butte et al. 1998).

During pregnancy, prolactin, growth hormone, placental lactogen, and the steroid hormones are all involved in mammary gland development, resulting in increased size of the breasts, nipples, glands of Montgomery and areolae, along with more pigmentation. Mammary growth begins by about 8 weeks pregnancy and is accompanied by an unpleasant, tense feeling, sometimes even painful, particularly during movement. This sensation is caused by hyperemia. In some cases, the nipples produce some yellowish secrete resulting from transudation towards the mammary ducts (Macias et al. 2012). Circulating prolactin levels, essential for milk production, increase with advancing pregnancy to peak at term, though, without resulting in any milk production before childbirth, as detailed above.

Postpartum, prolactin controls milk production, while oxytocin controls milk ejection from the gland, the release being triggered by stimulating myoepithelial cells in the mammary gland. The synthesis and release of prolactin and oxytocin depends on the sensory input produced by the infant's suckling as shown in ◘ fig. 1.26. Finally, the rate of breastfeeding and it's duration varies widely among women worldwide, due to psychological, socio-economic and cultural factors (Jonas et al. 2016).

1

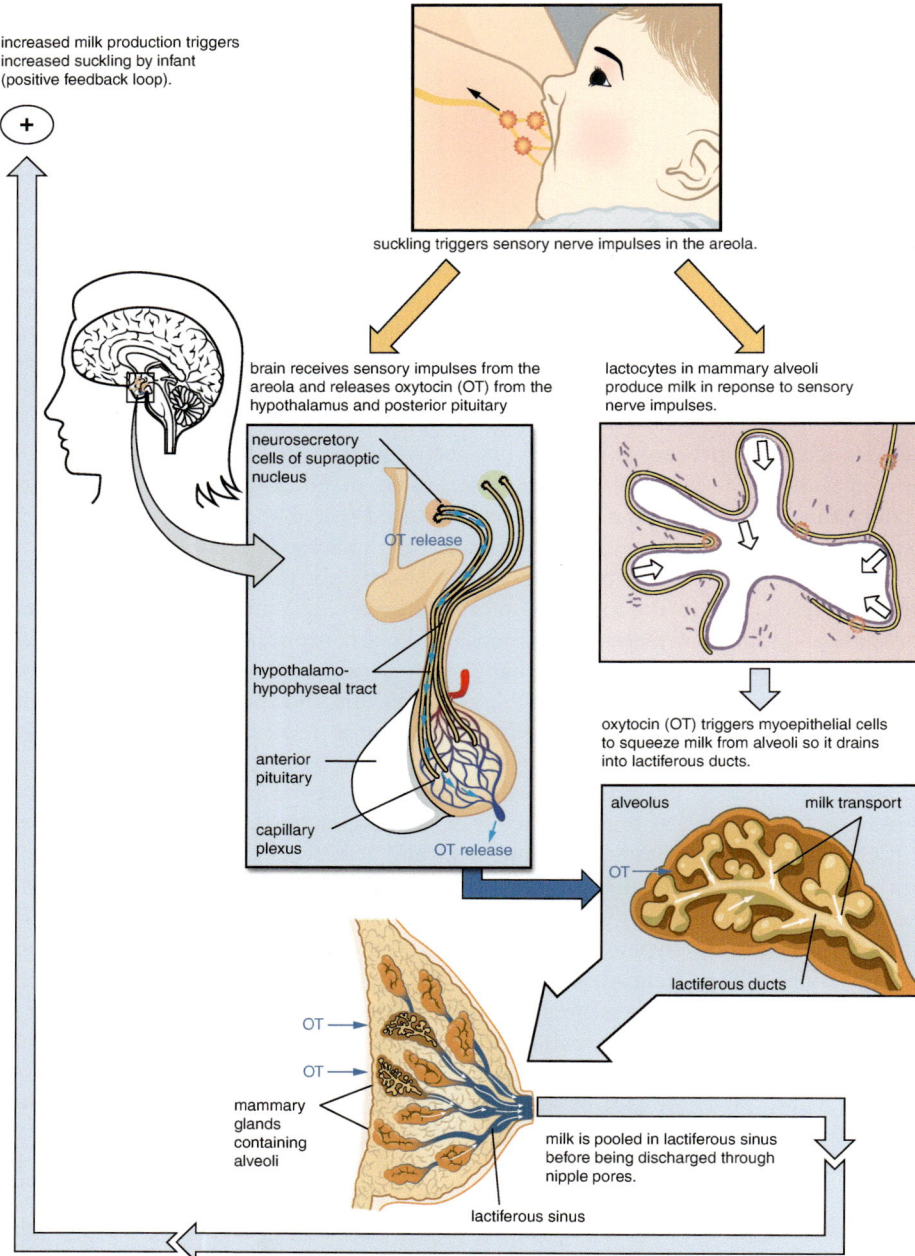

increased milk production triggers
increased suckling by infant
(positive feedback loop).

+

suckling triggers sensory nerve impulses in the areola.

brain receives sensory impulses from the
areola and releases oxytocin (OT) from the
hypothalamus and posterior pituitary

lactocytes in mammary alveoli
produce milk in reponse to sensory
nerve impulses.

neurosecretory
cells of supraoptic
nucleus

OT release

hypothalamo-
hypophyseal tract

anterior
pituitary

capillary
plexus   OT release

oxytocin (OT) triggers myoepithelial cells
to squeeze milk from alveoli so it drains
into lactiferous ducts.

alveolus   milk transport

OT

lactiferous ducts

OT

OT

mammary
glands
containing
alveoli

milk is pooled in lactiferous sinus
before being discharged through
nipple pores.

lactiferous sinus

■ Figure 1.26   Endocrine and mechanical triggers regulating lactation

References

Aardenburg R, Spaanderman MEA, Ekhart TH, et al. Low plasma volume following pregnancy complicated by pre-eclampsia predisposes to hypertensive disease in a next pregnancy. Brit J Obstet Gynaecol. 2003;110:1001–6.

Ander SE, Diamond MS, Coyne CB. Immune responses at the maternal-fetal interface. Sci Immunol. 2019;4. ► https://doi.org/10.1126/sciimmunol.aat6114.

Aplin JD, Ruane PT. Embryo-epithelium interactions during implantation at a glance. J Cell Sci. 2017;130:15–22.

Avsar AF, Keskin HL. Haemorrhoids during pregnancy. J Obstet Gynecol. 2010;30:231–7.

Baeyens L, et al. β-cell adaptations in pregnancy. Diabetes Obes Metab. 2016;18(suppl 1):63–70.

Bates SM. Pregnancy-associated venous thromboembolism: prevention and treatment. Semin Hematol. 2011;48:271–84.

Battaglia FC, Mechia G. Fetal nutrition. Ann Rev Nutr. 1988;8:43–61.

Battaglia FC, Meschia G. Principal substrates of fetal metabolism. Physiol Rev. 1978;58:499–527.

Battaglia FC, Meschia G. Foetal and placental metabolisms: their interrelationships and impact on maternal metabolism. Proc Nutr Soc. 1981;40:99–113.

Berlin DA, Bakker J. Understanding venous return. Intensive Care Med. 2014;40:1564–6.

Bertelli E and Bendayan M. Association between endocrine pancreas and ductal system. More than an epiphenomenon of endocrine differentiation and development? J Histochem Cytochem. 2005;53:1071–86.

Blaszczyk J, et al. Adaptive changes in spatiotemporal gait characteristics in women during pregnancy. Gait and Posture. 2016;43:160–4.

Bobrowski RA. Pulmonary physiology in pregnancy. Clin Obstet Gynecol. 2010;53:285–300.

Body C, Christie J. Gastrointestinal diseases in pregnancy: Review. Gastroenterol Clin North Am. 2016;45:267–83.

Bonney EA. Immune regulation in pregnancy. A matter of perspective? Obstet Gynecol Clin N Am. 2016;43:679–98.

Brenner B. Haemostatic changes in pregnancy. Thromb Res. 2004;114:409–14.

Brunton PJ. Endogenous opioid signalling in the brain during pregnancy and lactation. Cell Tissue Res. 2019;375:69–83.

Burton GJ, Hempstock J, Jauniaux E. Nutrition of the human fetus during the first trimester. A review. Placenta. 2001;22 Suppl. A Trophoblast Research 15:S70–6.

Burton GJ, Jauniaux E, Charnock-Jones DS. The influence of the intrauterine environment on human placental development. Int J Dev Biol. 2010;54:303–11.

Butte NF. Carbohydrate and lipid metabolism in pregnancy: normal compared with gestational diabetes. Am J Clin Nutr. 2000;71(5 suppl.):1256S–61S.

Butte NF, Hopkinson JM. Body composition changes during lactation are highly variable among women. J Nutr. 1998;128:285–381S.

Cakmak B, Ribeiro AP, Inanir A. Postural balance and the risk of falling during pregnancy. J Matern Fetal Neonatal Med. 2016;29:1623–5.

Cahill AG, Tuuli MG. Labor in 2013: the new frontier. Am J Obstet Gynecol 2013; 209: 531-4.

Caniggia I, Winter JL. Hypoxia inducible factor-1; oxygen regulation of trophoblast differentiation in normal and pre-eclamptic pregnancies – a review. Placenta. 2002;23(supplement A) Trophoblast Research 16:S47–57.

Carvalho LN, et al. Mesangial cell culture from pregnant rats display reduced reactivity to angiotensin II: the role of relaxin, nitric oxide and AT2 receptor. Cell Physiol Biochem. 2012;30:1456–64.

Challis JRG, Matthews SG, Gibb W, Lye SJ. Endocrine and paracrine regulation of birth at term and pre-term. Endocr Rev. 2000;21:514–50.

Chamley LW, Holland OJ, Chen Q et al. Review: where is the maternofetal interface? Placenta. 2014;35(suppl. A) Trophoblast Research 28:S74–80.

Chang S-R, Chen K-H, Ho H-N, et al. Depressive symptoms, pain, and sexual dysfunction over the first year following vaginal or cesarean delivery: a prospective longitudinal study. Int J Nurs Stud. 2015;52:1433–44.

Cheung KL, Lafayette RA. Renal physiology of pregnancy. Adv Chronic Kidney Dis. 2013;20:209–14.

Chung E, Leinwand LA. Pregnancy as a cardiac stress model. Cardiovasc Res. 2014;101:561–70.

Clark SL, et al. Am J Obstet Gynecol. 1989;161: 1439–42.

1

Cong J, Yang X, Zhang Y, et al. Quantitative analysis of left atrial volume and function during normotensive and preeclamptic pregnancy: a real-time three-dimensional echocardiography study. Int J Cardiovasc Imaging. 2015;31:805–12.

Conrad KP. Emerging role of relaxin in the maternal adaptations to normal pregnancy: Implications for preeclampsia. Semin Nephrol. 2011;31:15–32.

Conrad KP, Davison JM. The renal circulation in normal pregnancy and preeclampsia. Is there a place for relaxin? Am J Physiol Renal Physiol. 2014;306:F1121–35.

Conrad KP, Shroff SG. Effects of relaxin on arterial dilation, remodeling and mechanical properties. Curr Hypertens Rep. 2011;13:409–20.

Conrad KP, Graham GM, Chi YY, et al. Potential influence of the corpus luteum on circulating reproductive and volume regulatory hormones, angiogenic and immunoregulatory factors in pregnant women. Am J Physiol Endocrinol Metab. 2019;317:E677–85.

Cooklin AR, et al. Maternal physical health symptoms in the first 8 weeks postpartum among primiparous Australian women. Birth. 2015;42:254–60.

Costa MA. The endocrine function of the human placenta: an overview. Reprod Biomed Online. 2016;32:14–43.

Craciunas L, Gallos I, Chu J, et al. Conventional and modern markers of endometrial receptivity: a systematic review and meta-analysis. Hum Reprod Update. 2019;25:202–23.

Davison JM, Vallotton MB, Lindheimer MD. Plasma osmolality and urinary concentration and dilution during and after pregnancy: evidence that lateral recumbency inhibits maximal urinary concetration ability. Br J Obstet Gynaecol. 1981;88:472–9.

De Bari O, et al. Cholesterol, cholelithiasis in pregnant women: pathogenesis, prevention and treatment. Ann Hepatol. 2014;13:728–45.

De Haas S, Ghossein-Doha C, Van Kuijk SMJ, et al. Physiological adaptation of maternal plasma volume during pregnancy: a systematic review and meta-analysis. Ultrasound Obstet Gynecol. 2017;49:177–87.

Deryabin P, Griukova A, Nikolsky N et al. The link between endometrial stromal cell senescence and decidualization in female fertility: the art of balance. Cell Mol Life Sci. 2019. ► https://doi.org/10.1007/s00018-019-03374-0.

Druckmann R, Druckmann M. Progesterone and the immunology of pregnancy. J Steroid Biochem Mol. 2005;97:389–96.

Duvekot JJ, et al. Am J Obstet Gynecol. 1993;169: 1382–92.

Duvekot JJ and Peeters LL. Obstet Gynecol Surv. 1994;49: S1–14.

Erlebacher A. Immunology of the maternal-fetal interface. Annu Rev Immunol. 2013;31:387–411.

Faas MM, De Vos P. Uterine NK cells and macrophages in pregnancy. Placenta. 2017;56:44–52.

Feldt-Rasmussen U, Mathiesen ER. Endocrine disorders in pregnancy: Physiological and hormonal aspects of pregnancy. Best Pract Res Clin Endocrinol Metab. 2011;25:875–84.

Forsum E, Löf M. Energy metabolism during human pregnancy. Annu. Rev. Nutr. 2007;27:277–92.

Foti T, et al. A biomechanical analysis of gait during pregnancy. J Bone Joint Surg Am. 2000;82:625–32.

Fournier T, Guibourdenche J, Evain-Brion D. Review: hCGs: different sources of production, different glycoforms and functions. Placenta. 2015:36 (suppl. 1) vol. 29:S60–5.

Fowden AL et al. Review: endocrine regulation of placental phenotype. Placenta. 2015;(suppl. 1) Trophoblast Research vol 29:S50–9.

Galea LAM, Wainwright SR, Roes MM, et al. Sex, hormones and neurogenesis in the hippocampus: hormonal modulation of neurogenesis and potential functional implications. J Neuroendocrinol. 2013;25:1039–61.

Garlanda C, Maina V, Martinez de la Torre Y, et al. Inflammatory reaction and implantation: the new entries PTX3 and D6. Placenta. 2008;29:S129–34.

Gellersen B, Brosens JJ. Cyclic decidualization of the human endometrium in reproductive health and failure. Endocr. Rev. 2014;35:851–905.

Gellersen B, et al. Decidualization of the human endometrium: Mechanisms, functions and clinical perspectives. Semin Reprod Med. 2007;25:445–53.

Gelman S. Venous function and central venous pressure. Anesthesiology. 2008;108:735–48.

Geraghty LN, Pomeranz MK. Physiologic changes and dermatoses of pregnancy. Int J Dermatol. 2011;50:771–82.

Hadden DR, McLaughlin C. Normal and abnormal metabolism during pregnancy. Semin Fetal Neonatal Med. 2009;14:66–71.

Halligan A, et al. J Hypertens. 1993;11: 869–73.

Hanson L, VandeVusse L. Supporting labor progress towards physiologic birth. J Perinat Neonat Nurs. 2014;28:101–7.

Harris LK. IFPA Gabor than award lecture: transformation of the spiral arteries in human pregnancy: key events in the remodelling timeline. Placenta. 2011;32:S134–58.

Harris LK, Benagiano M, D'Elios, et al. Placental bed research: II. Functional and immunological investigations of the placental bed. Am J Obstet Gynecol. 2019;221:457–69.

Hegewald MJ, et al. Respiratory physiology in pregnancy. Clin Chest Med. 2011;32:1–13.

Hellgren M. Hemostasis during normal pregnancy and puerperium. Semin Thromb Hemost. 2003;29:125–30.

Huppertz B, Weiss G, Moser G. Trophoblast invasion and oxygenation of the placenta: measurements versus presumptions. J Reprod Immunol. 2014;101–102:74–9.

Hutchings G, Williams O, Cretoiu D, Ciontea SM. Myometrial interstitial cells and the coordination of myometrial contractility. J Cell Mol Med. 2009;13:4268–82.

James JL, Saghian R, Perwick R, et al. Trophoblastic plugs: impact on uteroplacental haemodynamic and spiral artery remodelling. Hum Reprod. 2018;33:1430–41.

Jensen D. Mechanical ventilation constraints during incremental cycle exercise in human pregnancy: implications for respiratory sensation. J Physiol. 2008;586:4735–50.

Jeyabalan A, Lain KY. Anatomic and functional changes of the upper urinary tract during pregnancy. Urol Clin N Am. 2007;34:1–6.

Jonas W, Woodside B. Physiological mechanisms, behavioral and psychological factors influencing the transfer of milk from mothers to their young. Horm Behav. 2016;77:167–81.

Kamel RM. The onset of human parturition. Arch Gynecol Obstet. 2010;281:975–82.

Keelan JA. Intrauterine inflammatory activation, functional progesterone withdrawal and the timing of term and preterm birth. J Reprod Immunol. 2018;125:89–99.

Kong S, Zhou C, Bao H, et al. Epigenetic control of embryo-uterine crosstalk at peri-implantation. Cell Mol Life Sci. 2019;76:4813–28.

Kühnert M, et al. Changes in the lymphocyte subsets during normal pregnancy. Eur J Obstet Gynecol Reprod Biol. 1998;76:147–51.

Lacroix M, et al. Maternal/fetal determinants of insulin resistance in women during pregnancy and in offspring over life. Curr Diab Rep. 2013;13:238–44.

Lammert E, Thorn P. The role of the island niche on beta cell structure and function. J Mol Biol. 2019. ▶ https://doi.org/10.1016/j.jmb.2019.10.032.

Larqué E, et al. Placental regulation of fetal nutrient supply. Curr Opin Clin Metab Care. 2013;16:292–7.

Leo CH, Jelinic M, Ng HH, Marshall SA, et al. Vascular actions of relaxin: nitric oxide and beyond (review article). Brit J Pharmacol. 2017;174:1002–14.

Li X et al. Modeling childbirth: elucidating the mechanisms of labor. WIREs Syst Biol Med. 2010:460–470.

Liao JB, Buhimschi CS, Norwitz ER. Normal labor: mechanism and duration. Obstet Gynecol Clin N Am. 2005;32:145–64.

Licht P, Fluhr H, Neuwinger J, et al. Is human chorionic gonadotropin directly involved in the regulation of human implantation? Mol Cell Endocrinol. 2007;269:85–92.

Lindheimer MD, Barron WM, Davison JM. Osmoregulation of thirst and vasopressin release in pregnancy. Am J Physiol. 1989;257:F159–69.

Liu H, Huang X, Mor G, Liao A. Epigenetic midifications in the decidualization and endometrial receptivity. Cell Mol Life Sci. 2020;77:2091–101.

Lockwood CJ. Pregnancy-associated changes in the hemostatic system. Clin Obstet Gynecol. 2006;49:838–43.

London V, et al. Hyperemesis gravidarum: a review of recent literature. Pharmacol. 2017;100:161–71.

Lonstein JS, Maguire J, Meinlschmidt G, et al. Emotion and mood adaptations in the peripartum female: Complementary contributions of GABA and oxytocin. J Neuroendocrinol. 2014;26:649–64.

Lotgering FK, Van Doorn M, Struijk PC, et al. Maximal aerobic exercise in pregnant women: Heart rate, O_2 consumption, CO_2 production and ventilation. J Appl Physiol. 1991;70:1016–23.

Lumbers ER, Pringle KG. Roles of the circulating renin-angiotensin-aldosterone system in human pregnancy. Am J Physiol Regul Integr Comp Physiol. 2014;306:R91–101.

Macias H, Hinck L. Mammary gland development. Wiley Interdiscip Rev Dev Biol. 2012;1:533–57.

Marques NR, et al. Passive leg raising during pregnancy. Am J Perinatol. 2015;32:393–8.

Melchiorre K, Sharma R, Thilaganathan B. Cardiac structure and function in normal pregnancy. Curr Opin Obstet Gynaecol. 2012;24:413–21.

Melchiorre K, Sharma R, Khalil A, Thilaganathan B. Maternal cardiovascular function in normal pregnancy; evidence of maladaptation to chronic volume overload. Hypertension. 2016;67:754–62.

Mendelson CR, Montalbano AP, Gao L. Fetal-to-maternal signaling in the timing of birth. J Steroid Biochem & Mol Biol. 2017;170:19–27.

Menon R, Mesiano S, Taylor RN. Programmed fetal membrane senescence and exosome-mediated signaling: a mechanism associated with timing of human parturition. Front Endocrinol. 2017;8:196. ► https://doi.org/10.3389/fendo.2017.00196.

Menon R, Bonney EA, Condon J, et al. Novel concepts on pregnancy clocks and alarms: redundancy and synergy in human parturition. Hum Reprod Update. 2016;22:535–60.

Meschia G. Fetal oxygenation and maternal ventilation. Clin Chest Med. 2011;32:15–9.

Moffett A, Colucci F. Uterine NK cells: active regulators at the maternal-fetal interface. J Clin Invest. 2014;124:1872–9.

Moses-Kolko EL, Horner MS, Phillips ML, et al. In search of neural endophenotypes of postpartum psychopathology and disrupted maternal caregiving. J Neuroendocrinol. 2014;26:665–84.

Murthi P. Review: placental homeobox genes and their role in regulating fetal growth. Placenta. 2014;28:S46–50.

Nama V, Antonios TF, Onwude J, et al. Mid-pregnancy drop in normal pregnancy: myth or reality? J Hypertens. 2011;29:763–8.

Nascimento SL, et al. Physical exercise during pregnancy: a systematic review. Curr Opin Obstet Gynecol. 2012;24:387–94.

Nelson DM. How the placenta affects your life, from womb to tomb. Am J Obstet Gynecol. 2015;213:S12–3.

Norwitz ER, Bonney EA, Snegovskikh VV, et al. Molecular regulation of parturition: the role of the decidual clock. Cold Spring Harb Perspect Med. 2015;5:1–21.

Odutayo A, Hladunewich M. Obstetric nephrology: Renal hemodynamics and metabolic physiology in normal pregnancy. Clin J Am Soc Nephrol. 2012;7:2073–80.

Okada H, Tsuzuki T, Murata H. Decidualization of the human endometrium. Reprod Med Biol. 2018;17:220–7.

Pang CC. Autonomic control of the venous system in health and disease; Effects of drugs. Pharmacol Ther. 2001;90:179–230.

Panicker VV, Riyaz N, Balachandran PK. A clinical study of cutaneous changes in pregnancy. J Epidemiol Global Health. 2017;7:63–70.

Racicot K, et al. Understanding the complexity of the immune system during pregnancy. Am J Reprod Immunol. 2014;72:107–16.

Ramin KD, et al. Disease of the gallbladder and pancreas in pregnancy. Obstet Gynecol Clin North Am. 2001;28:571–80.

Ravanos K, Dagklis T, Petousis S, et al. Factors implicated in the initiation of human parturition in term and preterm labor: a review. Gynecol Endocrinol. 2015;31:679–83.

Redman CWG, Dragovic DS, Gardiner RA, et al. Review: does size matter? Placental debris and the pathophysiology of pre-eclampsia. Placenta. 2012;(suppl. A) Trophoblast Research 26:548–54.

Reyes LM, Usselman CW, Davenport MH, Steinback CD. Sympathetic nervous system regulation in human normotensive and hypertensive pregnancies. Hypertension. 2018;71:793–803.

Robson SC, et al. Am J Physiol. 1989;256: H1060–5.

Romero R, et al. Preterm labor: one syndrome, many causes. Science. 2014;345:760–5.

Roth CJ, HaeussnerE, RuebelmanT et al. Dynamic modeling of uteroplacental blood flow in IUGR indicates vortices and elevated pressure in the intervillous space – a pilot study. Sci Rep (nature research). 2017;7:40771.

Saltzman W, Maestripieri D. The neuroendocrinology of primate maternal behavior. Prog Neuropsychopharmacol Biol Psychiatry. 2011;35:1192–204.

Sanghavi M, Rutherford JD. Cardiovascular physiology of pregnancy. Circulation. 2014;130:1003–8.

Savu O, et al. Morphologic and functional adaptation of the maternal heart during pregnancy. Circ Cardiovasc Imaging. 2012;5:289–97.

Schauberger CW, et al. Peripheral joint laxity increases during pregnancy but does not correlate with serum relaxin levels. Am J Obstet gynecol. 1996;174:667–71.

Schrier RW, Niederberger M. Paradoxes of body fluid volume regulation in Health and Disease – a unifying hypothesis. West J Med. 1994;161:293–408.

Schrier RW, Ohara M. Dilemmas in human and rat pregnancy: proposed mechanisms relating to arterial vasodilation. J Neuroendocrinol. 2010;22:400–6.

Schwartsburd P. Insulin resistance is a two-sided mechanism acting under opposite catabolic and anabolic conditions. Med Hypotheses. 2016;89:8–10.

Sharma S, Godbole G, Modi D. Decidual control of trophoblast invasion. Am J Reprod Immunol. 2016;75:341–50.

Shin GH, et al. Pregnancy and postpartum bowel changes: constipation and fecal incontinence. Am J Gastroenterol. 2015;110:521–9.

Shiri Rm Coggon D, Falah-Hassani K. Exercise for the prevention of low back and pelvic girdle pain in pregnancy: a meta-analysis of randomized controlled trials. Eur J Pain. 2018;22:19–27.

Solano ME. Decidual immune cells: guardians of human pregnancy. Best Pract Res Clin Obstet Gynaecol. 2019;60:3–16.

Spaanderman MEA, et al. Cardiac output increases independently of basal metabolic rate in early human pregnancy. Am J Physiol Heart Circ Physiol. 2000;278:H1585–8.

Spaanderman M, et al. Preeclampsia and maladaptation to pregnancy: A role for atrial natriuretic peptide? Kidney Int. 2001;60:1397–406.

Stolzenberg DS, Champagne FA. Hormonal and non-hormonal bases of maternal behavior: the role of experience and epigenetic mechanisms. Horm Behav. 2016;77:204–10.

Sunitha M, Chandrasekharappa S, Brid SV. Electrocardiographic QRS axis, Q-wave and T-wave changes in the 2nd and 3rd trimester of normal pregnancy. J Clin Diagn Res. 2014;8:BC 17–21.

Tan EK, Tan EL, Med M. Alterations in physiology and anatomy during pregnancy. Best Pract Res Clin Obstet Gynaecol. 2013;27:791–802.

Tessier DR, Yockell-Lelièvre J, Gruslin A. Uterine spiral artery remodeling: the role of uterine natural killer cells and extravillous trophoblasts in normal and high-risk human pregnancies. Am J Reprod Immunol. 2015;74:1–11.

Theofanakis C, Drakakis P, Besharat A, Loutradis D. Human chorionic gonadotrophin: the pregnancy hormone and more. Int J Mol Sci. 2017;18(1059):8. ▶ https://doi.org/10.3390/ijms18051059.

Tkachenko O, Shchekochikhin D, Schrier RW. Hormones and hemodynamics in pregnancy (review). Int J Endocrinol Metab. 2014;12:e14098.

Tyler K. Physiological skin changes during pregnancy. Clin Obstet Gynecol. 2015;58:119–24.

Vannuccini S, Bocchi C, Severi FM, et al. Endocrinology of human parturition. Ann Endocrinol. 2016;77:105–13.

Veenendaal MVE, Van Abeelen AFM, Painter RC, et al. Consequences of hyperemesis gravidarum for offspring: a systematic review and meta-analysis. Brit J Obstet Gynaecol. 2011;118:1302–13.

Vejrazkova D, et al. Steroids and insulin resistance. J Steroid Biochem Mol Biol. 2014;139:122–9.

Vink JY, Qin S, Brock CO, et al. A new paradigm for the role of smooth muscle cells in the human cervix. Am J Obstet Gynecol. 2016;215(478):e1–11.

Von Rango U. Fetal tolerance in human pregnancy – a crucial balance between acceptance and limitation of trophoblast invasion. Immunol Lett. 2008;115:21–32.

Weimar CH, Post Uiterweer ED, Teklenburg G, et al. In-vitro model systems for the study of human embryo-endometrial interactions. Reprod Biomed Online. 2013;27:461–76.

Weiss G, Sundl M, Glasner A, et al. The trophoblast plug during early pregnancy: a deeper insight. Histochem Cell Biol. 2016;146:749–56.

Young RC. Synchronization of regional contractions of human labor; direct effects of region size and tissue excitability. J Biomech. 2015;48:1614–9.

Zeng Z, et al. Metabolic adaptations in pregnancy. Ann Nutr Metab. 2017;70:59–65.

Pathophysiology of pregnancy complications in healthy women

Abstract

During pregnancy, the expectant mother provides a new human life with the ideal conditions to grow, mature and develop to its maximum genetic potential. This extra effort requires adaptive changes in her system, initially her immune function, but after embryo implantation, also various other organs, particularly in the cardiovascular/renal systems and metabolism. Some adaptations only consist of a reset of a particular setpoint (e.g. blood pressure and osmolality), whereas others (e.g. cardiovascular and metabolic adaptations) require the utilization of some of the maternal 'normal' reserve capacity (described in ▶ chap. 1). ▶ Chapter 2 consists of two sections. The first section describes frequently observed pathophysiologic developments in pregnancy in seemingly healthy women resulting from maladaptation of the maternal hemodynamic-, renal-, immune- and metabolic functions. The impact is usually a disruption of pregnancy course and outcome, because of the development of a (*1*) Placental syndrome, (*2*) Spontaneous preterm birth, or (*3*) Gestational diabetes. The second section describes less common pathophysiologic events that primarily affect maternal wellbeing, in conjunction with (*4*) side-effects of placental hormones, (*5*) abnormal placental morphology or insertion site in the uterus, and (*6*) distressing mechanical effects, caused by the rapidly growing pregnant uterus.

© Bohn Stafleu van Loghum is een imprint van Springer Media B.V., onderdeel van Springer Nature 2021
L. L. H. Peeters et al., *Pathophysiology of Pregnancy Complications*,
https://doi.org/10.1007/978-90-368-2571-9_2

> **Highlights**
>
> 1. Defective development of immunotolerance towards the embryo during the window of implantation can lead to implantation failure and early pregnancy loss.
> 2. The subnormal formation of hemodynamic reserves in early pregnancy predisposes to early-onset (< 34 weeks) placental syndromes (PS), presumably, because of the associated compensatory rise in cardiovascular sympathetic tone. The latter causes a rise in uterine vascular resistance, and with it, increases the risk of developing placental dysfunction.
> 3. Gradual developing placental dysfunction can lead to mild PS (pregnancy-induced hypertension). More rapid and/or severe development of placental dysfunction will likely lead to an earlier-onset and/or more severe form of PS (preeclampsia, HELLP syndrome or eclampsia).
> 4. Excessive maternal stress can disrupt the mechanism that triggers the onset of labor. It will not only accelerate fetal maturation and the senescence of placenta/membranes. It will also adversely impact the immune function, which has a negative effect on the composition of the microbiome in the birth canal. The latter most likely facilitates upstream colonization with pathogens, which is thought to be an important trigger for preterm birth.
> 5. Subnormal insulin reserves limit the maternal ability to raise insulin output in the second half of pregnancy. This predisposes a pregnant woman to develop gestational diabetes.

2.1 Pathophysiology of placental syndrome (PS)

Placental dysfunction is the final outcome of various different pathophysiological pathways, most of them still incompletely unravelled. Therefore, placental dysfunction has been used as common denominator for a set of widely varying pregnancy disorders, termed placental syndromes (PS), as metaphorically shown in ◘ fig. 2.1. The subtypes of PS have different sets of clinical symptoms requiring different management strategies. These strategies only have in common that they are supportive, focusing on the relief of symptoms, combined with maternal and fetal surveillance, but without direct actions to improve placental function (Myatt et al. 2014).

PS not only includes fetal growth restriction (FGR), preeclampsia (PE), HELLP syndrome and eclampsia, but also disorders, such as (late) spontaneous miscarriage, preterm labor, premature rupture of the membranes and placental abruption (Brosens et al. 2011). Although these disorders share placental dysfunction as a common denominator, their pathophysiology varies widely as reflected (for example), in the difference between early- (< 34 weeks) and late-onset PE. Early-onset PE begins with defective deep placentation shortly after implantation, whereas late-onset PE only develops in more advanced pregnancy, when even a perfectly normal placenta can become dysfunctional in response to maternal constitutive factors (e.g. obesity, chronic hypertension), known to predispose to vascular damage (Myatt et al. 2014). This pathophysiologic difference between early and late-onset PE is not absolute. Women that develop PE at for instance, circa 30 weeks often have pathophysiologic features of both early- and late-onset PE. Nevertheless, clinical presentation and management of that PE is the same. This example also

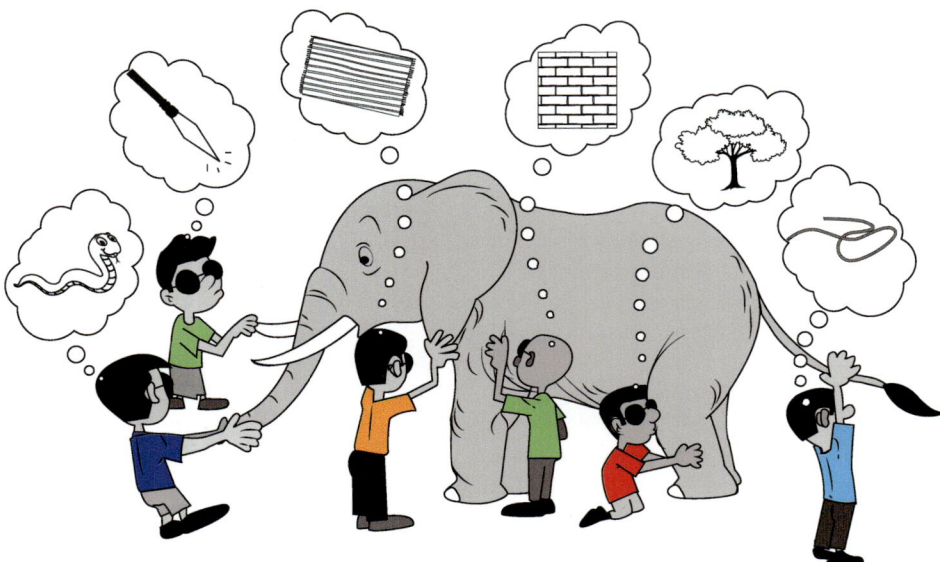

■ **Figure 2.1**   Placental syndrome (PS) refers to a set of disorders that share placental dysfunction as common denominator. A PS results from diverse, incompletely unraveled pathophysiology's. However, just knowing their phenotype is sufficient to institute the correct clinical management, which is only supportive without intention to remove its cause. One may compare PS with an elephant examined by a number of blind men, who all come to a 'correct', but different diagnosis depending on the phenotype they examined

shows that, because of the diverse, incompletely-unravelled pathophysiology of PS subtypes, it is virtually impossible to reliably identify women at risk for any subtype of PS by a single, all-inclusive algorithm. Also, it indicates that the gradually improving insight in the pathophysiology of each subtype of PS can be expected to lead to regular 'updates' in both definition of PS subtypes and their management, with the latter gradually shifting from supportive to causal treatment (Phipps et al. 2016).

Until a decade ago, PE was defined by the new onset of hypertension and proteinuria in the second half of pregnancy. However, the relevance of including these two clinical features in the definition of PE is gradually eroding and being replaced by placenta-derived toxic factors, such as sFlt-1 and endoglin. As a matter of fact, early investigators of PE focused on dysfunction of the cardiovascular system and kidneys. However, in the last decades it has become clear that other organ systems are more directly involved in the pathophysiology of PS (such as the decidua and maternal immune system).

The generally accepted and first-discernible abnormality in the pathophysiology of early-onset PS is 'shallow' placentation, which refers to spiral-artery (SA) remodeling restricted to its decidual portion. This indicates that the SA remodeling does not include a certain fragment of its myometrial portion as normally occurs (■ fig. 2.2). The more superficial SA remodeling is often accompanied by obstructive arterial lesions, such as thrombosis and acute atherosis, particularly if a PS includes FGR.

The wide phenotypical variation in early-onset PS relates to incomplete insight into the factors that may disrupt deep placentation. Presumably, the trigger is diverse and hard to identify as the set of synchronized events in the period from embryo implantation

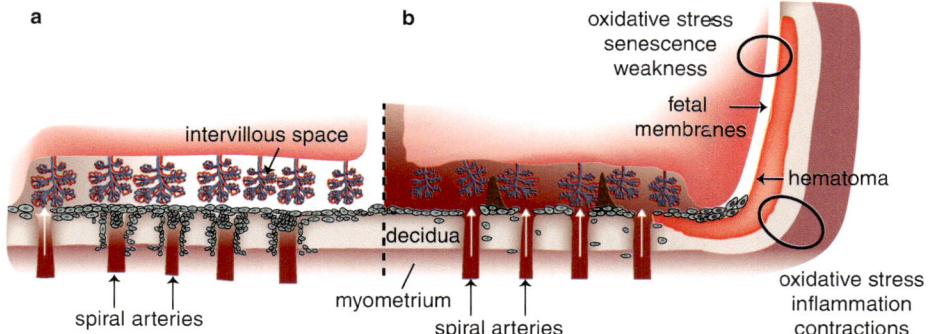

■ **Figure 2.2** **(a)** Normal placental bed with extravillous trophoblasts (green cells) orchestrating the remodeling of the spiral arteries across the decidua to as deep as the inner third of the myometrium along with their transient occlusion. **(b)** Shallow placentation as occurs in early-onset preeclampsia: Spiral artery remodeling is defective because of (1) Less spiral arteries being transformed, (2) Spiral artery remodeling being limited to its decidual portion, and (3) Spiral artery remodeling without accessory transient partial occlusion, which predisposes to both intrauterine hematoma formation and accelerated aging of the fetal membranes (upper circle), and increases the risk of premature rupture of the membranes or of an inflammatory response (*adopted from* Burton et al. 2017)

until fully developed placenta (midpregnancy), is almost entirely regulated by local, transiently-operating factors, most of them being sensitive to the impact of a wide range of external influences (Lash 2015). On the other hand, when PS only becomes symptomatic in *late* pregnancy (e.g. > 34 weeks pregnancy), the prolonged subclinical phase enables the development of systemic, recognizable and interrelated effects, that facilitate the interpretation of the pathophysiology of that particular PS.

The prevalence of PS is higher in developing- than in developed countries, because of inadequate (access to) health care services, along with cultural and poverty-related factors, such as teenage pregnancy, promiscuity, undiagnosed or poorly-managed chronic diseases, nutritional deficiencies, excessive survival stress and a higher chance of exposure to a polluted environment. In developed countries, other unfavorable external factors prevail, such as obesity, excessive alcohol consumption, unhealthy food habits, sedentary lifestyle and poor stress management. These factors undermine the health state and wellbeing of pregnant women, and with it, their ability to complete a pregnancy uneventfully. PS in general, and PE and eclampsia in particular, are worldwide the most important causes of maternal morbidity and mortality. In spite of a marked fall in PS-related maternal mortality in developed countries in the last decades, morbidity remains high and is still the leading cause of intensive care admissions during pregnancy (Myatt et al. 2014).

A precondition for a normal pregnancy is the presence of a number of key local and systemic factors. Poor insight into events during early placentation also explains the modest success of pregnancy achieved by in-vitro fertilization techniques, with only about 40 % of fertilized oocytes surviving implantation and only one-third of these 'early-survivors' eventually resulting in a life birth (Larsen et al. 2013). About 2 to 5 % of the latter group develops PS in their pregnancy (Norwitz 2001; Lash 2015). Factors or events, identified as potential disruptors of placental development are summarized in ■ fig. 2.3 and discussed in more detail below.

2

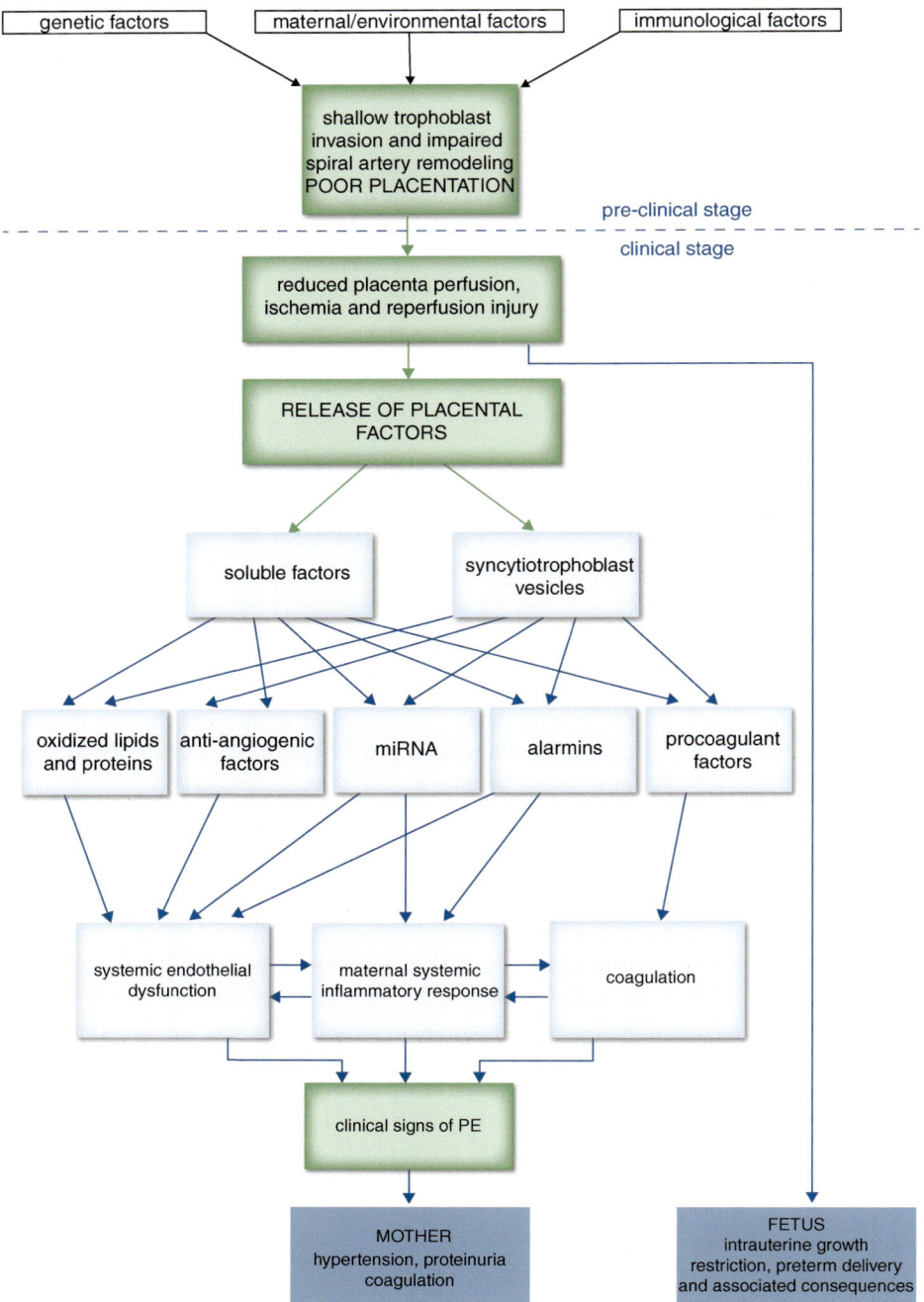

□ **Figure 2.3**   Pathogenesis of PE and the involvement of factors that may contribute to disease progression. The interrelation between the events indicated in the upper 2 green boxes are yet to be unveiled. They are assumed to cause the release of the toxic placental factors responsible for maternal symptoms (*adopted from* Tannetta and Sargent 2013)

2.1.1 **Pathophysiology of the PS subtypes**

Genetic or immunologic defects may disrupt early placentation, often acting in concert with unfavorable extrinsic factors, such as chronic latent disorders, obesity and poor stress management. Placental damage in this process results from endoplasmic-reticulum stress and inflammatory/oxidative damage causing syncytial necrosis, autophagy/apoptosis and excessive shedding of syncytial knots and micro-vesicles (Redman et al. 2012 *and* 2014). The poor predictive capacity of various early biomarkers (Kleinhouweler et al. 2016; Gaccioli et al. 2018) indicates that the early abnormal events at the F-M interface are strictly localized with insufficient spill into the circulating blood to cause a detectable rise in the blood levels of locally produced abnormal molecules. It follows, that the pathophysiologic chain of events that begins shortly after embryo implantation and eventually results in a dysfunctional placenta, still contains several undetermined mechanisms, particularly in the first half of pregnancy. Afterwards, it becomes easier to determine the type and severity of placental dysfunction based on clinical signs, such as disrupted transplacental metabolic exchange, endocrine 'control' of maternal adaptations, and peripheral effects triggered by excessive oxidative stress and accumulation of metabolic waste products at the F-M interface. Presumably, the subtype of PS that develops in the second half of pregnancy depends on firstly, the gestational age, when the disease becomes manifest and secondly, on the mix of clinical signs, severity and rate of deterioration of the three placental functions, mentioned in the previous sentence. The epidemiology and pathophysiology of each PS subtype will be discussed below in order of the severity of the clinical presentation.

1. *FGR* refers to the failure of the fetus to reach its full genetic growth potential. The severity of this particular PS increases with earlier onset, which may even begin as early as in the embryonic period. Ideally, the definition of FGR should include – besides current fetal size and growth rate – information on fetal and placental health, which is often difficult to obtain (Zhang et al. 2010; Gaccioli et al. 2018). On the other hand, the cause of FGR is often multifactorial, which complicates the differentiation between constitutionally small infants and PS-induced FGR. Therefore, the definition of FGR should also consider the contribution of constitutional features to the estimated fetal weight. Some years ago, a customized estimate of fetal growth potential was developed using software to calculate "term optimal weight" adjusted for maternal height, weight, ethnicity, parity and the infant's gender (Gardosi 2012). It is a simple and practical assessment, particularly useful for clinical purposes.
   FGR caused by placental dysfunction, primarily results from inadequate transplacental metabolic exchange. The latter is the consequence of the combination of subnormal intervillous blood flow and subnormal villous exchange area. After the first trimester, fetal growth rate accelerates and with it, the demands for metabolic substrates to sustain the higher growth rate. Obviously, an earlier onset of FGR in pregnancy implies a more severe impairment of the placental metabolic exchange function. The imbalance in fetal nutrient supply and demand can develop gradually or in flares. A more gradual development enables the fetus to adapt to a prolonged state of intrauterine starvation by minimizing tissue accretion, using all its available reserves to improve the chance of survival. If the disrupted placental exchange already begins in midpregnancy, FGR will affect all tissues equally, resulting in proportional FGR. However, if the disruption develops in the last trimester, the

2

fetal stress response will be sufficiently matured to minimize the adverse effects of deficient nutrients supply on the growth and development of brain and heart by preferentially imposing the shortage of metabolic substrates on nonvital organs, such as skeletal tissues, skin, kidneys and visceral organs. This will result in disproportional FGR. Absence of maternal symptoms usually indicates a low risk of an adverse impact on her postpartum health.

In most cases of early-onset FGR, the disrupted exchange function is an aftereffect of defective spiral artery remodeling during early placental development. This defect leads to the development of a relatively small placenta with subnormal perfusion capacity and villous exchange area. The vascular origin of placental insufficiency implies that the eventual compromised blood supply does not develop gradually, but in flares. Occasionally, a flare may be complicated by the development of a placental infarction. If so, that particular flare can be expected to predispose to fetal asphyxia or even fetal death, because of the concomitant severe compromise of the fetal O_2 supply.

2. *PIH* refers to gestational hypertension defined by *de-novo* hypertension developing after the 20th week of pregnancy, and resolving again before the 12th week postpartum. This definition ignores the wide variety in clinical presentation of PIH, as it does not include any of the other possible clinical signs, such as persistent severe headache, new-onset epigastric tenderness or pain, visual disturbances (blurred vision, diplopia, floating spots), edema of the face, hands and feet, and hyperreflexia. Therefore, it is not surprising that this definition has been updated several times, with the NICE guideline of 2011 being accompanied by an excellent expert comment (Redman 2011).

   PIH develops because of excess oxidative stress at the F-M interface, but usually leads to a relatively mild clinical appearance. The disorder may develop secondary to the placental release of the antiangiogenic factors sFlt-1α and endoglin, combined with the shedding of syncytiotrophoblast cells (usually in the third trimester of pregnancy) (Redman et al. 2012). These placental products may trigger a systemic stress response, raising the cardiovascular sympathetic tone and with it, the resistance in the already compromised uteroplacental vascular bed. The endothelial dysfunction also impacts the fluid distribution between the intra- and extravascular compartments, clarifying part of the clinical signs mentioned above. PIH affects about 10 % of all pregnancies, with 1 in 4 affected women deteriorating to PE (Brown et al. 2018).

3. *PE* refers to a PIH-affected pregnancy, complicated by the *de-novo* development of proteinuria or other signs of maternal organ-/uteroplacental dysfunction (Poon et al. 2019). PE develops, when toxic products of oxidative stress accumulate at the F-M interface, spilling over into the maternal blood to trigger the abnormalities, specified in ◘ figs. 2.4 and 2.5.

   The prevalence of PE among pregnant women is 2 to 3 %, with 0.4 % (about 1 in 6 PE-affected women) experiencing early-onset PE (◘ fig. 2.6). Obviously, the prevalence of PE will be higher in a population with overrepresentation of risk patients, such as nulliparas, women older than 35 years and women with chronic hypertension, diabetes or obesity (Lisonkova et al. 2013). Early-onset PE occurs more often in black women, women with chronic hypertension or women carrying a child with specific chromosomal anomalies. On the other hand, late-onset PE is overrepresented in nulliparas and in women with a relatively large placenta

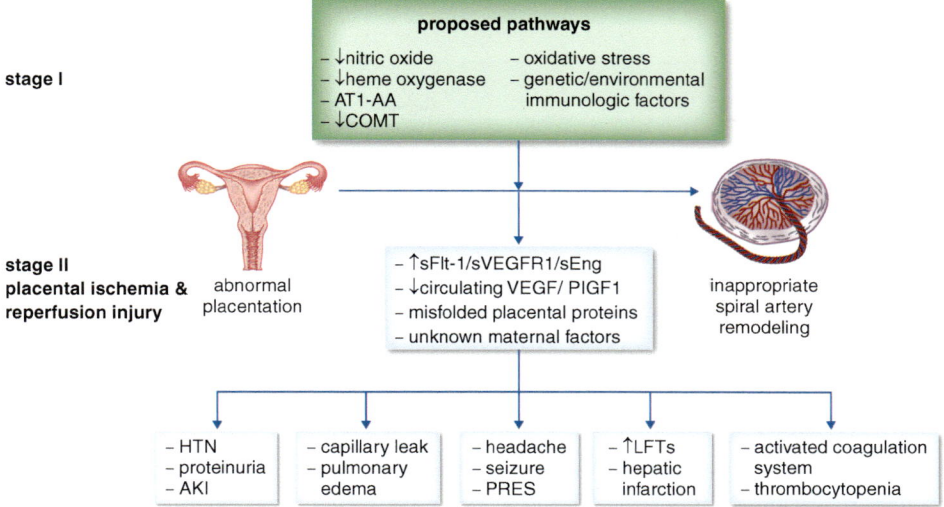

proposed pathways

- ↓nitric oxide   – oxidative stress
- ↓heme oxygenase   – genetic/environmental
- AT1-AA   immunologic factors
- ↓COMT

stage I

stage II
placental ischemia &   abnormal   – ↑sFlt-1/sVEGFR1/sEng   inappropriate
reperfusion injury   placentation   – ↓circulating VEGF/ PlGF1   spiral artery
                                                – misfolded placental proteins remodeling
                                                – unknown maternal factors

- HTN   – capillary leak   – headache   – ↑LFTs   – activated coagulation
- proteinuria   – pulmonary   – seizure   – hepatic   system
- AKI   edema   – PRES   infarction   – thrombocytopenia

◾ **Figure 2.4**   Pathogenesis of preeclampsia: two-stage model. *Abbreviations*: AT1-AA, autoantibodies to angiotensin receptor 1; COMT, catechol-O-methyltransferase; HTN, hypertension; AKI, acute kidney injury; LFT, liver function test; PlGF1, placental growth factor-1; PRES, posterior reversible encephalopathy syndrome; sEng, soluble endoglin; sFlt-1, soluble fms-like tyrosine kinase-1; sVEGFR1, soluble endothelial growth factor receptor 1; VEGF, vascular endothelial growth factor (*adopted from* Phipps et al. 2016)

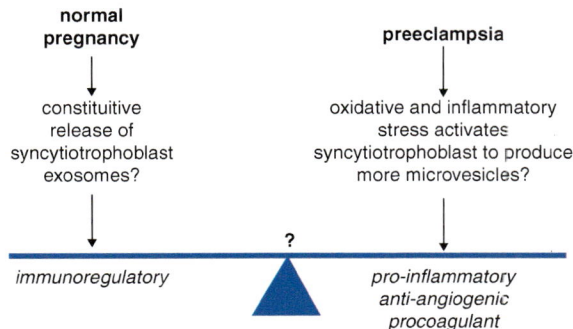

**normal
pregnancy**   **preeclampsia**

constituitive   oxidative and inflammatory
release of   stress activates
syncytiotrophoblast   syncytiotrophoblast to produce
exosomes?   more microvesicles?

                          ?

immunoregulatory   *pro-inflammatory
                                        anti-angiogenic
                                        procoagulant*

◾ **Figure 2.5**   The placenta of women with PE releases antiangiogenetic factors as shown in ◾ fig. 2.4, but also micro-vesicles with pro-inflammatory, anti-angiogenic and pro-coagulant properties, as opposed to a normal placenta that releases micro-vesicles with only immunoregulatory effects (*adopted from* Redman et al. 2012)

(e.g. multiple pregnancy, gestational diabetes, severe anemia, and women living at high altitude). Also, a history of PE or having limited functional reserves due to chronic cardiovascular-, renal-, metabolic- or autoimmune disorders predisposes to (both early- and late-onset) PE. The impact of chronic disorders on pregnancy and vice versa has been elaborated in ▶ chaps. 3 and 4. The subdivision of PE in early- and late-onset disease is primarily motivated by the impact on the unborn infant (prematurity, FGR).

rate per 1000
ongoing pregnancies

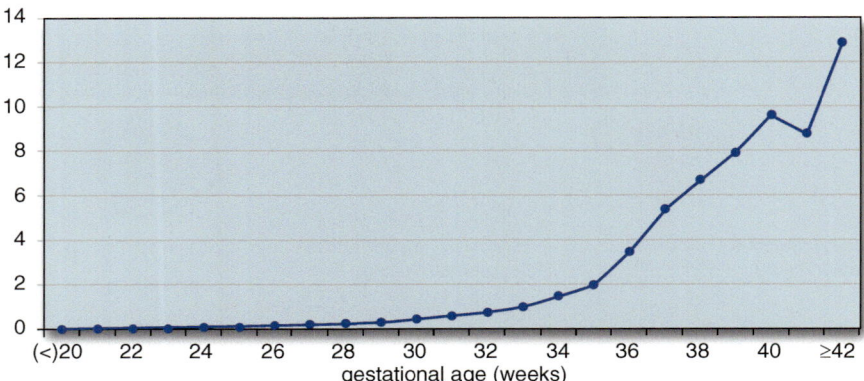

Figure 2.6 Gestational-age-specific incidence of preeclampsia in singleton pregnancies in Washington state, USA (about 450,000 women) between 2003 and 2008 (*adopted from* Lisonkova et al. 2013)

Structure and function of the placenta in women developing late-onset PE, may have been normal until the third trimester. With pregnancy approaching term, the loss of STBMs with a certain fraction being 'activated', can be expected to rise and with it, the chance that the number of activated cells exceeds the clearing capacity of the maternal lungs (Redman et al. 2012). In both early- and late-onset PE, the placental release of anti-angiogenic factors together with activated STBMs may challenge the maternal circulatory integrity, inducing a rise in the maternal cardiovascular sympathetic activity. This effect contributes to the development of part of the clinical symptoms (such as the hypertension and cardiac output redistribution in favor of heart and brain).

The renal lesions that develop in conjunction with the albuminuria (■ fig. 2.7) are typical for PE. Various studies in the last two decades provide evidence for these lesions to result from an angiogenic imbalance in the maternal blood due to excessive clearance of placental growth factor (PlGF) and vascular endothelium growth factor A (VEGF-A) by the raised circulating levels of placental sFlt-1α and endoglin (Turner et al. 2015).

The antiangiogenic factors sFlt-1α and endoglin not only activate glomerular endothelial cells and with it, their release of endothelin-1 (ET-1). These factors also eliminate most of the VEGF generated in the glomerulus, mostly produced by the podocytes (Eremina et al. 2007). This source of VEGF is key in maintaining the glomerular filtration barrier by both paracrine interaction with the glomerular endothelium and autocrine interaction with podocytes (Henao et al. 2010). The concomitant presence of high local levels of ET-1 also damages the podocytes' actin cytoskeleton and foot-process structure, and accelerates their release of nephrin, a transmembrane protein involved in the protection of the glomerular filtration barrier. It follows that podocyte damage impairs the protection of the glomerular filtration barrier resulting in the development of proteinuria. The unfavorable local endocrine conditions also cause glomerular endothelial swelling, termed 'glomeruloendotheliosis', which is considered typical for PE

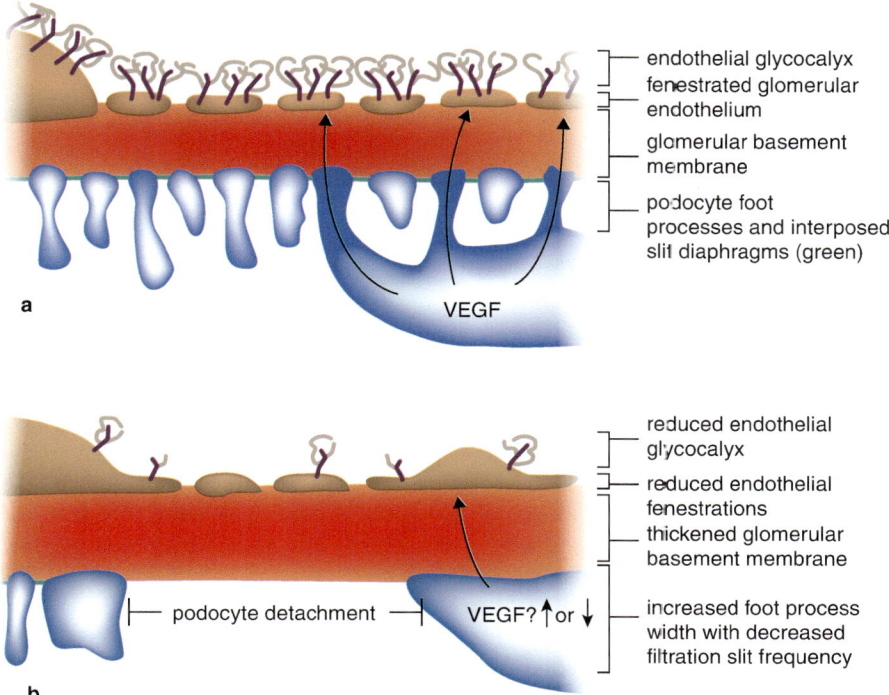

a

endothelial glycocalyx
fenestrated glomerular
endothelium

glomerular basement
membrane

podocyte foot
processes and interposed
slit diaphragms (green)

VEGF

b

reduced endothelial
glycocalyx

reduced endothelial
fenestrations
thickened glomerular
basement membrane

podocyte detachment — VEGF? ↑ or ↓

increased foot process
width with decreased
filtration slit frequency

■ **Figure 2.7**   Mechanism that leads to the proteinuria in preeclampsia. (**a**) In healthy conditions with balanced availability of pro- and anti-angiogenic factors, podocytes represent the main glomerular source of VEGF, also supplying VEGF to the glomerular endothelium. (**b**) In PE, excessive circulating Flt-1α and endoglin induce angiogenic imbalance, leading to VEGF shortage in the glomerulus. This enables endothelin-1 (ET-1) to interact with its receptor on the podocytes, resulting in endothelial swelling, reduced endothelial fenestrations, thickening of the basement membrane (BM) and detachment of the podocytes' foot-processes from the BM. This leads to widening of the pores in between them allowing albumin to pass (see Turner et al. 2015)

(Hennessy et al. 2011). Endothelial swelling in the glomerulus increases the intraglomerular pressure and resistance to flow, that may result in local ischemia. This effect may explain the urinary loss of (apoptotic) podocytes.

These inferences indicate that excessive oxidative stress at the M-F interface initiates the pathophysiology of both PIH and PE with that of PE resulting in a more severe placental dysfunction. PE seems to differ from PIH by a larger and a more rapidly rising spill of the same placental endotheliotoxic factors into the maternal blood. The concomitant rise in the sympathetic contribution to the autonomic control of the circulation raises uteroplacental vascular resistance, and with it, the risk of further worsening of the placental injury. All PE symptoms relate to placenta-induced endothelial dysfunction.

4. The *HELLP syndrome* – acronym for hemolysis (H), elevated liver enzymes (EL), and low platelets (LP) -, is a subtype of PS associated with relatively high maternal and perinatal morbidity and mortality rates. It is usually diagnosed based on the widely-used 'Tennessee classification' (Abildgaard et al. 2013). Maternal symptoms

are often vague, although many patients experience right-sided upper-abdominal pain or vague tenderness due to stretch exerted upon the liver capsule caused by liver congestion. This complaint is often accompanied by raised circulating levels of ALAT, ASAT, LDH and uric acid, along with reduced levels of haptoglobin and low platelet count, the latter two effects being caused by systemic thrombotic microangiopathy (TMA) (Kappler et al. 2014). The F-M exchange capacity is also compromised in many HELLP patients, which increases the risk of FGR and fetal asphyxia. The prevalence of HELLP in an unselected pregnant population is just 0.2–0.8 %, in most cases developing superimposed on PE. As many as 10 % of HELLP patients remain normotensive or do not develop proteinuria, indicating only partial overlap of the pathophysiology of HELLP and PE (Abildgaard et al. 2013).

The early stages of the pathophysiology of early-onset PE and HELLP is probably the same: post-implantation shallow placentation resulting in poorly remodeled spiral arteries. As a consequence, these arteries achieve insufficient perfusion capacity to meet the uteroplacental flow demands in the second half of pregnancy. The absence of the trumpet-shaped outlets of these arteries also affects their ability to dampen shear forces in the intervillous space exerted upon both maternal blood cells and placental villi (Burton et al. 2019). These adverse rheological effects raise the risk of villous damage and excessive shedding of villous debris (Redman et al. 2015). In fact, indirect evidence suggests that HELLP differs from PE by the shedding of larger amounts of villous debris into the maternal blood with the latter also containing cell-free DNA and necrotic material. This toxic mix triggers a systemic inflammatory response (Tranquilli et al. 2007; Polsani et al. 2013; Von Salmuth et al. 2020) reflected in placental overexpression of NF-kappa-B (Simsek et al. 2013). An inflammatory response that develops in a vascular bed already affected by endothelial dysfunction can be expected to (1) increase vascular permeability, (2) enhance the release of prothrombotic and antifibrinolytic factors, (3) trigger the expression of adhesion molecules, and (4) interfere with endothelial renewal. Particularly the latter effect is typical for HELLP as it affects the smoothness of the vascular endothelial lining, thus increasing the risk of developing TMA and activation of platelets, effects that promote vasoconstriction and microthrombi formation (Kazmi et al. 2011).

A chronic condition characterized by a thrombophilic phenotype predisposes to HELLP syndrome and confirms the role of a pro-coagulant state in the pathophysiology of HELLP. Liver sinusoidal endothelial cells (LSECs) are most vulnerable to the toxic mix released by the HELLP placenta (Van Lieshout 2019). This mixture contains – besides pro-inflammatory mediators (Abildgaard et al. 2013) – Fas-ligand, a protein that accelerates apoptosis, particularly of hepatocytes (Strand et al. 2004). Interaction of these mediators with activated LSECs in the hepatic sinusoids, where the prevailing shear forces are low, facilitates the development of sinusoidal TMA. These events will gradually evolve to sinusoidal obstruction by micro-thrombi and fibrin deposits, hypoxic demise of hepatocytes, necrosis and hemorrhage, eventually triggering periportal inflammatory infiltration with neutrophilic granulocytes (Abildgaard et al. 2013; Westbrook et al. 2016; Von Salmuth et al. 2020). Sinusoidal obstruction leads to upstream congestion and downstream ischemia, thus threatening the hepatic filter function for toxins reaching the liver by the portal vein. The pathophysiology of HELLP is illustrated in ◘ fig. 2.8.

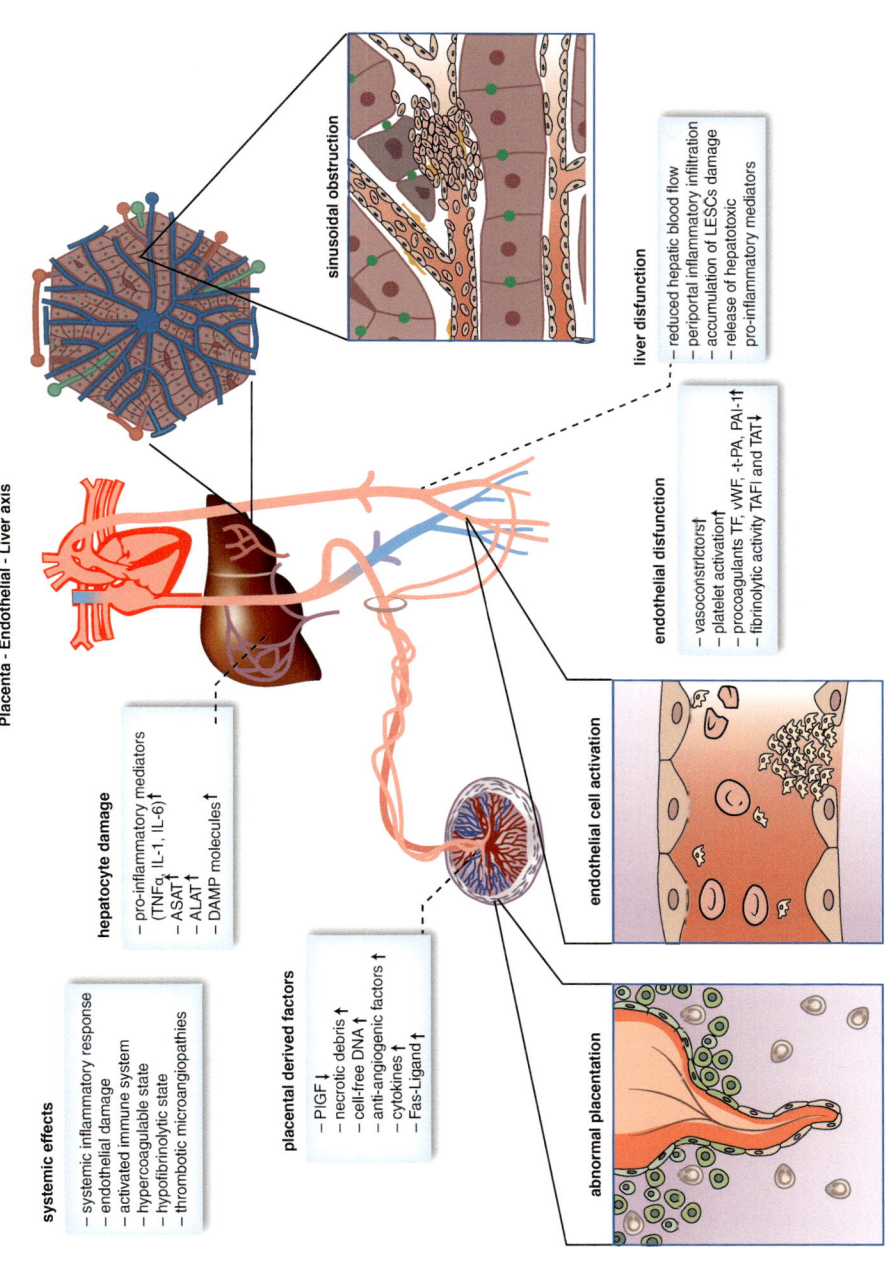

Placenta - Endothelial - Liver axis

sinusoidal obstruction

liver disfunction
- reduced hepatic blood flow
- periportal inflammatory infiltration
- accumulation of LESCs damage
- release of hepatotoxic pro-inflammatory mediators

endothelial disfunction
- vasoconstrictors↑
- platelet activation↑
- procoagulants TF, vWF, -t-PA, PAI-1↑
- fibrinolytic activity TAFI and TAT↓

hepatocyte damage
- pro-inflammatory mediators (TNFα, IL-1, IL-6)↑
- ASAT↑
- ALAT↑
- DAMP molecules↑

endothelial cell activation

systemic effects
- systemic inflammatory response
- endothelial damage
- activated immune system
- hypercoagulable state
- hypofibrinolytic state
- thrombotic microangiopathies

placental derived factors
- PlGF↓
- necrotic debris↑
- cell-free DNA↑
- anti-angiogenic factors↑
- cytokines↑
- Fas-Ligand↑

abnormal placentation

Figure 2.8 Interacting pathway of the placenta-endothelial-liver axis in the development of the HELLP syndrome. The dysfunctional placenta not only releases anti-angiogenic factors, but also necrotic debris, cell free DNA, cytotoxic cytokines and Fas-L. These compounds induce a systemic inflammatory response, that is particularly toxic for the liver (see text for details) (*adopted from* Von Salmuth et al. 2020)

It is not only women with a preexistent thrombophilia that are predisposed to develop HELLP in pregnancy. Women whose fetus suffers from a genetic defect in the fatty acid oxidation (Browning et al. 2006) and women with an autoimmune disorder, such as the antiphospholipid syndrome (Appenzeller et al. 2011) or an overactivated complement system (Baines et al. 2017) are also at increased risk. *Eclampsia* is to be considered a default diagnosis in pregnant or postpartum women with generalized seizures, until proven otherwise. In most cases, the seizures develop in women diagnosed with PE, without history of other conditions that may cause seizures. In most cases, eclampsia is superimposed on PE. The endothelial dysfunction in PE causing enhanced capillary leakage and a higher sympathetic contribution to the autonomic control of the circulation, plays also a key role in the pathophysiology of eclampsia. The clinical presentation of eclampsia (Sibai 2005) resembles that of the so-called Posterior Reversible Encephalopathy Syndrome (PRES), which is characterized by headache, vomiting, confusion, reduced alertness and behavioral changes, ranging from drowsiness to stupor, slowing of mental functions, generalized seizures, cortical blindness, other visual abnormalities and motor signs (Hinchey et al. 1996). Findings with neuroimaging resemble those of hypertensive encephalopathy and are consistent with extensive bilateral white matter abnormalities. These are most likely related to edema formation in the posterior regions of the cerebral hemispheres and are often accompanied by impact to other cerebral areas, brainstem and cerebellum (Fugate et al. 2015). Therefore, it has been suggested that eclampsia is triggered by a rapid *and* large rise in arterial pressure to a level above the autoregulatory range for cerebral blood flow. This leads to hyperperfusion and with it, vasogenic edema along with interstitial extravasation of plasma and macromolecules, consistent with a 'disrupted blood-brain-barrier (BBB) permeability'. On the other hand, eclampsia may also develop *without* appreciable rise in blood pressure (Cipolla 2007), which is in line with the view that the disorder resembles PRES rather than hypertensive encephalopathy and therefore, looks more like a 'brain-capillary-leak syndrome' resulting from an abnormal interplay between blood pressure, fluid retention and endothelial dysfunction (◘ fig. 2.9). This alternative interpretation of the pathogenesis of eclampsia is supported by both the raised circulating anti-angiogenic factors in eclamptic women and the genetic predisposition for eclampsia via several gene variants involved in thrombophilia, inflammation, oxidative stress and the RAAS (Aya et al. 2016). In this context, it is interesting to note that one-third of all cases of eclampsia occur within two days postpartum (Abalos et al. 2013) and coincide with the marked volume redistribution between extra- and intravascular compartments to eliminate the extra fluid accumulated during pregnancy. This mechanism may be defective in women, at increased risk of developing postpartum eclampsia, because of the coinciding endothelial dysfunction.

The incidence of eclampsia is about 50 cases per 10,000 pregnancies worldwide. Significant regional variation exists, ranging from 2.7 cases in the UK (Schaap et al. 2014) to almost 300 cases in sub-Saharan Africa (Abalos et al. 2013). This huge variation is due to differences in both access and quality of health care systems along with variability in early diagnosis, important for the timely and vigorous treatment of newly onset hypertension. Usually, eclampsia develops acutely in patients suffering from PE, with two-thirds of the cases occurring in (late) pregnancy or during labor, and one-third postpartum.

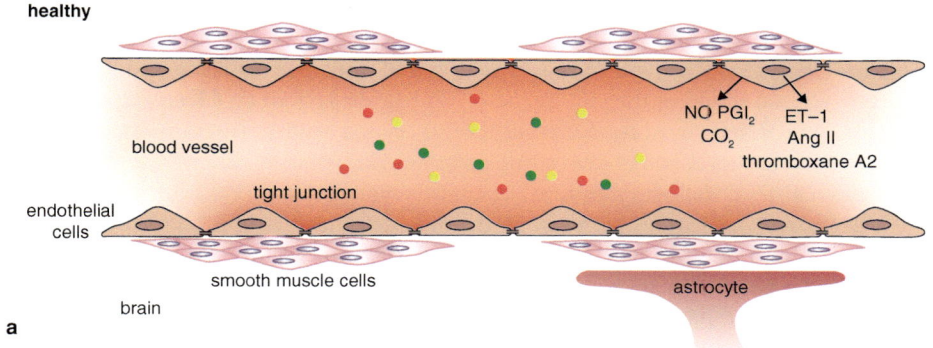

healthy

NO PGI$_2$ ET–1
CO$_2$ Ang II
thromboxane A2

blood vessel

tight junction

endothelial cells

smooth muscle cells

astrocyte

brain

a

posterior reversible encephalopathy syndrome

↑ET-1, ↓NO, TNFα,
↑VEGF IL-1

endothelial secretion

leukocyte interaction

increased permeability

disrupted tight junctions

ICAM–1 VCAM–1 E-selectin

astrocyte injury

interstitial edema

↑cytokine release

b

🔲 **Figure 2.9** Role of endothelial dysfunction in pathophysiology of posterior reversible encephalopathy syndrome (PRES). (**a**) *Healthy blood brain barrier (BBB)*. Tight junctions connect vascular endothelium. Various vasodilators (NO, CO$_2$, PGI$_2$) and – constrictors (thromboxane A2, endothelin-1, angiotensin-II) regulate vascular tone. (**b**) *Disrupted BBB in PRES*. Endothelial dysfunction leads to extravasation of fluid and macromolecules into the interstitium. Raised blood levels of cytotoxic cytokines (TNFα, IL-1, ET-1) activate endothelial cells, increasing the expression of adhesion molecules (e.g. intracellular adhesion molecule-1 [ICAM-1]). This enables them to interact/adhere to circulating leukocytes, which disrupts the integrity of the connections between tight junctions. Activated endothelial cells also display increased VEGF expression, that also raises vascular permeability and interstitial brain edema (*adopted from Fugate et al. 2015*)

Finally, normal pregnancy-induced cardiovascular adaptations may also contribute to the risk of eclampsia, as they cause both a downward shift of the cerebral blood flow autoregulatory interval (Cipolla 2007) and a rise in BBB permeability, which is probably related to a lower threshold for vasogenic edema formation (Chapman-Johnson et al. 2015). These adaptations reduce cerebral vascular resistance, though, at the cost of cerebral blood flow autoregulation and a lower threshold at which to develop cerebral edema (Faraci 2011; Chapman-Johnson et al. 2015).

In summary, the common denominator of PS is placental dysfunction with a variable adverse impact on fetal growth/wellbeing and maternal involvement.

Differences in (1) severity of placental dysfunction and deterioration rate, (2) maternal intrinsic susceptibility and (3) presence of extrinsic factors, are responsible for the diversity in type and severity of the PS subtypes. Because of poor insight into the initial stages of the pathogenesis of PS and a lack of an effective management strategy that could restore placental function, clinical care is limited to symptomatic treatment aimed at alleviating symptoms in combination with surveillance of maternal/fetal wellbeing. In most cases, this management reduces the chance of PS deterioration. However, at present, the only definite cure of PS is termination of pregnancy and removal of the dysfunctional placenta. The overall recurrence rate of PS in the next pregnancy is about 10 %, which is slightly higher, when the previous PS had developed at an earlier gestational age or was characterized by a more severe hypertension (Bernardus et al. 2018). Last but not least, PS predisposes former patients to future cardiovascular morbidity (Wu et al. 2017).

2.2 Pathophysiology of spontaneous preterm birth (SPTB)

SPTB, defined as pregnancy ending in spontaneous birth before 37 completed pregnancy weeks (Esplin 2014), is the most important cause of perinatal morbidity and mortality worldwide (Lockwood et al. 2001). Worldwide, it affects up to 15 million women (over 11 % of all livebirths) annually, with wide variations between countries (Cappelletti et al. 2016). The highest rates are observed in low-income countries, such as India, China, Nigeria and Pakistan, but also in the US (Purisch et al. 2017). More than one-third of the annual 3 million neonatal deaths worldwide result from complications from SPTB, making it one of the most common causes of death in infants below the age of 5 (Blencowe et al. 2012).

About 1 in 6 cases of SPTB occurs before the 32nd pregnancy week (◘ fig. 2.10). Infants born from these pregnancies are at highest risk of severe prematurity-related complications. Obviously, morbidity and mortality fall rapidly with childbirth occurring closer to term. SPTB is associated with a wide range of fetal, medical, obstetric, sociodemographic and environmental risk factors. However, these are absent in two-thirds of the cases (Vogel et al. 2018). SPTB may begin with spontaneous preterm premature rupture of the membranes (PPROM), uterine contractions, or cervical insufficiency.

The mechanism of normal term labor has been detailed in ▶ chap. 1 and serves as a reference for the pathophysiologic events resulting in SPTB. In short, the currently accepted concept is that fetal maturity, particularly that of the hypothalamic-pituitary-adrenal (HPA) axis, triggers the term onset of labor (Liao et al. 2005). This event coincides with the aging of fetal membranes, decidua and placenta, and together these events enhance the release of inflammatory mediators (Menon et al. 2017a). These mediators raise the inflammatory load in the myometrium, cervix and decidua and with it, amplify the effect of the coinciding fall in progesterone-related inhibition of immune-driven responses (Romero et al. 2014). As soon as the inflammatory load exceeds a certain threshold, uterine tissues switch from their quiescent state to the active state of labor, as illustrated in ◘ fig. 2.11 and detailed elsewhere (Liao et al. 2005; Romero et al. 2014; Menon et al. 2017a; Shynlova et al. 2020).

Yet, there are still important gaps in our understanding of the onset of normal term labor. It is generally accepted that throughout pregnancy, inflammatory stimuli interact with the progesterone/progesterone-receptor signaling to control labor. Inherent

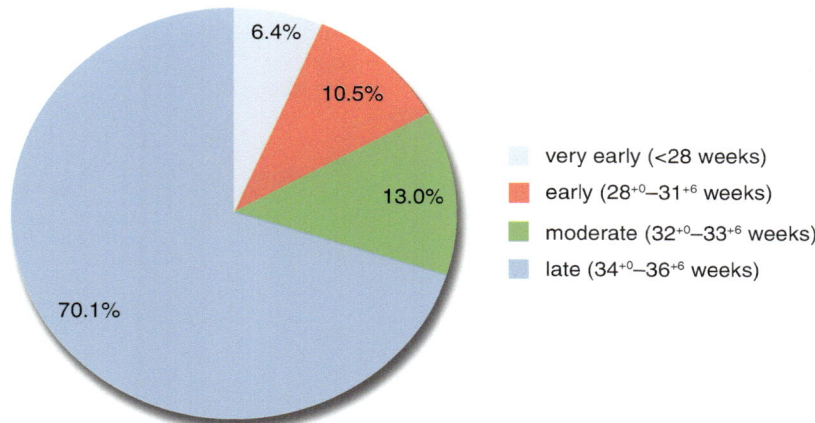

Figure 2.10   Distribution of spontaneous preterm births in the USA in 2013 (*adopted from* Frey and Klebanoff 2016)

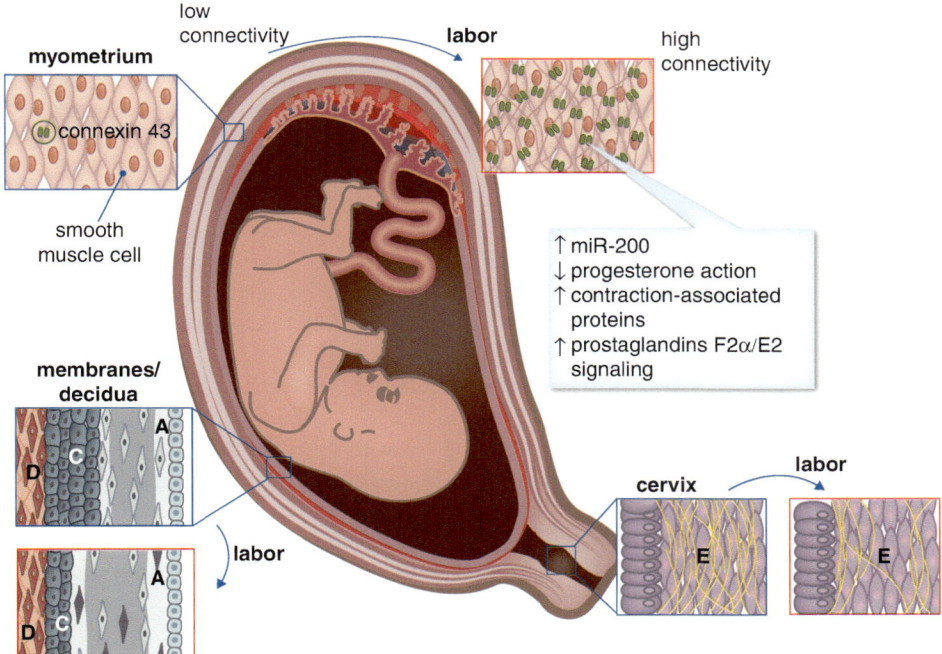

Figure 2.11   Labor is characterized by increased myometrial contractility, cervical ripening and rupture of the membranes. A decline in progesterone action on the myometrium induced by the local rise in MiR-200 activity, in concert with other local activities, such as rises in local estrogen receptor signaling and prostaglandins levels, lead to a myometrial switch from the quiescent to the contractile state. In the meantime, cervical ripening is mediated by changes in extracellular matrix (E) proteins, along with a change in its barrier and immune surveillance properties. Decidual (D) and chorion (C)/amnion (A) membrane activations close to the cervix occur in preparation for membrane rupture (*adopted from* Romero et al. 2014)

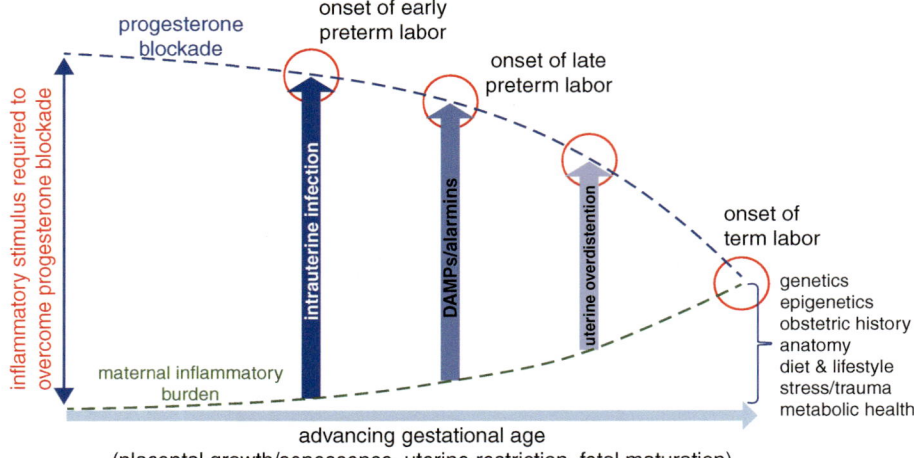

Figure 2.12   In near-term pregnancy, the progesterone-related inhibition of myometrial contractility declines, while the degree of inflammatory activity in the birth canal increases gradually. These two events act in concert to trigger the onset of labor. The gap between these activities narrows near-term. The inflammatory activation is driven by both physiological and pathological stimuli, but earlier in pregnancy, the likelihood of a pathological trigger is greater. The maternal inflammatory burden consists of: tissue aging, telomere shortening, low-level microbial exposure, placental cytokines/lipids/reactive oxygen species, syncytiotrophoblast membrane microparticles, fetal endocrine maturation, maternal oxidative stress, uterine distension, obesity/insulin resistance and environmental factors (*adopted from Keelan 2018*)

to this concept is the fact that the uterus and cervix are continuously exposed to pro-labor stressor signals from intrinsic – (e.g. uterine distension) and extrinsic sources (e.g. intrauterine infection). With advancing pregnancy these pro-labor stressors gradually increase the 'inflammatory load' imposed upon the uterine tissues, but until late pregnancy, are antagonized by the anti-inflammatory actions of progesterone. As soon as the anti-inflammatory activity of progesterone is overruled, the inflammatory response at the tissue level not only converts the uterus to the labor state, but also raises the local production of prostaglandins (PGs). According to this model, the onset of labor is determined by the trajectory of rise in inflammatory load on the one hand and decline in inflammatory-load threshold on the other hand, as shown in ◘ fig. 2.12. This concept would explain the increased risk of PTB in case of intrauterine infection, uterine overdistension, cervical disease, etc. as summarized in ◘ fig. 2.13 (Esplin 2014) and discussed below.

2.2.1 Pathophysiology of SPTB

SPTB is defined by gestational age rather than by clinical phenotype. Therefore, SPTB is the common endpoint of different pathophysiologic pathways, an aspect that complicates its classification. SPTB phenotypes share part of a specific set of biochemical and physical features already present in the subclinical phase, particularly shortly before its

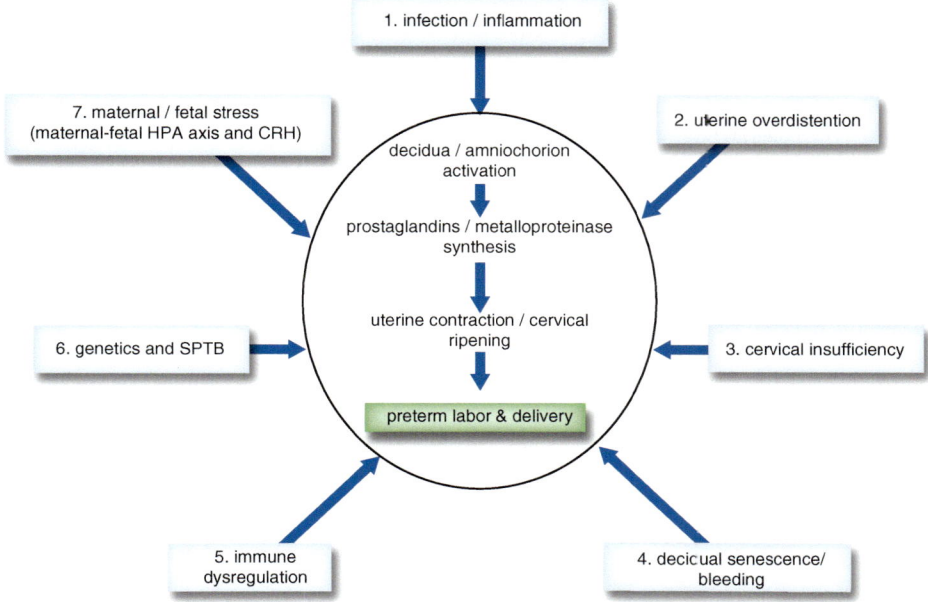

Figure 2.13   Pathophysiological pathways of spontaneous preterm birth (SPTB). A wide range of known risk factors, including genetic, biological, behavioral, social, and environmental factors influence multiple molecular mechanisms ultimately resulting in SPTB

onset (Esplin 2016), which enables subdividing phenotypes based on underlying mechanism. SPTB develops as a consequence of one (or a combination) of the conditions listed in ▢ fig. 2.13:

(1) Infection/inflammation, (2) Uterine overdistention, (3) Cervical insufficiency, (4) Decidual senescence/bleeding, (5) Immune dysregulation/genetics, (6) Genetic predisposition and (7) Maternal and/or fetal stress. These seven conditions develop in response to variable input from maternal, fetal and external sources. The pathophysiology of these conditions is as follows:

1. *Infection/inflammation.* The surface of micro-organisms in the vagina and cervix contains so-called 'pathogen-associated molecular patterns' (PAMPs). These PAMPs can bind to so-called 'toll-like receptors' (TLR) on leukocytes, epithelial cells, and thus also cytotrophoblast cells (CTBs). Binding leads to activation of the innate immune system, which induces an inflammatory response (Koga et al. 2010) and consists of the release of inflammatory cytokines, chemokines, interferons and other effectors. It follows that these TLR receptors play a key role in the defense against pathogens. Presumably, these TLR receptors at the F-M inferface also contribute to the acceptance of a normal pregnancy by already being bound to commensal bacteria in the reproductive tract. This bond averts their post-conceptional binding to these PAMPs, thus preventing activation of the innate immune system in early pregnancy. Whether this mechanism operates normally in infection-induced SPTB, is unknown. It is possible that in these women cervical shielding against colonization by micro-organisms that reside in the vagina may be defective, or the composition of the vaginal microbiome may be more toxic. At any

rate, it may trigger an inflammatory response and with it, induce SPTB. Already for decades, it has been recognized that SPTB is linked to infection/inflammation, an association based on epidemiological studies showing signs of infection amongst almost half of SPTB cases (Lamont 2015) with infection prevalence inversely related to gestational age (◘ fig. 2.14).

Recently, the underlying mechanism has become more clear (◘ fig. 2.15), even though there are still important gaps in our understanding of the cascade of events between the moment of acquiring the infection/inflammation and the onset of SPTB (Agrawal and Hirsch 2012).

Inflammation is a physiologic defense mechanism against harmful stimuli. However, the processes in labor-associated inflammation lack the combination of pain, heat, redness, swelling and loss of function, that are part of the classic definition of inflammation. Instead, these processes are controlled by activation of inflammatory gene expression in the fetal membranes, myometrium and cervix, eventually leading to labor contractions, membrane rupture and cervical effacement and dilation. Pro-inflammatory mediators and signaling cascades, that prevail in these processes are best described by the term "inflammatory activation" (Keelan 2018). Whether the physiological processes typical for normal term labor are also operative in SPTB, is still unknown. Current evidence suggests that the onset of normal term

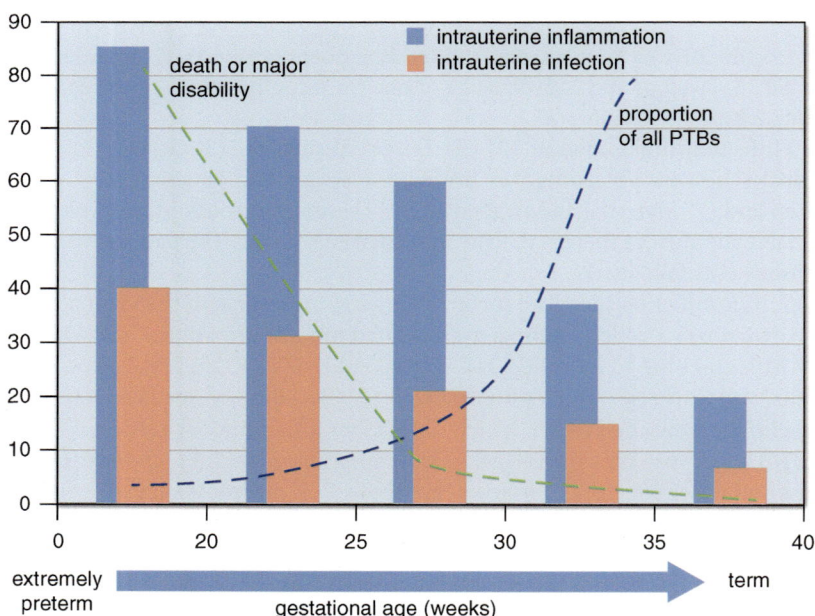

◘ **Figure 2.14** The relation of gestational age at birth between infection/inflammation and neonatal outcome. Gestational age relates inversely with the prevalence of intra-uterine infection/ inflammation and risk of neonatal morbidity. The rate of 'sterile' inflammation is more than twice that of infection-driven intra-uterine inflammation (based on analysis of amniotic fluid microbial content (reported by Keelan 2018)

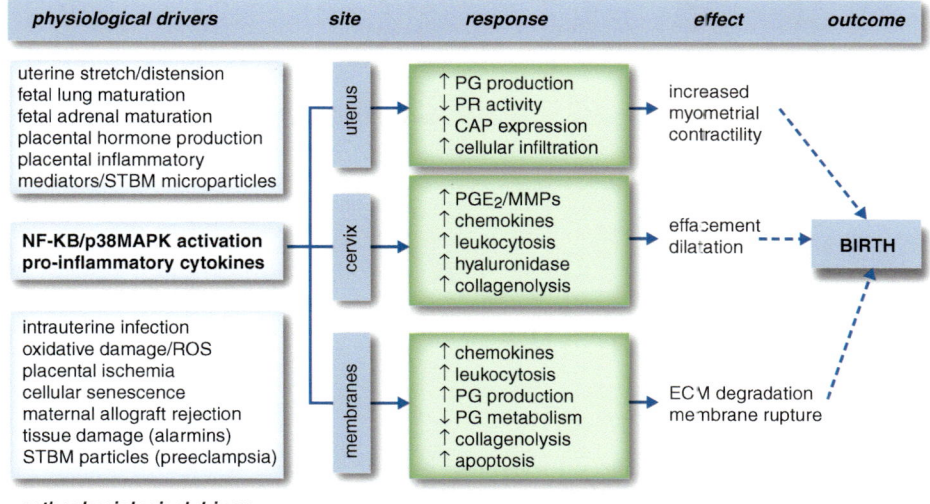

physiological drivers	site	response	effect	outcome
uterine stretch/distension fetal lung maturation fetal adrenal maturation placental hormone production placental inflammatory mediators/STBM microparticles	uterus	↑ PG production ↓ PR activity ↑ CAP expression ↑ cellular infiltration	increased myometrial contractility	
NF-ΚB/p38MAPK activation pro-inflammatory cytokines	cervix	↑ PGE₂/MMPs ↑ chemokines ↑ leukocytosis ↑ hyaluronidase ↑ collagenolysis	effacement dilatation	**BIRTH**
intrauterine infection oxidative damage/ROS placental ischemia cellular senescence maternal allograft rejection tissue damage (alarmins) STBM particles (preeclampsia)	membranes	↑ chemokines ↑ leukocytosis ↑ PG production ↓ PG metabolism ↑ collagenolysis ↑ apoptosis	ECM degradation membrane rupture	

pathophysiological drivers

⬛ Figure 2.15 Biochemical mechanisms linking inflammation with parturition. Inflammatory activation plays a key role in all 3 major tissue sites (uterus, cervix, membranes) needed for coordinated processes during labor. The drivers of inflammation include both maturational and pathophysiological factors. In the uterus, pre-labor changes (phase 1) start at about 37 weeks. In the fetal membranes/cervix, the activity of the drivers of inflammation begins to increase by about 25 weeks. *Abbreviations.* STBM, syncytiotrophoblast membrane; PG, prostaglandin; PGE₂, prostaglandin E₂; PR, progesterone receptor; MMPs, matrix metalloproteinases; CAP, contractile-associated proteins; ROS, reactive oxygen species, ECM, extra-cellular matrix *(adopted from* Keelan 2018)

labor is characterized by a decline in anti-inflammatory actors (progesterone) that coincides with the onset of inflammatory activation (⬛ fig. 2.12). This synchronicity is absent in SPTB.

2. *Uterine overdistention.* During pregnancy the uterus grows in line with its contents. Until mid-pregnancy, the uterus mostly grows by hyperplasia, induced by estrogen-dependent growth factors, such as Insulin-like Growth Factor-1 (IGF-1) and its binding proteins (Shynlova et al. 2009). Afterwards, the myometrium mostly grows by hypertrophy and synthesis of the extracellular matrix. The trigger for this switch is increasing stretch exerted upon the uterine wall by the rapidly growing conceptus hindering the synchronous rise in myometrial blood supply, and with it, giving rise to ischemic episodes in varying regions of the myometrium. This produces a mechanoreceptor-mediated stimulus to switch the myometrial phenotype from a proliferative into a synthetic one (Shynlova et al. 2009), which – importantly – requires both a degree of tension on the uterine wall and the presence of progesterone.

Uterine overdistention, as in multiple pregnancies, induces a pro-inflammatory stretch response (⬛ fig. 2.16), that links the onset of SPTB to a finite uterine capacity. Overdistention of amnion and myometrium also induces the release of inflammatory cytokines by mechanotransduction (Kendal-Wright 2007) and its downstream signaling (Langevin 2006; Chiquet et al. 2009). It also enhances the release of prostaglandins, which is also observed in other subtypes of SPTB

2

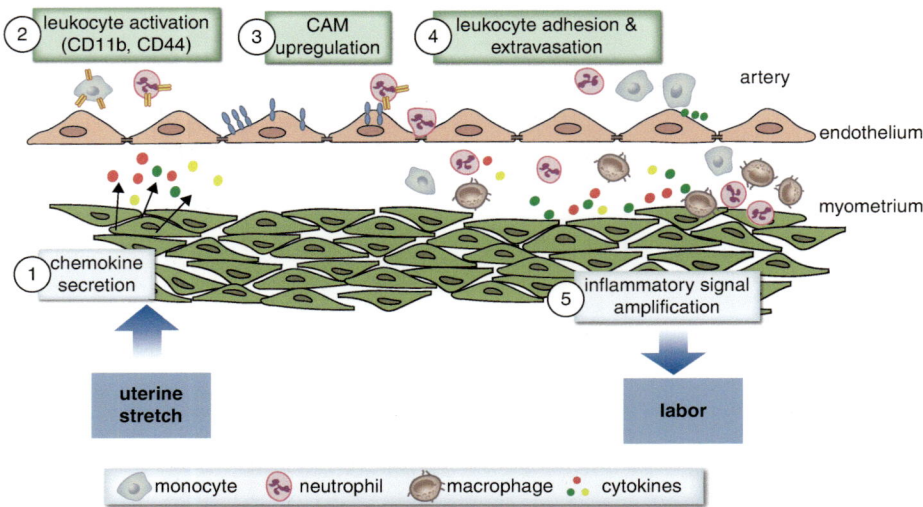

Figure 2.16 Mechanical stretch of the myometrium by the growing conceptus induces uterine chemokine secretion (1). These chemokines activate peripheral immune cells (2) and the expression of endothelial cell adhesion molecules (CAM) (3). Within the myometrium, immune cells differentiate, producing additional cytokines and chemokines that contribute to a cycle of more inflammation (4, 5) eventually inducing labor (Shynlova et al. 2013)

(Adams Waldorf et al. 2015). Even though myometrial overdistention is generally thought to be key in the onset of SPTB in multiple pregnancies, the higher risk of SPTB in these pregnancies compared to singleton pregnancies may in part be related to factors coinciding with multiple pregnancies, such as a short cervix that facilitates the upward migration of micro-organisms into the birth canal, and/or the presence of more than one fetus in the uterus resulting in a higher total fetal cortisol output at an earlier gestational age than in a singleton pregnancy.

3. *Cervical insufficiency.* Intrauterine infection caused by bacteria, that trigger the production of pro-inflammatory cytokines, plays a key role in the mechanism of SPTB. Most microbes reach the uterus by ascending in the female reproductive tract in cases, where the cervical mucosa provides insufficient protection. Prior to conception, the endocervical canal forms a mucus plug that acts like an anatomical and immunological barrier against ascending infection. This plug contains antimicrobial peptides with potent antimicrobial activity (Racicot et al. 2014). If this mucus plug is expelled or the cervical length is short, the risk of an ascending uterine infection increases (◨ figs. 2.17 and 2.18).

The fetal membranes surround the intrauterine cavity, providing a physical barrier to contain amniotic fluid for the growing fetus. Senescence or aging of these membranes is now recognized as a contributor to the onset of term and preterm labor (◨ fig. 2.19), as it leads to oxidative stress in the membranes and with it, the production of inflammatory mediators that reach the adjacent cervix, decidua and myometrium, packaged in exosomes. Here, they increase the overall inflammatory load and with it, contribute to the onset of labor. About half of SPTB

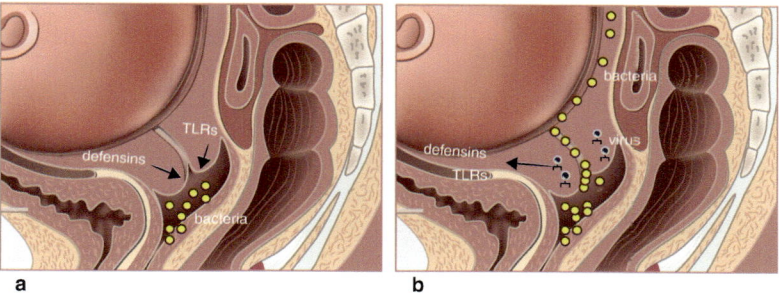

□ **Figure 2.17** **a**: Role of the cervix in controling bacterial migration to the upper reproductive tract. **b**: A viral infection of the cervix alters the expression and function of toll-like receptors (TLRs) and defensins and with it, undermines the protective role of the cervix against bacterial colonization (*adopted from* Racicot et al. 2014)

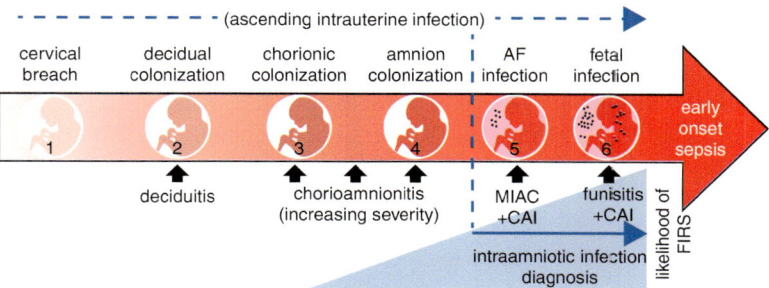

□ **Figure 2.18** The transient relationship of the fetal inflammatory response with ascending intra-uterine infection, chorioamnionitis (CAI). Infection of the fetal membranes triggers CAI. However, the infection only becomes detectable after penetration of the amniotic membrane and colonization of the amniotic cavity (dotted line) and is associated with an increased risk of fetal inflammation (funisitis), sepsis and fetal inflammatory response syndrome (FIRS). *Abbreviations*: MIAC, microbial invasion of the amniotic cavity; AF, amniotic fluid (*adopted from* Keenan 2018)

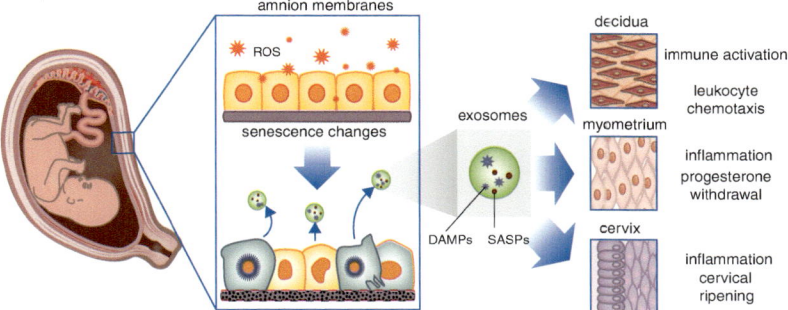

□ **Figure 2.19** In late pregnancy, cumulative exposure of the fetal membranes to oxidative stress causes them to release reactive oxygen species (ROS). Senescent fetal cells respond with releasing damage-associated molecular patterns (DAMPs) and senescence-associated secretory proteins (SASPs). These are *sterile* inflammatory mediators that pass over to the uterine wall in exosomes, where they raise the local inflammatory load, thus contributing to the transition of the uterus from a quiescent state to active labor (*adopted from* Menon et al. 2017a)

2

cases, are preceded by preterm premature rupture of the membranes (pPROM) (Menon et al. 2017b). In these cases, exposure during pregnancy to extrinsic factors, such as poor nutrition, environmental pollutants, high/low BMI, etc., leads to raised levels oxidative stress weakening the membranes, eventually resulting in pPROM (Menon 2017b).

4. *Decidual senescence/bleeding*. Bleeding in the decidual layer underneath or adjacent to the site of placental attachment to the uterine wall, may also lead to SPTB. This applies particularly to placental abruption, which is defined by the premature (in) complete separation of the normally-adhered placenta from its decidual implantation site. This serious complication of advanced pregnancy develops – together with placental syndromes – as a complication of defective spiral artery remodeling in early pregnancy (Romero et al 2011; Morgan 2016). Spiral arteries with a subnormal blood flow capacity, may also be more rigid because of structural lesions, such as atherosis and fibrin deposition (Brosens et al. 2011). Rigid spiral arteries, perpendicularly crossing the decidual-placental interface, are likely to be more vulnerable to wear-and-tear as a consequence of the mechanical forces exerted upon them by the oscillating blood pressure. Indirect evidence for this concept comes from epidemiologic studies indicating an increased risk of placental abruption in women with a relatively high pulse pressure or a less compliant vascular bed due to chronic hypertension, smoking or cocaine use (Romero et al. 2011). Rupture of a spiral artery may lead to partial or complete placental abruption (◨ fig. 2.20). The clinical impact of spiral artery damage or rupture may well remain limited to a minor subchorionic bleeding, occasionally accompanied by some vaginal blood loss and transient uterine contractions. These cases only occasionally advance to SPTB. The associated uterine contractions are caused by the trauma-induced local release of factors with thrombotic, inflammatory or uterotonic properties. A spiral artery may also be ripped as a result of the development of a retroplacental hematoma. Obviously, the clinical impact of such an event is usually much larger, as the often-concealed hematoma formation can be massive, resulting in acute fetal asphyxia/demise along with disseminated intravascular coagulopathy, which may also threaten maternal health (Oyelese et al. 2006).

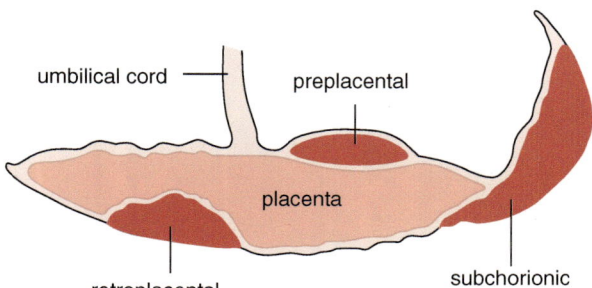

◨ **Figure 2.20**   Concealed *retroplacental hematoma:* no vaginal blood loss, acute and serious clinical presentation. *Subchorionic hematoma:* vaginal blood loss and increased risk of spontaneous preterm birth. *Preplacental hematoma:* no vaginal blood loss, only minor risk of clinical consequences

5. *Immune dysregulation.* There is convincing evidence for the nature and intensity of an inflammatory response in adults and children to be under genetic control. Inflammation is often presented as an etiologic factor in SPTB. Yet, it is still unclear, whether a genetic predisposition to SPTB relates to some pathological form of inflammation. In a recent editorial, it was suggested that rare mutations or damaging-missense variants in innate immunity genes could be involved in the etiology of PPROM. Also, an overlapping genetic substrate may contribute to the development of inflammatory conditions, such as inflammatory bowel syndrome (IBS) and periodontal disease, in causing SPTB (Strauss et al. 2018).

6. *Genetics and SPTB.* The genomic landscape of SPTB is complex. Family and twin-based studies support a significant contribution of maternal and fetal genetics to the onset of (not only) normal term labor, but also SPTB (Strauss et al. 2018). The increased odds ratio between the offspring of sisters was independent of other well-known maternal risk factors for SPTB, which emphasizes the importance of maternal genetics in the pathophysiology of SPTB. As a matter of fact, a large epidemiologic study indicated that maternal genetic factors explain about a quarter of the variation in SPTB, with only marginal influence from fetal and paternal genetic factors (Svensson et al. 2009). Unfortunately, this has not yet resulted in the identification of genes that clearly predispose to SPTB. This effect seems to be mediated by the nature and intensity of the inflammatory response, a key component in initiating labor. Genome-wide association studies designed to identify chromosomal loci responsible for complex traits, have yet to provide convincing evidence for DNA variants that predispose to SPTB.

7. *Maternal and/or fetal stress.* SPTB may also result from maternal/fetal stress caused by placental dysfunction. These events not only accelerate fetal maturation, but also produce an earlier survival-signal to initiate labor by using the same mechanism as detailed previously for normal term labor. Depression, anxiety or perceived stress, severe enough to require either medication or the use of illicit drugs/binge alcohol consumption during pregnancy are often signs of excessive maternal stress. This may also apply to socioeconomic risks factors, such as having an income below poverty level or an education below high-school level. These conditions have been found to predispose to both SPTB (Staneva et al. 2015) and low birth weight (Liou et al. 2016; Molina Lima et al. 2018). Presumably, these adverse effects on pregnancy are mediated by activation of the maternal hypothalamic-pituitary-adrenal axis resulting in higher circulating levels of cortisol and catecholamines, along with a rise in the sympathetic contribution to the autonomic regulation of the cardiovascular function (■ fig. 2.21). These effects not only raise the sympathetic tone in the uteroplacental vascular bed. They also suppress the maternal immune function, as indicated by elevated circulating levels of pro-inflammatory cytokines (Coussons-Read et al. 2005).

2

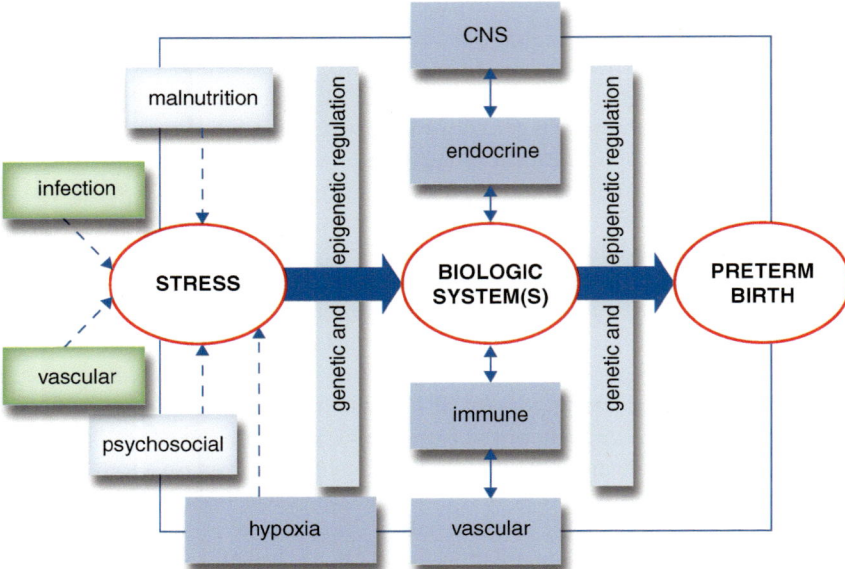

◘ **Figure 2.21**   The contribution of maternal stress and stress biology to spontaneous preterm birth is a matter of context, as the impact of psychosocial stress on stress-sensitive biology is complex and may operate in concert with other stressors, such as infection, malnutrition and hypoxia. Its impact also relates to nature, magnitude and duration of the stressor (*adopted from* Wadhwa et al. 2011)

Causality between depression, anxiety and stress perceived during pregnancy on the one hand, and SPTB and LBW on the other hand, is supported by the beneficial effects of medical and social support measures intended to ameliorate these unfavorable psychological conditions (Straub et al. 2014). Obviously, some of the causality is related to confounders, such as smoking, unhealthy eating habits, and the use of drugs and/or alcohol.

Conclusion. SPTB is a common pregnancy complication, responsible for a large fraction of perinatal morbidity and mortality. Maternal genetic factors contribute to the risk of SPTB by their influence on the degree of inflammatory activation, which is a key component in initiating labor. Meanwhile, non-genetic causes of SPTB are insufficient protection against upstream colonization of the cervix and excessive maternal stress. Still, important gaps in our understanding of the cascade of events that leads to the onset of SPTB, limit the early identification of the majority of patients at extra risk of SPTB.

2.3 Pathophysiology of gestational diabetes mellitus (GDM)

GDM is defined as hyperglycemia diagnosed for the first-time during pregnancy. This definition includes not only true GDM typically developing after the first trimester in concert with the normal pregnancy-related circa 60 % fall in insulin sensitivity (Catalano 2014). It also includes women with yet undiagnosed type-2 diabetes mellitus (T2DM), for the first time identified in early pregnancy. GDM predisposes to various pregnancy complications, with – after childbirth – mother and infant being at increased risk of developing obesity (defined as BMI in excess of 35 kg/m²), T2DM and cardiovascular disorders (Chiefari et al. 2017).

An important drawback in studying GDM is the absence of a universally accepted gold standard for its diagnosis, a shortcoming that challenges the value and comparability of both epidemiologic data and reported data on efficacy of various clinical management strategies. To overcome this weakness, the Federation of Gynecology and Obstetrics (FIGO) has developed a global strategy to diagnose GDM by combining fasting plasma glucose (FPG) with both the glycated hemoglobin level (HbA1c) and an oral glucose tolerance test (oGTT) as detailed in ☐ fig. 2.22 (American Diabetes Association 2018). For the time being, this lack of uniformity in diagnosing GDM demands for extra caution in judging reported epidemiologic data. Nevertheless, reported trends and comparisons of patient groups selected by the same diagnostic criteria, can be expected to provide more reliable results.

GDM is a serious pregnancy disorder affecting 15–20 % of all pregnancies worldwide, comprising circa 85 % of all diabetic pregnancies (Cho et al. 2018). By 2040, its prevalence is expected to have risen by 50 % in concert with the expected global increase in the incidence of obesity (Ogurtsova et al. 2017). In any (sub)population or ethnic group, the prevalence of GDM correlates with that of T2DM. Women of non-white ethnicity have a higher risk of GDM compared to their Caucasian counterparts (Alfadhli 2015). Risk factors for GDM include a family history of diabetes mellitus (DM), a sister or first-degree relative with GDM, obesity, a sedentary lifestyle, advanced maternal age (≥ 40 years), polycystic ovary syndrome and persistent glucosuria. Also, pregnant women with an obstetric history of GDM, unexplained stillbirths, recurrent abortions or

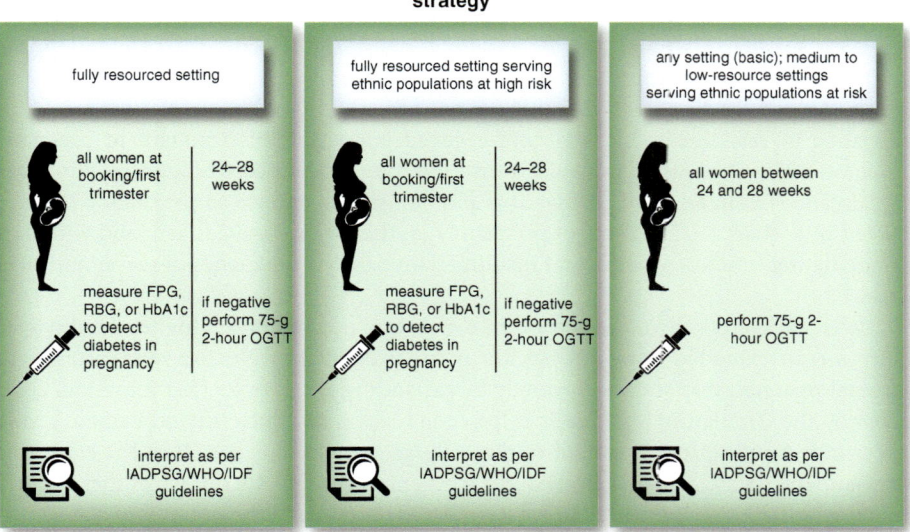

☐ **Figure 2.22** Proposal for diagnosing GDM by the Federation of Gynecology and Obstetrics (FIGO). *Abbreviations*: FPG: fasting plasma glucose, RBG: random blood glucose, HbA1c: glycated hemoglobin, OGTT: oral glucose tolerance test (*adopted from* Lapolla et al. 2018)

birth of a macrosomic infant (≥ 4.5 kg) are at increased risk of having their pregnancy complicated by GDM (Zhang et al. 2016).

Women with true GDM have a normal pre-pregnancy glucose tolerance, and no postprandial hyperglycemia in the first trimester of pregnancy. Yet, these women elicit some signs of insulin resistance (IR) and altered insulin response already in the 1st trimester (Catalano 2014). Therefore, the observed normal glucose tolerance in early pregnancy in these women may mask subclinical impairment of the glucose metabolism, which could still expose the embryo to abnormal genetic imprinting.

2.3.1 Pregnancy-induced adaptation of the maternal glucose metabolism

In early pregnancy, glucose tolerance is normal or slightly improved relative to that of before pregnancy (Butte 2000). In the second half of pregnancy, maternal insulin sensitivity declines gradually to a near-term low of about 60 % below pre-pregnancy levels (Catalano et al. 1993; Catalano 2014). This adaptive response enables a larger fraction of the maternal glucose pool to be preferentially taken up by the maternal brain with glucose utilization being dependent on blood level rather than insulin. The fall in insulin sensitivity in advanced pregnancy is favorable for fetal glucose availability, as transplacental glucose transfer is gradient-dependent (McGowan and McAuliffe 2010). A lower insulin sensitivity forces insulin-dependent maternal organs to utilize alternative substrates, such as fatty acids, glycerol and amino acids to fuel their oxidative metabolism (Lain and Catalano 2007). Meanwhile, the pregnancy-related decline in maternal glucose level is small, probably benefiting from the preserved hepatic gluconeogenesis, altered β-cell responsiveness and elevated circulating lipolytic products (Butte 2000; Petersen et al. 2017). This adaptation, combined with relatively low fetal glucose levels, preserves the transplacental glucose gradient enabling the fetus to preferentially utilize glucose, the most important metabolic substrate of its oxidative metabolism and growth (Mottola et al. 2016). The pregnancy-induced IR develops in the second half of pregnancy in response to the placenta-induced endocrine environment of pregnancy (Catalano 2010) and seems to result from inhibition of the post-receptor insulin signaling cascade (Catalano 2010, 2014). This physiological response to pregnancy has been detailed in ▶ chap. 1. The effects of pregnancy on the glucose metabolism and with it, on the circulating levels of glucose and insulin relative to pre-pregnancy are summarized in ▢ tab. 2.1.

The IR that develops in the second half of pregnancy requires a higher insulin availability for an extended period to secure optimal control of glucose homeostasis. The maternal pancreas responds accordingly by expanding β-cell mass (Baeyens et al. 2016), driven by the circulating high levels of placental lactogen, prolactin and hepatic growth factor, and stimuli directly related to intracellular glucose shortage (Baeyens et al. 2016; Wortham and Sander 2016). Placental detachment interrupts the release of these stimuli, signaling to the β-cell mass to dissolve again so as to return to the pre-gravid state.

□ **Table 2.1** Changes in carbohydrate metabolism in uneventful pregnancy relative to pre-pregnant estimates (*adopted from* Lain and Catalano 2007)

	early pregnancy	late pregnancy
basal metabolism		
fasting glucose	↔	↓ (0.9×)
fasting insulin	↔	↑ (1.7×)
hepatic metabolism		
– basal hepatic glucose production	↔	↑ (1.3×)
– hepatic insulin sensitivity		↓
– glucose suppression	↓ (0.9×)	↓ (0.9×)
insulin metabolism		
insulin secretion		
– first phase insulin response	↑ (2.0×)	↑ (3×)
– second phase insulin response	↑ (1.5×)	↑ (3×)
insulin sensitivity	↓ (0.7×)	↓ (0.4×)

2.3.2 Pathophysiology of GDM

GDM is a disorder resulting from the inability of β-cells to meet the higher insulin demands of pregnancy. This defect leads to periods of abnormal hyperglycemia accompanied by elevated circulating levels of non-carbohydrate metabolic substrates. The impaired glucose handling and relative insulin deficiency interferes with pregnancy course and outcome, as indicated by the increased incidence of fetal macrosomia, polyhydramnios, preterm birth, intrauterine fetal asphyxia and demise, and hypertensive complications. These complications predispose to cesarean birth and birth trauma, postnatally followed by a high incidence of adverse prematurity-related as well as metabolic effects in the newborn. Last but not least, intra-uterine exposure to impaired glucose homeostasis predisposes to epigenetic imprinting, which alters the memory of the β-cells. This effect may explain the increased risk of the infant to develop obesity and/or T2DM in later life.

GDM is caused by a pregnancy-induced rise in IR to a level that exceeds the reserve capacity of the β-cells, needed to compensate for the higher insulin demands. GDM resembles subclinical T2DM that becomes overt in response to the more than twice as high insulin demands in the second half of pregnancy relative to pre-pregnancy (Catalano et al. 1993, Garcia-Patterson et al. 2010). Insight in the pathophysiology of GDM is still incomplete. Factors involved in the etiology are genetic predisposition, (intra-uterine) epigenetic imprinting and external factors related to overnutrition and lifestyle. □ Figure 2.23 illustrates the general concept of the pathogenesis of GDM.

Often, obesity plays an important role, usually combined with an unhealthy lifestyle. It is now well-established that adipocytes are active cells producing a wide range of signaling proteins or hormones, so-called 'adipokines'. Obesity induces dysregulation of their production and release, which affects various regulatory functions in metabolic

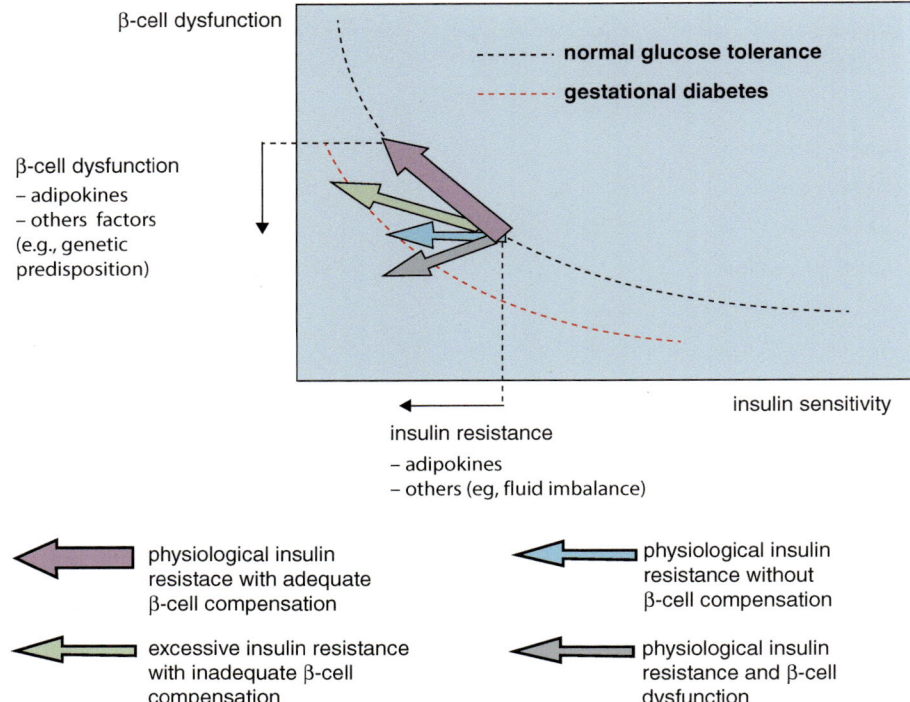

β-cell dysfunction

------- **normal glucose tolerance**

------- **gestational diabetes**

β-cell dysfunction
– adipokines
– others factors
(e.g., genetic
predisposition)

insulin sensitivity

insulin resistance
– adipokines
– others (eg, fluid imbalance)

physiological insulin
resistace with adequate
β-cell compensation

physiological insulin
resistance without
β-cell compensation

excessive insulin resistance
with inadequate β-cell
compensation

physiological insulin
resistance and β-cell
dysfunction

■ **Figure 2.23**   Presumed mechanism of the pathophysiology of gestational diabetes mellitus (GDM). In the 2nd half of pregnancy, insulin resistance (IR) increases to a level close to that in diabetes mellitus type 2. Yet, most women remain normoglycemic, because of a compensatory rise in β-cell functional capacity (dotted blue line, purple arrow). GDM (dotted red line) develops, if IR exceeds insulin reserve capacity (green arrow), β-cell compensation is absent (blue arrow), β-cell insulin output declines (grey arrow), or a combination of these. These defects result from (a combination of) modifiable & non-modifiable factors as detailed in the text. (*Redrawn from* Fasshauer et al. 2014)

processes. The development of low-grade inflammation is particularly relevant for GDM as it amplifies the IR as illustrated in ■ fig. 2.24 (Fasshauer et al. 2014).

The placenta is also a site of production and release of adipokines into both the uterine and umbilical veins. Besides increasing maternal IR, these proteins also influence trophoblast proliferation and invasion. Whether they play a role in fetal growth and metabolism, is not clear (D'Ippolito et al. 2012).

Chronic emotional or physical stress may also magnify the pregnancy-induced rise in IR on top of the rise caused by maternal obesity as shown in ■ fig. 2.25 (Tsatsoulis et al. 2013) probably by boosting the rise in the peripheral levels of inflammatory cytokines or stress hormones (Lionetti et al. 2009).

■ Figure 2.26 summarizes, how modifiable and non-modifiable factors in variable combinations may contribute to the pathophysiology of GDM.

In GDM pregnancies, episodes of extreme hyperglycemia are accompanied by transient glucose spill-over to the fetus, where it triggers fetal β-cells to accelerate their

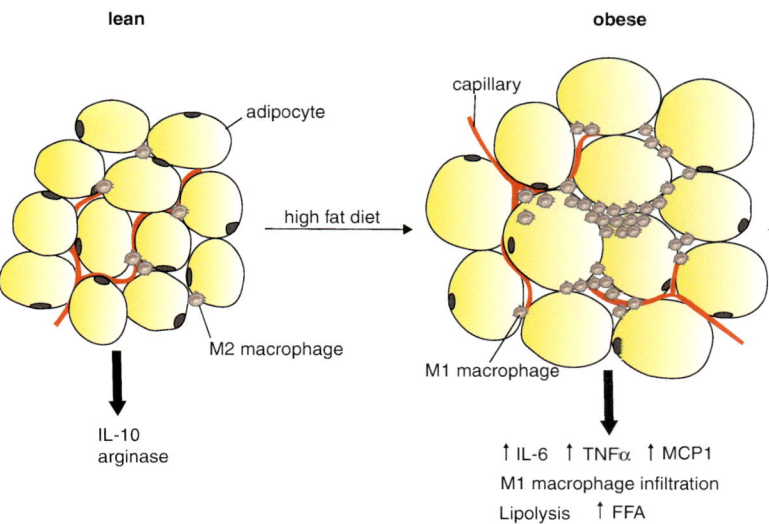

🔲 **Figure 2.24**　Adipose tissue macrophages (ATMs) in the lean state show features of 'alternative' or M2 activation with raised output of e.g. the anti-inflammatory cytokine IL-10. These ATMs participate in tissue repair, e.g. by mitigating inflammatory processes. Excessive accumulation of adipocytes leads to their hypertrophy and with it, their release of chemokines that accelerate recruitment of M1 macrophages. These cells produce the pro-inflammatory cytokines TNFα and IL6 that enhance insulin resistance (IR) in adipocytes, changes the composition of produced adipokine and accelerate both lipolysis and the output of non-esterified fatty acids

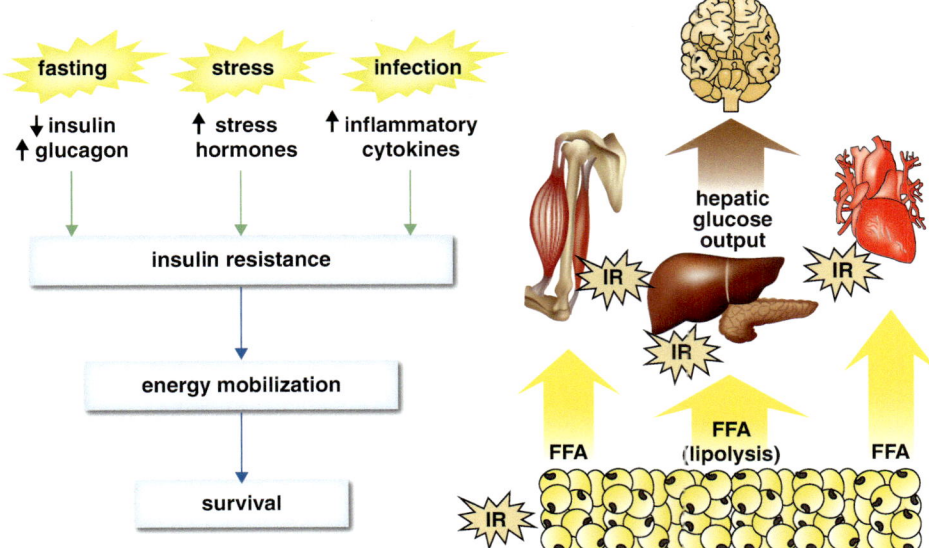

🔲 **Figure 2.25**　Increased physical and/or emotional stress raise circulating levels of inflammatory cytokines. These promote insulin resistance (IR), enhancing the mobilization of free fatty acids (FFAs) and glycerol from fat stores, thus raising circulating FFAs levels. The FFAs replace glucose as metabolic substrate to cover the peripheral energy demands, thus preserving a larger fraction of the available glucose pool to be utilized by the brain for survival (*adopted from* Tsatsoulis et al. 2013)

2

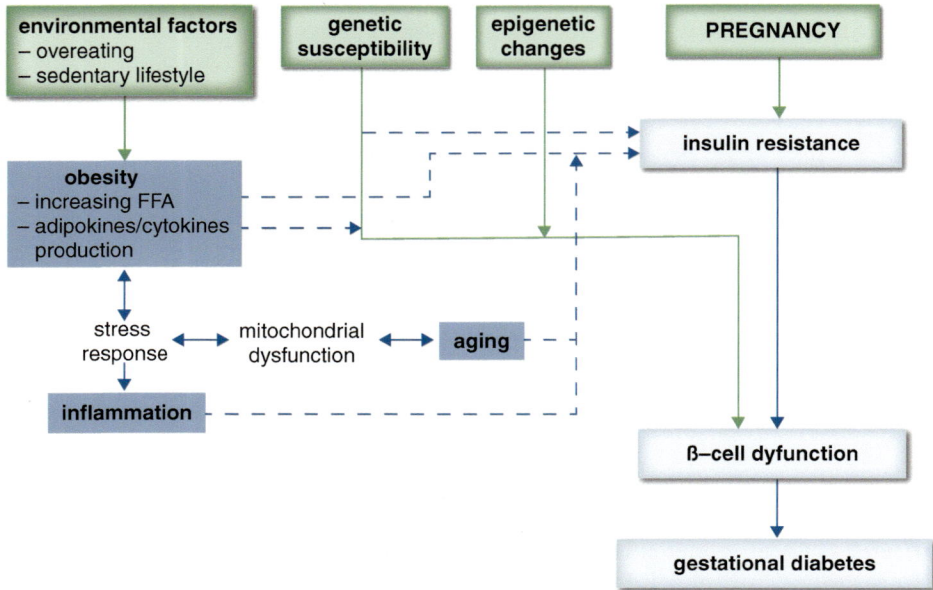

■ **Figure 2.26**   Interaction during pregnancy of environmental factors with genetic susceptibility and epigenetic modulation. The environmental factors are capable of magnifying the physiologic pregnancy-specific insulin resistance and worsening β-cell dysfunction, increasing the risk of developing gestational diabetes mellitus (*adopted from* Chiefari et al. 2017)

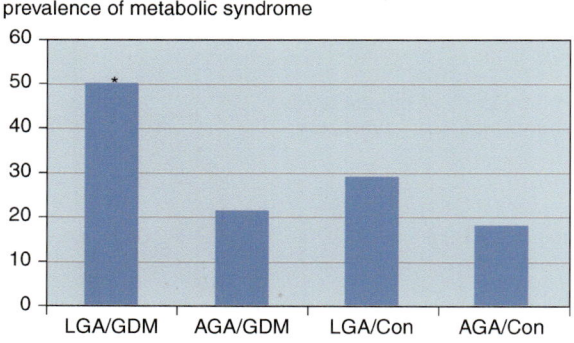

■ **Figure 2.27**   Prevalence of metabolic syndrome among children (n = 175) divided into 4 groups based on birthweight (LGA or AGA) with type of pregnancy (GDM or control). Definition metabolic syndrome (MS): presence of at least 2 of the 4 typical risk factors: obesity, hypertension, high triglycerides or low HDL levels, glucose intolerance. Children were counted once during the 5-years study period. The risk of an infant to develop MS was 2-3 times higher in the LGA/GDM subgroup than in the 3 other subgroups (p < 0.01). *Abbreviations*. LGA, large for gestational age; AGA, appropriate for gestational age; GDM, gestational diabetes mellitus (*adopted from* Boney et al 2005)

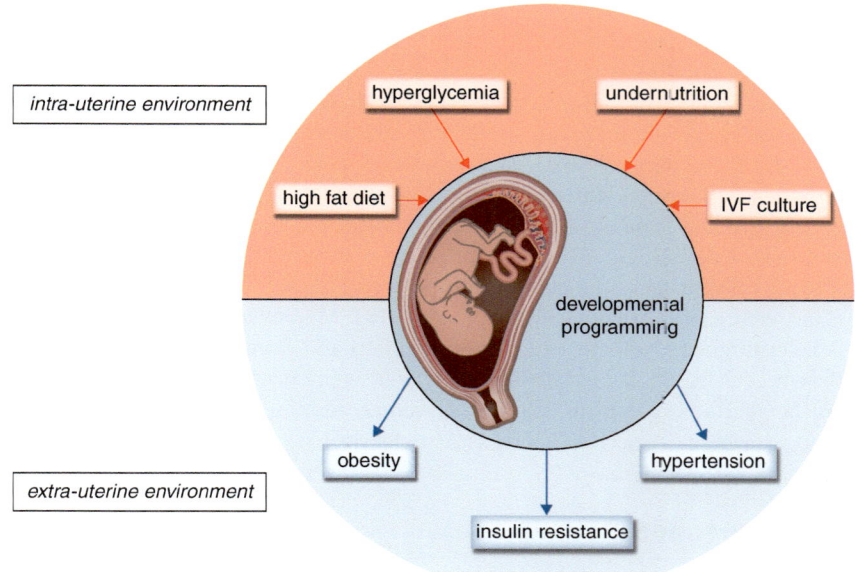

□ Figure 2.28 Proposed model of intra-uterine perturbances that alter normal fetal programming, predisposing the infant to adult metabolic syndrome (MS). Maternal factors, such as chronic undernutrition, lead to adaptive epigenetic programming in the fetus towards nutritional thrift to survive. These adaptations persist postnatally into adulthood, predisposing offspring to metabolic syndrome (*adopted from* Block and El-Osta 2017)

insulin output, in order to deposit the extra glucose into fat and glycogen. The latter may have a transgenerational effect as suggested by a higher rate of obesity and T2DM in adulthood of the offspring (Devlieger et al. 2008). The latter is supported by a study relating GSM with/without macrosomia, to the risk of metabolic syndrome in the infant (□ fig. 2.27) (Boney et al. 2005).

Animal studies provided convincing evidence for the concept that the distorted metabolic profile in a GDM pregnancy induces epigenetic changes that affect the postnatal β-cells' reserve capacity to produce insulin (Devlieger et al. 2008; Block and El-Osta 2017) as shown in □ fig. 2.28. Yet, this concept still awaits experimental proof in sufficiently powered human studies (Moen et al. 2017).

2.3.3 Prevention, early detection and clinical management of GDM

GDM is a multi-causal pregnancy disorder with variable input of modifiable – (epigenetic reprogramming, obesity, lifestyle and nutritional habits) and non-modifiable factors (genetic predisposition based on family history, parity, age and ethnicity). Obviously, the subgroup of women, that are at high risk because of the presence of modifiable factors and/or obesity can be expected to benefit most.

2

Exercise increases the insulin sensitivity of skeletal muscles by enhancing transloca-tion of the glucose transporter GLUT4 to the cell membrane, thus raising the insulin-independent cellular glucose uptake (Mottola and Artal 2016; Bird and Hawley 2017). The same holds for adjustments in the composition and quantity of food intake, that has the additional advantage of improving pregnancy outcome (Zhang et al 2016, Mijatovic-Vucas et al. 2018) including a lower risk of unfavorable epigenetic metabolic programming of the embryo/fetus (Duque-Guimarães and Osanne 2013). There is accumulating evidence for the view that the primary strategy in the clinical management of *healthy* women at increased risk of developing GDM, is a program of supervised lifestyle interventions, as this approach prevents almost a quarter of these women from developing GDM in the first place (Guo et al. 2019; Mijatovic-Vucas et al. 2018). Moreover, such a program reduces the risk of both giving birth to a macrosomic infant and developing postpartum depres-sion (Brown et al. 2017). If lifestyle adjustments in women with confirmed GDM do not result in the satisfactory control of normoglycemia, additional treatment will be needed, as detailed elsewhere. (American Diabetes Association 2018; Simmons et al. 2010).

2.3.4 Postpartum follow-up

A GDM pregnancy predisposes to various health issues later in life due to the chronic, often subclinical, metabolic dysfunction. The severity of these medical issues depends on a combination of (1) persistence of the limited reserve capacity of β-cells to produce insu-lin, (2) obesity, preexistent or retained after the GDM-pregnancy, and (3) the postpar-tum inability of β-cells to restore their pre-pregnant endocrine functional capacity. The chance of developing GDM in a next pregnancy is about 40 %, which is tenfold higher than in women with a history of only non-GSM pregnancies. Former patients also have a seven-fold higher risk of developing T2DM later in life and are at increased risk of devel-oping a cardiovascular disorder (Kim 2014). The latter is a consequence of the damaging effects of the abnormal profile of metabolic substrates in the circulating blood, which low-ers vascular compliance and interferes with endothelial function (Khurana et al. 2014).

Postpartum, GDM patients should be urged to breastfeed for at least three months, as this lowers the risk of developing T2DM (Kim 2014). The reserve capacity of their β-cells should be assessed around six weeks postpartum, as detailed in ▢ tab. 2.2. It's also recommended that these women have their vascular function checked at least once a year.

2.4 Pregnancy discomforts, that may deteriorate to relevant morbidity

Pregnancy induces various changes in the maternal body that may cause discomfort, such as (*1*) Side effects caused by placental hormones; (*2*) Complications related to abnormal placental morphology with respect to depth of its invasion into the uterine wall and uterine site of its insertion, and (*3*) Mechanical discomforts due to the growing uterus. The focus of this section is on side effects, that may deteriorate into a medical condition requiring clinical management (Body et al. 2016).

■ **Table 2.2** Postpartum diabetes screening guidelines for women after a GDM pregnancy from the National Institute for Health and Clinical Excellence (NICE), the World Health Organization (WHO), the American Diabetes Association (ADA), and the Canadian Diabetes Association (CDA) (*adopted from* Kim 2014)

	NICE	WHO	ADA	CDA
when?	6 weeks post-partum, if normal, annually	6 weeks post-partum	6–12 weeks postpartum, if normal, every 3 years; if impaired or elevated 2-h glucose, annually	6 weeks post-partum if normal, repeat 6 months post-partum
which test?	fasting blood glucose	fasting blood glucose or 75-g 2-h oral glucose test	75-g 2-h glucose tolerance test (*HbA1c not rec-ommended*)	75-g 2-h oral glucose tolerance test

2.4.1 Side effects induced by placental hormones

The gastrointestinal (GI) tract

The incidence of nausea, vomiting, gastroesophageal reflux, constipation and diarrhea is higher in pregnant women than in the general population.

Between 70 and 85 % of women experience *pregnancy sickness*, usually limited to the first trimester of pregnancy. The condition refers to nausea, vomiting and food aversions (Cardwell 2012). In the past, pregnancy sickness was attributed to emotional factors, as it was more common in women with negative family relationships or with an unwanted pregnancy. However, current insights suggest that this discomfort could be an embryo-protective mechanism to minimize its exposure to phytotoxins and other environmental perils. In most cases, the pathophysiology of pregnancy sickness seems to relate to the inhibiting effects of hCG, progesterone and estrogen on gastric emptying and gastrointestinal (GI) contractility and motility. About 1.2 % of pregnant women require medical intervention due to dehydration, the result of severe vomiting. These women have developed so-called '*hyperemesis gravidarum*' (HG), a condition of extreme dehydration leading to weight loss and metabolic changes reflected in ketoacidosis, abnormal liver function tests and hypokalemia (Body et al. 2016; London et al. 2017). HG primarily affects maternal wellbeing, but – if not properly managed – may also have a negative impact on pregnancy as indicated by a higher rate of preterm birth and low birthweight (Veenendaal et al. 2011). Diagnosing HG requires exclusion of other causes of vomiting, such as preexistent maternal GI conditions, including gastric colonization with helicobacter pylori (Body et al. 2016).

Ptyalism or sialorrhea of pregnancy is an oral pathological condition characterized by excessive salivation that typically begins in the first trimester and may also be accompanied by esophageo-salivary reflux. Sialorrhea is considered an effect that serves to protect the esophageal mucosa against damage by gastric reflux (Pedersen et al. 2002). The discomfort is difficult to manage (Van Dinter 1990). Symptoms usually diminish in the second trimester of pregnancy, although they can persist until term.

2

Gastroesophageal reflux disease (GERD) is a clinical diagnosis of a GI motility disorder that leads to reflux of stomach contents into the esophagus or oral cavity. GERD can cause damage of the mucosal lining of the esophagus and disrupt its motility, resulting in the symptoms, listed in ◘ tab. 2.3.

GERD affects quality of life and may lead to erosive esophagitis and esophageal strictures. It also predisposes to cancer (Kellerman and Kintanar 2017). Reflux symptoms are often observed in pregnancy, typically manifesting as heartburn. These symptoms develop because of the combination of altered visceral anatomy and reduced GI motility (Ali and Egan 2007). Clinical management of GERD in pregnancy depends on the frequency and severity of the symptoms and needs to consider the potential teratogenic effects of medication (Boeckstaens et al. 2014; Body et al. 2016).

Intrahepatic cholestasis of pregnancy (ICP) usually develops in the third trimester in 1 to 2 % of pregnant women in the developed Western world. However, worldwide, the incidence varies widely and may be as high as 27 % in certain ethnic groups. This aspect together with the high recurrence rate in their next pregnancy in ICP-affected women suggests an important contribution of genetic susceptibility, possibly in combination with specific environmental factors (Smith and Rood 2019). Primary bile acids are end-products of cholesterol catabolism and already highly cytotoxic at low levels. Therefore, both their synthesis in the liver and clearance via the biliary ductal system are tightly regulated by homeostatic mechanisms. Besides, over 90 % of the bile acids remains within the 'close circuit' of enterohepatic circulation (shown in ◘ fig. 2.29).

◘ **Table 2.3**   Symptoms triggered by gastroesophageal reflux

typical symptoms	heartburn, acid regurgitation and nausea
atypical symptoms	Dysphagia, painless sensation of having a food bolus in the throat, non-cardiac chest pain, hypersalivation, dyspepsia and abdominal pain.
extra-esophageal symptoms	Husky voice, sore throat, sinusitis, chronic dry cough, laryngitis, dental erosions, non-atopic asthma, and recurrent choking

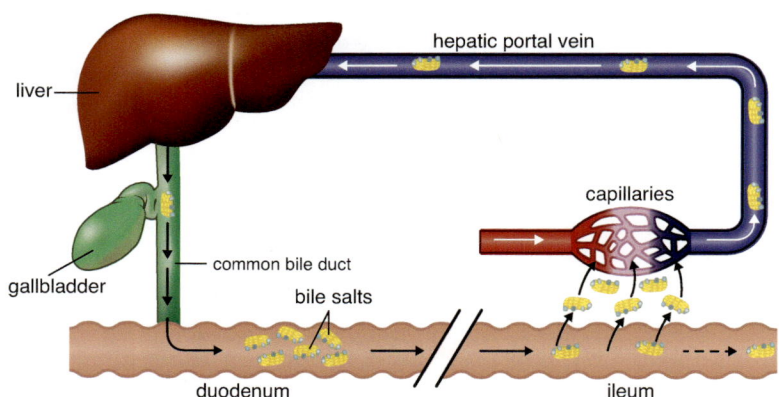

◘ **Figure 2.29**   The enterohepatic circulation of bile acids enables 95 % of body's bile acids to be conserved during each passage cycle

At formation, primary bile acids are already conjugated to prevent them from damaging hepatocytes and the biliary lining during their passage through the biliary ductal system. Cholestasis may challenge this adaptive capacity and lead to higher serum and tissue levels of highly toxic hydrophobic bile acids that can cause mitochondrial damage, apoptosis and necrosis of susceptible cell types. Therefore, the pregnancy-induced lower motility of both the GI tract and its tubular derivatives, such as the biliary duct, may cause a certain degree of cholestasis that deteriorates into ICP. However, this will only occur in the presence of high circulating levels of steroid hormones and in genetically susceptible women (Smith and Rood 2019). The exact etiology of ICP is still not completely elucidated, although a genetic mutation in one of the proteins involved in securing the sophisticated damage-control system is likely to be key as recently reported (Smith and Rood 2019). Typical for ICP is the otherwise unexplained generalized pruritus, which seems to result from increased circulating levels of bile acids (Maillette et al. 2010). The pruritus is probably mediated by a raised opioidergic tone (Bergasa 2018), and easily manageable by the scavenger ursodeoxycholic acid. However, this drug does *not* lower the ICP-related increased risk of fetal asphyxia and demise, particularly after the 34th week of pregnancy (Ovadia et al. 2019; Chappell et al. 2019). Therefore, ICP management should include the timely elective birth of the infant after carefully weighing the risks of prematurity against those of intra-uterine fetal asphyxia/demise with a continuing pregnancy (Dixon and Williamson 2016).

Between 3.5 % and 10 % of pregnant women have *gallstones*, that are in most cases asymptomatic. Because of the lower motility of the biliary duct, their risk of developing gallstone-related complications during pregnancy, such as acute cholecystitis, pancreatitis and ileus, is higher than in the nonpregnant state. Although, the absolute rate of these complications in pregnant women is low, these options ought to be considered in pregnant women with an abdominal emergency, as diagnosing these complications in pregnancy is more difficult than in the nonpregnant state (Bouyou et al. 2015).

Constipation is usually described by subjective definitions. However, a widely accepted definition of constipation is the presence of at least two of the following six symptoms during at least a quarter of defecations: (1) having less than three bowel movements per week, (2) straining, (3) Hard, lumpy stools, (4) sensation of anorectal obstruction, (5) sensation of incomplete emptying and (6) using manual actions to assist with defecation. Using this definition, between 25 to 40 % of pregnant women experience constipation during their pregnancy, most commonly in the first and second trimester, gradually diminishing in the third trimester (Body et al. 2016). ◘ Table 2.4 summarizes the possible causes of constipation in pregnancy (Bonapace and Fisher 1998). In most cases this annoyance can be managed adequately using non-pharmacolocal means as detailed elsewhere (Body et al. 2016).

◘ **Table 2.4**　Pregnancy-related causes of constipation

behavior changes	hormonal effects	obstructive
stool dehydration/fluid intake ↓	delayed gastro-intestinal transit	hemorrhoids/anal fissure
dietary changes (fibre intake ↓; iron suppl.)		compression by pregnant uterus
physical activity ↓		
psychosocial stress		

2

Table 2.5	Pregnancy-induced urinary-tract changes (Glaser and Schaeffer et al. 2015)
kidneys	↑ Renal length; ↑ Glomerular filtration rate (30–50 %).
collecting system	↓ Peristalsis.
ureters	↓ Peristalsis; Mechanical obstruction.
bladder	Displaced anteriorly and superiorly; Smooth muscle relaxation; ↑ Capacity.

The cause of *diarrhea* in pregnancy is usually similar as in the nonpregnant state, with rarely any contribution of pregnancy to its pathogenesis (Bonapace and Fisher 1998). It follows that diarrhea in pregnancy can to be managed similarly as in the non-pregnant state.

The urinary tract is sterile under normal circumstances. Also, the urinary tract responds to pregnancy with a lower motility, and this alters its physiology (see ◻ tab. 2.5) in such a way, that the risk of *urinary tract infections (UTIs)* is increased. UTIs can be classified as asymptomatic bacteriuria (ASB), infections of the lower urinary tract (cystitis) or infections of the upper urinary tract (pyelonephritis). ASB usually develops, when ascending bacteria from the fecal reservoir or the vaginal/perineal skin flora colonize the urinary bladder. ASB and cystitis are associated with a 20 to 30 % increase in the risk of developing pyelonephritis in pregnancy (Glaser and Schaeffer 2015). In pregnancy, ASB impacts both maternal and fetal outcomes adversely, the latter particularly due to the higher risk of preterm birth. Therefore, screening and treatment of ASB during pregnancy is the currently recommended standard care in the clinical guidelines of most professional organizations.

2.4.2 Complications of abnormal placental shape, invasion depth and insertion site

The placenta is a transient organ, only functional during pregnancy, when it serves to enable the fetus to grow and mature. Its positioning as an interface between the fetal and maternal compartments is ideal to control and manage the exchange of gases, nutrients and waste products between mother and fetus. Placental dysfunction due to defective placentation, has been described in detail in the first section of this chapter, as it plays a key role in the pathophysiology of placental syndromes. The section below describes the pathophysiology and functional consequences of the following defects of an otherwise normally-functioning placenta:

a. *Abnormal shape*, as shown in ◻ fig. 2.30;
b. *Abnormally deep invasion*, as shown in ◻ fig. 2.31;
c. *Abnormal site of attachment*, as shown in ◻ fig. 2.33.

An atypical placental shape refers to the forms illustrated in ◻ fig. 2.30. The common denominator of the *succenturiate-, Battledore-* and *velamentous placentas* is an increased risk of *vasa previa*, and with it, an increased risk of some umbilical vessels running over

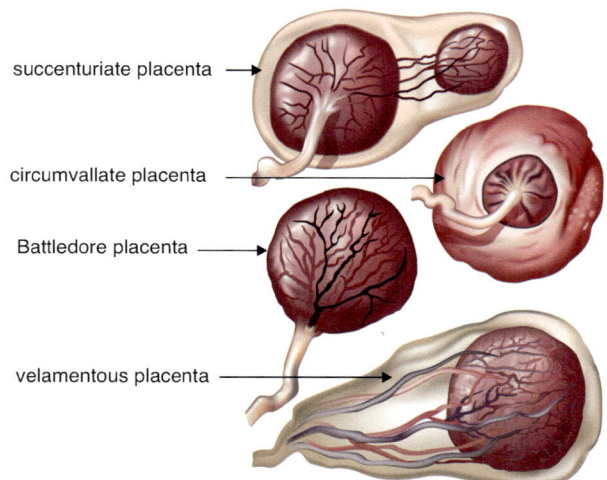

Figure 2.30 Various forms of abnormal placental shape. The *succenturiate* placenta refers to the presence of an extra lobe. In the *circumvallate* placenta, the membranes of the chorion leave are inserted between the placental margin and the umbilical cord. In the *Battledore* placenta, the umbilical cord is inserted in the placental margin. Finally, in the *velamentous* placenta the umbilical vessels merge into the umbilical cord, somewhere in the fetal membranes

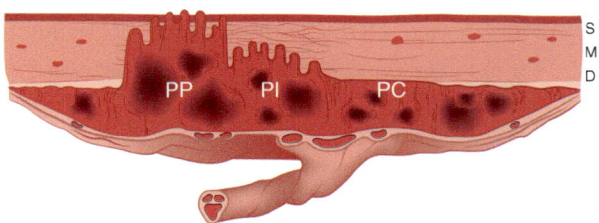

Figure 2.31 Various forms of abnormally deep placental invasion into the uterine wall. *Abbreviations*: S: serosa; M: myometrium, D: decidua, PC: placenta accreta, PI: placenta increta, PP: placenta percreta (*adopted from* Jauniaux et al. 2018)

the internal ostium of the cervix (Ismail et al. 2017). This anomaly is associated with an increased risk of the fetus suffering from a life-threatening hemorrhage in the event that the fetal membranes rupture spontaneously. The presence of umbilical vessels located between the fetal membranes, implies that they are exposed to pressure fluctuations in the uterine cavity, potentially increasing the resistance in the fetal umbilical circulation, and with it, increasing the risk of fetal growth restriction. Finally, a *circumvallate pla-centa*, (observed in about 1 % of all pregnancies), predisposes to fetal growth restriction, preterm labor, oligohydramnios and placental abruption (Suzuki 2008).

Placental accreta spectrum (PAS) is defined as implantation of anchoring villi on the uterine myometrium without an interjacent layer of decidua. PAS results in a morbidly adherent placenta, the extend of adherence varying from placenta accreta, via increta, to percreta, as shown in fig. 2.31 (ACOG guideline 2018).

There are no reliable data on prevalence, because of the high heterogeneity in qualitative and diagnostic criteria between studies (Jauniaux et al. 2019). Nevertheless, in a recent retrospective analysis of 2,219 cases from China, the prevalence had increased more than four-fold between 2011 and 2015, from 0.18 to 0.78 % of all pregnancies, presumably in line with the increasing rate of cesarean births (Zhang et al. 2019). PAS develops in pregnant women with a damaged endometrium-myometrial interface of the uterine wall, usually after a previous cesarean section, but sometimes also after a previous manual placental removal, curettage or endometritis. When these women also have a placenta previa in their current pregnancy, they are at highest risk of developing PAS.

The most favored hypothesis on the etiology of PAS is that a defect of the endometrial-myometrial interface obstructs normal decidualization in the area of the uterine scar, allowing abnormally deep infiltration of placental anchoring villi and trophoblast (Jauniaux et al. 2018). Absent endometrial re-epithelialization of the scar area, allows the trophoblast and villous tissue to invade deeply into the myometrium and its vasculature, and may even reach the surrounding pelvic tissues. Presumably, the absence of a normally functioning decidua leads to loss of control of the migratory and invasive properties of EVT cells, possibly due to the local absence of dNK cells (Erlebacher 2013). Therefore, the interstitial EVT cells invade deeper than usual into the myometrium with the endovascular EVT cells also invading more deeply into the myometrial portions of the spiral arteries, possibly up to the radial arteries or even arcuate arteries. Although this excessively deep intravascular invasion and following arterial remodeling has no apparent impact on placental function during pregnancy, it does disrupt the normal uterine functions immediately after childbirth, by blocking both the spontaneous placental detachment and the inability to limit blood loss through uterine involution and contraction. Therefore, PAS is a severe pregnancy complication associated with massive immediate postpartum hemorrhage, often only manageable by emergency hysterectomy.

Abnormal intra-uterine site of attachment. The site of embryo implantation determines the location of the placenta in the uterus. It is a carefully orchestrated process involving intense pre-implantation crosstalk between embryo and receptive endometrium as illustrated in ◘ fig. 2.32.

The most common abnormal placental insertion site is a placenta previa, defined as a placenta implanted in the lower uterine segment, partially or completely covering the internal cervical ostium as illustrated in ◘ fig. 2.33 (Abduljabbar et al. 2016).

The worldwide prevalence of placenta previa is about 1 case in 250 births. Smoking, a high parity, advanced maternal age and multiple pregnancy are associated with a higher risk of placenta previa. The same applies to a history of cesarean section, termination of pregnancy or intrauterine instrumentation, such as is associated with in-vitro fertilization followed by embryo transfer (Grady et al. 2012). The pathophysiology is not clear, but it is plausible that in some cases the normal pre-implantation crosstalk between blastula and endometrium to identify an optimal implantation site is defective. Placenta previa predisposes to fetal growth restriction, abnormal fetal presentation, but most important, to an increased risk of massive maternal hemorrhage during labor. Obviously, if the placenta completely covers the internal cervical ostium, safe birth of the infant is only possible by cesarean section.

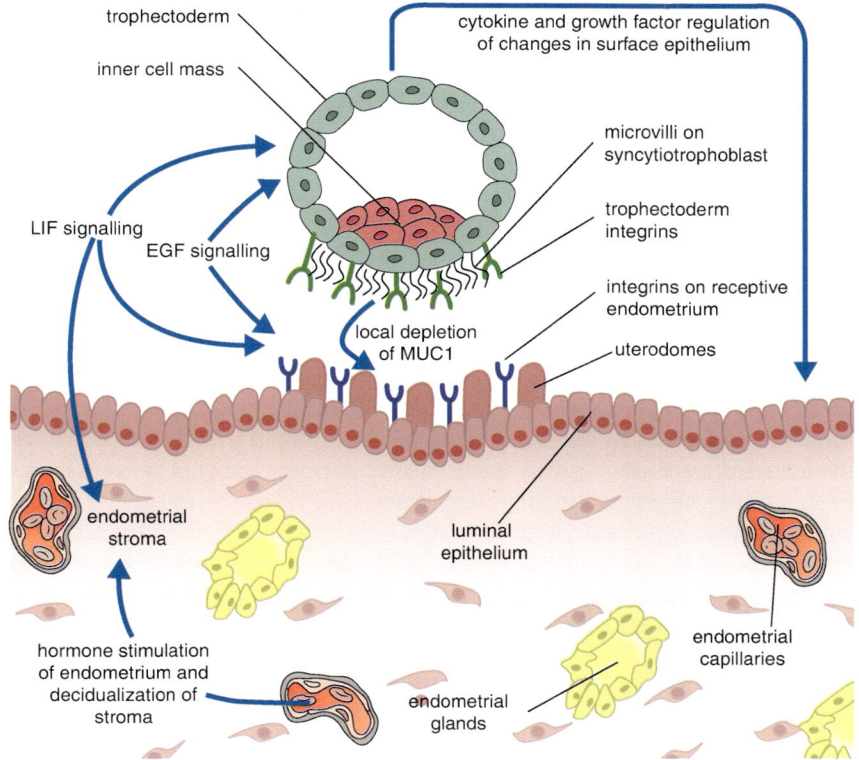

■ Figure 2.32 Schematic illustration of the pre-implantation signaling between embryo and endometrium. The blastocyst approaches the receptive endometrium, defined by the appearance of uterodomes and integrin profiles. Abbreviations: LIF: leukemia inhibitory factor; EGF: epidermal growth factor; MUC1: mucin-1 (*adopted from* Davison and Coward 2016)

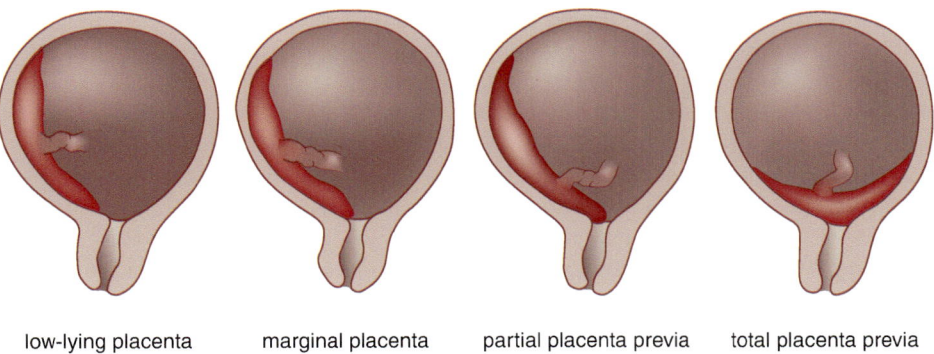

low-lying placenta   marginal placenta   partial placenta previa   total placenta previa

■ Figure 2.33 Various types of placenta previa

2.4.3 Mechanically induced issues caused by the growing pregnant uterus

Throughout pregnancy, women experience physical, physiological and hormonal changes that affect their postural control (▣ fig. 2.34). Particularly in the second trimester, the maternal body undergoes major anthropometric and physiologic changes that challenge its balance (McCrory et al. 2010). This may explain, why falls are the most common cause of minor injury during pregnancy, making up 25 % of all trauma-related visits to hospital emergency departments.

Falls during pregnancy may result in maternal injury, such as fractures, sprains/strains, head injury and the rupture of internal organs. The consequences for pregnancy may also be serious, as indicated by the occurrence of placental abruption, rupture of the uterus or membranes (Dunning et al. 2010). Interestingly, most falls in pregnant women have been observed in the second trimester, when the changes in body shape and stature are not yet as explicit as in the third trimester (Dunning et al. 2003). It is conceivable that the maternal response to preserve her balance during walking or otherwise moving, are a measure of sensory processing capacity resulting from the integrated input from vestibular, proprioceptive and visual information. Actually, women in the last trimester of pregnancy are likely to be at greater risk of falling, because of these biomechanical and physiologic changes (Inanir et al. 2014), but seem to fall less often, because of maternity leave and unintentionally curtailing physical activities in late pregnancy. Posturography could be a screening tool to identify postural instability and fall risk in pregnant women (Danna-Dos Santos et al. 2018). Women at risk of falling during pregnancy are expected to benefit from exercise participation that helps them to adapt to their altered body shape and better able to prevent a fall, should a trip or slip occur (McCrory et al. 2020).

The postural changes inherent to pregnancy, together with the higher laxity of the joints and greater body weight, may also cause other mechanically-induced discomfort, such as low back pain (LBP) and pain in the knees, ankles and feet. LBP often develops together with pelvic girdle pain (PGP), which refers to pain between the posterior iliac crest and the gluteal fold, particularly near the sacroiliac joint. PGP tends to radiate to the thighs and hips and may also be accompanied by a separate pain in the pubic symphysis (Walters et al. 2018). The pathophysiology of PGP in pregnancy is multifactorial with presumably a most important role for pregnancy-specific hormonal (e.g. relaxin) and biomechanical factors. The latter factors relate to the already maximally stressed lumbar spine to preserve balance, while the uterus is markedly enlarged, shifting the maternal center of gravity anteriorly. This leads to more stress in the lower back and pelvic girdle. The induced compensatory postural changes magnify the lumbar lordosis. Women with PGP often have increased pelvic, thoracic and lumbar joint mobility, predisposing them to pelvic instability and pain. The most favorable management consists of a strategic approach for activity modification, pelvic support garments, management of acute exacerbations, physiotherapy and exercise programs to prevent progression of symptoms. In most cases, the pain gradually disappears within three months postpartum.

During pregnancy, the sacroiliac joints often relax, an effect that is accompanied by widening of the pubic symphysis in most pregnant women. In pregnancy and during childbirth, the pubic ligaments can be stretched up to 1.5 cm without rupture

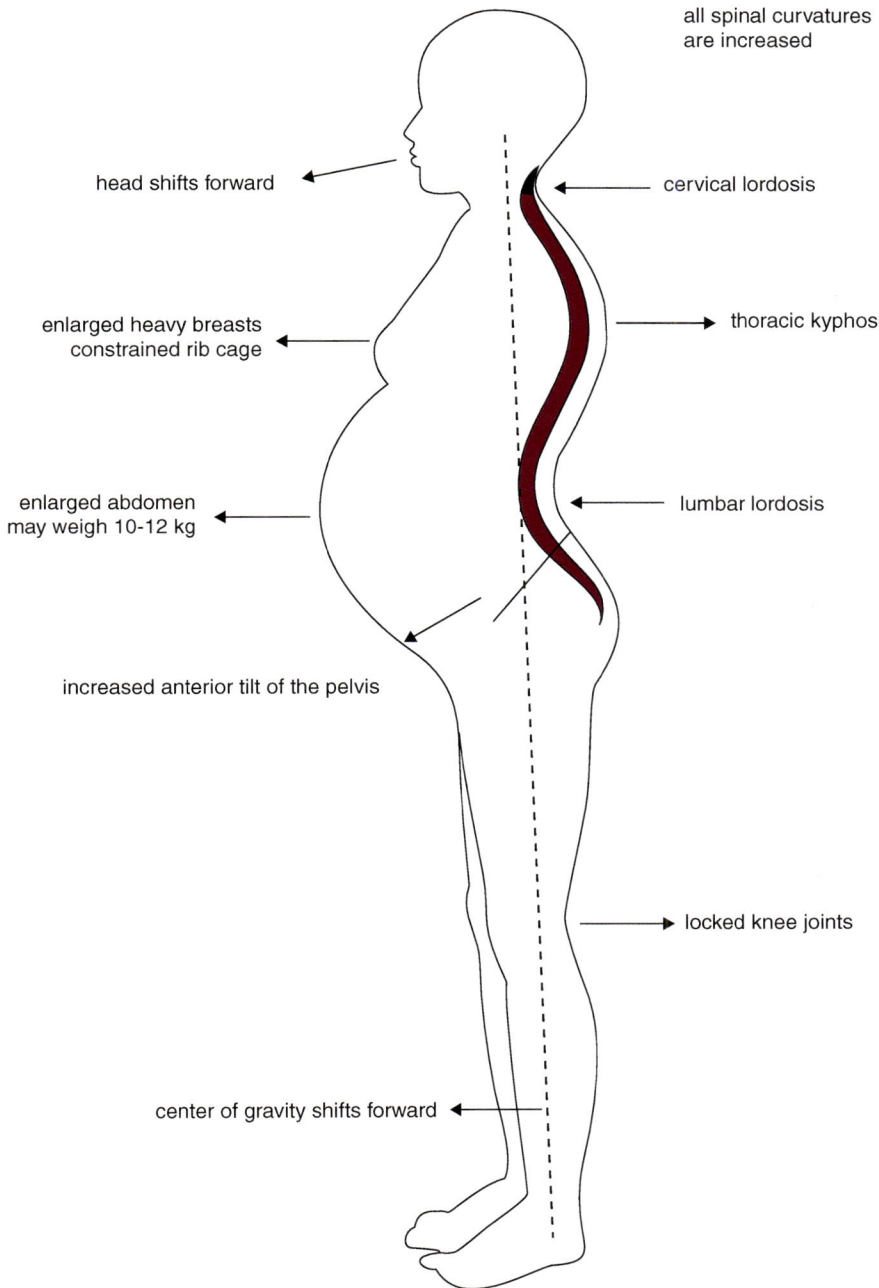

all spinal curvatures
are increased

head shifts forward

cervical lordosis

enlarged heavy breasts
constrained rib cage

thoracic kyphosis

enlarged abdomen
may weigh 10-12 kg

lumbar lordosis

increased anterior tilt of the pelvis

locked knee joints

center of gravity shifts forward

◘ Figure 2.34   Pregnancy-induced postural changes: With advancing pregnancy, the center of gravity shifts more anteriorly giving rise to more anterior pelvic tilt

2

(Jain and Sternberg et al. 2005). This ability results from the increased elasticity of the pubic ligaments in response to exposure to the elevated peripheral levels of progesterone and relaxin. Postpartum, this effect rapidly decreases enabling the return of pelvic stability. Separation of the pubic symphysis is usually asymptomatic to resolve postpartum without treatment. However, in rare cases it may deteriorate into pubic symphysis rupture, a serious complication as detailed elsewhere (Shnaeckel et al. 2015)

References

Abalos E, Cuesta C, Grosso AL, et al. Global and regional estimates of preeclampsia and eclampsia: a systematic review. Eur J Obstet Gynecol Reprod Biol. 2013;170:1–7.

Abduljabbar HS, Bahkali NM, Al-Basri SF, et al. Placenta previa: A 13 years' experience at a tertiary care center in Western Saudi Arabia. Saudi Med J. 2016;37:742–66.

Abildgaard U, Heimdal K. Pathogenesis of the syndrome of hemolysis, elevated liver enzymes, and low platelet count (HELLP): a review. Eur J Obstet Gynecol Reprod Biol. 2013;166:117–23.

ACOG. Obstetric care consensus no 7. Placenta accreta spectrum. Obstet Gynecol. 2018;132:e259–275.

Adams Waldorf KM, Singh N, Mohan AR, et al. Uterine overdistention induces preterm labor mediated by inflammation: observations in pregnant women and nonhuman primates. Am J Obstet Gynecol. 2015;213(830):e1–19.

Agrawal V, Hirsch E. Intrauterine infection and preterm labor. Semin Fetal Neonatal Med. 2012;17:12–9.

Alfadhli EM. Gestational diabetes mellitus. Saudi Med J. 2015;36:399–406.

Ali RAR, Egan LJ. Gastroesophageal reflux disease in pregnancy. Best Pract Res Clin Gastroenterol. 2007;21:793–806.

American Diabetes Association. Management of diabetes in pregnancy: standards of medical care in diabetes-2018. Diabetes Care. 2018;41(Suppl. 1):S137–43.

Appenzeller S, Souza FHC, Silva de Souza AW et al. HELLP syndrome and its relationship with antiphospholipid syndrome and antiphospholipid antibodies. Semin Arthritis Rheum. 2011;41:517–23.

Aya AGM, Ondze B, Ripart J, Cuvillon P. Seizures in the peripartum period: Epidemiology, diagnosis, and management. Anaesth Crit Care Pain Med. 2016;35S:S13–21.

Baeyens L et al. β-cell adaptation in pregnancy. Diabetes Obes Metab. 2016;18(suppl. 1):63–70.

Baines AC, Brodsky RA. Complementopathies. Blood Rev. 2017;31:213–23.

Bergasa NV. The pruritus of cholestasis: from bile acids to opiate agonists: relevant after all these years. Med Hypotheses. 2018;110:86–9.

Bernardus TP, Mol BW, Ravelli ACJ, et al. Recurrence risk of preeclampsia in a linked population-based cohort: Effects of first pregnancy maximum diastolic blood pressure and gestational age. Pregnancy Hypertens. 2018;15:32–6.

Bird SR, Hawley JA. Update on the effects of physical activity on insulin sensitivity in humans. BMJ Open Sport Exerc Med. 2017;2:1–26.

Blencowe H, Cousens S, Oestergaard MZ, et al. National, regional and worldwide estimates of preterm birth rates in the year 2010 with time trends since 1990 for selected countries: a systematic analysis and implications. Lancet. 2012;379:2162–72.

Block T, El-Osta A. Epigenetic programming, early life nutrition and the risk of metabolic disease. Atherosclerosis. 2017;266:31–40.

Body C, Christie JA. Gastrointestinal diseases in pregnancy. Nausea, vomiting, gastrointestinal reflux disease, constipation and diarrhea. Gastroenterol Clin N Am. 2016;45:267–83.

Boeckxstaens G, El-Serag H, Smout AJPM, et al. Symptomatic reflux disease: the present, the past and the future. Gut. 2014;63:1185–93.

Bonapace ES Jr, Fisher RS. Constipation and diarrhea in pregnancy. Gastroenterol Clin North Am. 1998;27:197–211.

Boney CM, et al. Metabolic syndrome in childhood: association with birth weight, maternal obesity and gestational diabetes mellitus. Pediatrics. 2005;115:e290–6.

Bouyou J, Gaujoux S, Marcellin L, et al. Abdominal emergencies during pregnancy. J Visc Surg. 2015;152:S105–15.

Brosens I, Pijnenborg R, Vercruysse L, Romero R. The "Great Obstetrical Syndromes" are associated with disorders of deep placentation. Am J Obstet Gynecol. 2011;193–201.

Brown J et al. Lifestyle interventions for the treatment of women with gestational diabetes. Cochrane Database Syst Rev. 2017;(5): Art. No: CD011970.

Brown MA, Magee LA, Kenny LC et al. Hypertensive disorders of pregnancy. ISSHP classification, diagnosis, and management recommendations for international practice. Hypertension. 2018;72:24–43.

Browning MF, Levy HL, Wilkins-Haug LE, et al. Fetal fatty acid oxidation defects and maternal liver disease in pregnancy. Obstet Gynecol. 2006;107:115–20.

Burton GJ, Jauniaux E. The cytotrophoblastic shell and complications of pregnancy. Placenta. 2017;60:134–9.

Burton GJ, Redman CW, Roberts JM, Moffett A. Pre-eclampsia: pathophysiology and clinical implications. BMJ. 2019;366. ▶ https://doi.org/10.1136/bmj.l2381.

Butte NF. Carbohydrate and lipid metabolism in pregnancy: normal compared with gestational diabetes mellitus. Am J Clin Nutr. 2000;71(suppl):1256–61(S).

Cappelletti M, Della Bella S, Ferrazzi E, et al. Inflammation and preterm birth. J Leukoc Biol. 2016;99:67–78.

Cardwell MS. Pregnancy sickness: a biopsychological perspective. Obstet Gynecol Surv. 2012;67:645–52.

Catalano PM. Obesity, insulin resistance and pregnancy outcome. Reproduction. 2010;140:365–71.

Catalano PM. Review article: trying to understand gestational diabetes. Diabet Med. 2014;31:273–81.

Catalano PM et al. Carbohydrate metabolism during pregnancy in control subjects and women with gestational diabetes. Am J Physiol. 1993;264(Endocrinol Metab 27):E60–7.

Chapman-Johnson A, Nagle KJ, Tremble SM, Cipolla MJ. The contribution of normal pregnancy to eclampsia. PLOS One. 2015. ▶ https://doi.org/10.1371/journal.pone.0133953.

Chappell LC, Bell JL, Smith A, et al. Ursodeoxycholic acid versus placebo in women with intrahepatic cholestasis of pregnancy (PITCHES): a randomized controlled trial. Lancet. 2019;394:849–60.

Chiefari E, Arcidiacono B, Foti D, Brunetti A. Gestational diabetes mellitus: An updated overview. J Endocrinol Invest. 2017;40:899–909.

Chiquet M, Gelman L, Lutz R, et al. From mechanotransduction to extracellular matrix gene expression in fibroblasts. Biochim Biophys Acta. 2009;1793:911–20.

Cho NH, et al. IDF Diabetes Atlas: global estimates of diabetes prevalence for 2017 and projections for 2045. Diabetes Res Clin Pract. 2018;138:271–81.

Cipolla MJ. Cerebrovascular function in pregnancy and eclampsia. Hypertension. 2007;50:14–24.

Coussons-Read ME, Okun ML, Schmitt MP. Prenatal stress alters cytokine levels in a manner that may endanger human pregnancy. Psychosom Med. 2005;67:625–31.

D'Ippolito S, et al. Adipokines, an adipose tissue and placental product with biological functions in pregnancy. Review article. Biofactors. 2012;38:14–23.

Danna-Dos-Santos A, Magalhães AT, Silva BA, et al. Gait Posture. 2018;66:7–12.

Davison LM, Coward K. Review: molecular mechanisms of membrane interaction at implantation. Birth Defects Research (part C). 2016;108:19–32.

Devlieger R, et al. Reduced adaptation of the pancreatic B-cells during pregnancy is the major causal factor for gestational diabetes: current knowledge and metabolic effects on the offspring. Acta Obstet Gynaecol. 2008;87:1266–70.

Dixon P, Williamson C. The pathophysiology of intrahepatic cholestasis of pregnancy. Clin Res Hepatol Gastroenterol. 2016;40:141–53.

Dunning K, LeMasters G, Levin L, et al. Falls in workers during pregnancy risk factors, job hazards and high-risk occupations. Am J Ind Med. 2003;44:664–72.

Dunning K, LeMasters G, Bhattacharrya A. A major public health issue: the high incidence of falls during pregnancy. Matern Child Health J. 2010;14:720–5.

Duque-Guimarães DE, Osanne SE. Nutritional programming of insulin resistance: causes and consequences. Trends Endocrinol Metab. 2013;24:525–35.

Eremina V, Baelde HJ, Quaggin SE. Role of the VEGF-A signaling pathway in the glomerulus: evidence for crosstalk between components of the glomerular filtration barrier. Nephron Physiol. 2007;106:32–7.

Erlebacher A. Immunology of the maternal-fetal interface. Annu Rev Immunol. 2013;31:387–411.

Esplin MS. Overview of spontaneous preterm birth: a complex and multifactorial phenotype. Clin Obstet Gynecol. 2014;57:518–30.

Esplin MS. The importance of clinical phenotype in understanding and preventing spontaneous preterm birth. Am J Perinatol. 2016;33:236–44.

Faraci FM. Leaky vessels: how the brain deals with pregnancy under pressure. J Appl Physiol. 2011;110:305–6.

Fasshauer M. Adipokines in gestational diabetes. Lancet Diabetes Endocrinol. 2014;2:488–99.

Frey HA, Klebanoff MA. The epidemiology, etiology and costs of preterm birth. Semin Fetal Neonatal Med. 2016;21:68–73.

Fugate JE, Rabinstein AA. Posterior reversible encephalopathy syndrome: clinical and radiological manifestations, pathophysiology and outstanding questions. Lancet Neurol. 2015;14:914–25.

Gaccioli F, Aye ILMH, Sovio U, Charnock-Jones DS, Smith GCS. Screening for fetal growth restriction using fetal biometry combined with maternal markers. Am J Obstet Gynecol febr. 2018:S725–37.

Garcia-Patterson, et al. Insulin requirements throughout pregnancy in women with type 1 diabetes mellitus: three changes of direction. Diabetologia. 2010;53:446–51.

Gardosi J. Customised assessment of fetal growth potential: implications for perinatal care. Arch Dis Child Fetal Neonatal. 2012;97:F314–7.

Glaser AP, Schaeffer AJ. Urinary tract infection and bacteriuria in pregnancy. Urol Clin N Am. 2015;42:547–60.

Grady R, Alavi N, Vale R, et al. Elective single embryo transfer and perinatal outcomes: a systematic review and meta-analysis. Fertil Steril. 2012;97:324–31.

Guo X-Y, Shu J, Fu X-H, et al. Improving the effectiveness of lifestyle interventions for gestational diabetes prevention: a meta-analysis and meta-regression. Brit J Obstet Gynaecol. 2019;126:311–20.

Henao DE, Saleem MA, Cadavid AP. Glomerular disturbances in preeclampsia: disruption between glomerular endothelium and podocyte symbiosis. Hypertens Pregnancy. 2010;29:10–20.

Hennessy A, Makris A. Preeclamptic nephropathy (review). Nephrology. 2011;16:134–43.

Hinchey J, Chaves C, Appignani B, et al. A reversible posterior leukoencephalopathy syndrome. N Engl J Med. 1996;334:494–500.

Inanir A, Cakmak B, Hisim Y, et al. Evaluation of postural equilibrium and fall risk during pregnancy. Gait Posture. 2014;39:1122–5.

Ismail KI, Hannigan A, O'Donoghue K et al. Abnormal placental cord insertion and adverse pregnancy outcomes: a systematic review and meta-analysis. Syst Rev. 2017;6:242(11 pages).

Jain N, Sternberg LB. Symphysial separation. Obstet Gynecol. 2005;105:1229–32.

Jauniaux E, Collins S, Burton GJ. Placenta accreta spectrum: pathophysiology and evidence-based anatomy for prenatal ultrasound imaging. Am J Obstet Gynecol. 2018;218:75–87.

Jauniaux E, Bunce C, Gronbeck L, et al. Prevalence and main outcomes of placenta accreta spectrum: a systematic review and meta-analysis. Am J Obstet Gynecol. 2019;221:2018–218.

Kappler S, Ronan-Bentle S, Graham A. Thrombotic microangiopathies (TTP, HUS, HELLP). Emerg Med Clin N Am. 2014;32:649–71.

Kazmi RS, Cooper AJ, Lwaleed BA. Platelet function in pre-eclampsia. Semin Thromb Hemost. 2011;37:131–6.

Keelan JA. Intrauterine inflammatory activation, functional progesterone withdrawal, and timing of term and preterm birth. J Reprod Immunol. 2018;125:89–99.

Kellerman R, Kintanar T. Gastroesophageal reflux disease. Prim Care Clin Office Pract. 2017;44:561–73.

Kendal-Wright CE. Stretching, mechanotransduction and proinflammatory cytokines in the fetal membranes. Reprod Sci. 2007;14:35–41.

Khurana R, et al. The effect of hyperinsulinemia and hyperglycemia on endothelial function in pregnant patients with type-2 diabetes. Diabetes Res Clin Pract. 2014;103:311–3.

Kim C. Maternal outcomes and follow-up of gestational diabetes mellitus. Diabet Med. 2014;31:292–301.

Kleinhouweler CE, Cheong-See FM, Collins GS et al. Prognostic models in obstetrics: available, but far from applicable. Clinical opinion. Am J Obstet Gynecol. January 2016;79–90.

Koga K, Mor G. Toll-like receptors at the maternal-fetal interface in normal pregnancy and pregnancy disorders. Am J Reprod Immunol. 2010;63:587–600.

Lain KY, Catalano PM. Metabolic changes in pregnancy. Clin Obstet Gynecol. 2007;50:938–48.

Lamont RF. Advances in the prevention of infection-related preterm birth. Front Immunol. 2015;6:art 566.

Langevin HM. Connective tissue: a body-wide signaling network? Med Hypotheses. 2006;66:1074–7.

Lapolla A and Metzger BE. The post-HAPO situation with gestational diabetes. The bright and dark sides. Acta Diabetologica. 2018;55:885–92.

Larsen E, Christiansen OB, Kolte AM, Macklon N. New insights into mechanisms behind miscarriage. BMC Med. 2013;11:154(10 pages).

Lash GE. Molecular cross-talk at the feto-maternal interface. Cold Spring Harb Perspect Med. 2015;5(12):(14 pages).

Liao JB, Buhimschi CS, Norwitz ER. Normal labor: mechanism and duration. Obstet Gynecol Clin N Am. 2005;32:145–64.

Lionetti L, et al. From chronic overnutrition to insulin resistance: the role of fat-storing capacity and inflammation. Nutr Metab Cardiovasc Dis. 2009;19:146–52.

Liou S-R, Wang P, Cheng C-Y. Effects of maternal mental stress on birth outcomes. Women Birth. 2016;29:376–80.

Lisonkova S, Joseph KS. Incidence of preeclampsia: risk factors and outcomes associated with early- versus late-onset disease. Am J Obstet Gynecol. 2013;209:544.e1–12.

Lockwood CJ, Kuczynski E. Risk stratification and pathological mechanisms in preterm delivery. Paediatr Perinat Epidemiol. 2001;15(Suppl 2):78–89.

London V, Grube S, Sherer DM, et al. Hyperemesis gravidarum: a review of recent literature. Pharmacology. 2017;100:161–71.

Maillette de Buy Wenniger L, Beuers U. Bile salts and cholestasis. Dig Liver Dis. 2010;42:409–18.

McCrory JL, Chambers AJ, Daftary A, et al. Dynamic postural stability during advanced pregnancy. J Biomechanics. 2010;43:2434–9.

McCrory JL, Chambers AJ, Daftary A, et al. Torso kinematics during gait and trunk anthropometry in pregnant fallers and non-fallers. Gait Posture. 2020;76:204–9.

McGowan CA, McAuliffe FM. The influence of maternal glycaemia and dietary glycaemic index on pregnancy outcome in healthy mothers. Brit J Nutr. 2010;104:153–9.

Menon R, Mesiano S, Taylor RN. Programmed fetal membrane senescence and exome-mediated signaling: a mechanism associated with timing of human parturition. Front Endocrinol. 2017a;8:article 196.

Menon R, Richardson LS. Preterm prelabor rupture of the membranes: a disease of the fetal membranes. Semin Perinatol. 2017b;41:409–19.

Mijatovic-Vukas J, et al. Associations of diet and physical activity with risk for gestational diabetes mellitus: a systematic review and meta-analysis. Nutrients. 2018;10:1–19.

Moen G-H, et al. Epigenetic modifications and gestational diabetes: a systematic review of published literature. Eur J Endocrinol. 2017;176:R247–67.

Molina Lima SA, Paolucci El Dib R, Rossetto M, et al. Is the risk of low birth weight or preterm labor greater when maternal stress is experienced during pregnancy? A systematic review and meta-analysis of cohort studies. PLoS ONE. 2018;13:e0200594.

Morgan TK. Role of the placenta in preterm birth: a review. Am J Perinatol. 2016;33:258–66.

Mottola MF, Artal R. Fetal and maternal metabolic responses to exercise during pregnancy. Early Human Dev. 2016;94:33–41.

Myatt L, Redman CW, Staff AC, et al. Strategy for standardization of preeclampsia research study design. Hypertension. 2014;63:1293–301.

Myatt L, Roberts JM. Preeclampsia: syndrome or disease? Curr Hypertens Rep. 2015;17:83(8 pages).

Norwitz ER, Schust DJ, Fisher SJ. Implantation and the survival of early pregnancy. N Engl J Med. 2001;345:1400–8.

Ogurtzova K, et al. IDF Diabetes Atlas: global estimates for the prevalence of diabetes for 2015 and 2040. Diabetes Res Clin Pract. 2017;128:40–50.

Ovadia C, Seed PT, Sklavounos A, et al. Association of adverse perinatal outcomes of intrahepatic cholestasis of pregnancy with biochemical markers: results of aggregate and individual patient data meta-analysis. Lancet. 2019;393:899–909.

Oyelese Y, Ananth CV. Placental abruption. Obstet Gynecol. 2006;108:1005–16.

Pedersen AM, Bardow A, Beier S, et al. Saliva and gastrointestinal functions of taste, mastication, swallowing and digestion. Oral Diseases. 2002;8:117–29.

Petersen MC, et al. Regulation of hepatic glucose metabolism in health and disease. Nat Rev Endocrinol. 2017;13:572–87.

Phipps E, Prasanna D, Brima W, et al. Preeclampsia: updates in pathogenesis, definitions, and guidelines. Clin J Am Soc Nephrol. 2016;11:1102–13.

Polsani S, Phipps E, Jim B. Emerging new biomarkers of preeclampsia. Adv Chronic Kidney Dis. 2013;20:271–9.

Poon LC, Shennon A, Hyett JA, et al. The International Federation of Gynecology and Obstetrics (FIGO) initiative on pre-eclampsia: A pragmatic guide for first-trimester screening and prevention. Int J Gynecol Obstet. 2019;145(suppl 1):1–33.

Purish S, Gyamfi-Bannerman C. Epidemiology of preterm birth. Semin Perinatol. 2017;41:387–91.

Racicot K, Kwon J-Y, Aldo P, et al. Understanding the complexity of the immune system during pregnancy. Am J Reprod Immunol. 2014;72:107–16.

Redman CWG. Hypertension in pregnancy: the NICE guidelines. Heart. 2011;97:1967–9.

Redman CW, Sargent IL, Staff AC. IFPA senior award lecture: making sense of pre-eclampsia – two placental causes of preeclampsia? Placenta. 2014;35(Suppl. A Trophoblast Research Vol 28):S20–25.

Redman CWG, Tannetta DS, Dragovic RA et al. Review: Does size matter? Placental debris and the pathophysiology of pre-eclampsia. Placenta. 2012;33 Suppl. A. Trophoblast Research Vol 26:S48–54.

Redman CWG, Staff AC. Preeclampsia, biomarkers, syncytiotrophoblast stress and placental capacity. Am J Obstet Gynecol. 2015;213(4 Suppl):S9–11.

Romero R, Kusanovic JP, Chaiworapongsa T, et al. Placental bed disorders in preterm labor, preterm PROM, spontaneous abortion, and abruptio placentae. Best Pract Res Clin Obstet Gynecol. 2011;25:313–27.

Romero R, Dey SK, Fisher SJ. Preterm labor: one syndrome, many causes. Science. 2014;345:760–4.

Schaap TP, Knight M, Zwart JJ, et al. Eclampsia, a comparison within the international network of obstetric survey systems. BJOG. 2014;121:1521–9.

Shnaeckel KL, Magann EF, Ahmadi S. Pubic symphysis rupture and separation during pregnancy. Obstet Gynecol Surv. 2015;70:713–8.

Shynlova O, Tsui P, Jaffer S, Lye SJ. Integration of endocrine and mechanical signals in the regulation of myometrial functions during pregnancy and labour. Eur J Obstet Gynecol Reprod Biol. 2009;144S:S2–10.

Shynlova O, Lee Y-H, Srikhajon K, et al. Physiologic uterine inflammation and labor onset: Integration of endocrine and mechanical signals. Reprod Sci. 2013;20:154–67.

Shynlova O, Nadeem L, Zhang J, et al. Myometrial activation: Novel concepts underlying labor. Placenta. 2020;92:28–36.

Sibai BM. Diagnosis, prevention, and management of eclampsia. Obstet Gynecol. 2005;105:402–10.

Simmons D, et al. Gestational diabetes mellitus: nice for the US? Diabetes Care. 2010;33:34–7.

Simsek Y, Gul M, Celik O, et al. Nuclear transcription factor-kappa beta-dependent ultrastructural alterations within the placenta and systemic inflammatory activation in pregnant patients with hemolysis, elevated liver functions and low thrombocyte count (HELLP) syndrome: a case-control study. Hypertens Pregnancy. 2013;32(3):281–91.

Smith DD, Rood KM. Intrahepatic cholestasis of pregnancy. Clin Obstet Gynecol. 2019;63:134–51.

Staneva A, Bogossian, Pritchard M, et al. The effects of maternal depression, anxiety, and perceived stress during pregnancy on preterm birth: a systematic review. Women Birth. 2015;28:179–93.

Strand S, Strand D, Seufert R, et al. Placenta-derived CD95 ligand causes liver damage in hemolysis, elevated liver enzymes and low platelet count syndrome. Gastroenterol. 2004;126:849–58.

Straub H, Qadir S, Miller G, et al. Stress and stress reduction. Clin Obstet Gynecol. 2014;57:579–606.

Strauss III, JF, Romero R, Gomez-Lopez N et al. Spontaneous preterm birth: advances towards discovery of genetic predisposition. Am J Obstet Gynecol. March 2018:294–314.

Suzuki S. Clinical significance of pregnancies with circumvallate placenta. J Obstet Gynecol Res. 2008;34:51–4.

Svensson AC, Sandin S, Cnattingius S, et al. Maternal effects for preterm birth: a genetic epidemiologic study of 630,000 families. Am J Epidemiol. 2009;170:1365–72.

Tannetta D, Sargent I. Placental disease and the maternal syndrome of preeclampsia: missing link? Curr Hypertens Rep. 2013;15:590–9.

Tranquilli AL, Landi B, Corradetti A, et al. Inflammatory cytokines patterns in the placenta of pregnancies complicated by HELLP (hemolysis, elevated liver enzymes, and low platelet) syndrome. Cytokine. 2007;40:82–8.

Tsatsoulis A, et al. Insulin resistance: an adaptive mechanism becomes maladaptive in the current environment – an evolutionary perspective. Metabolism. 2013;62:622–33.

Turner RJ, Bloemenkamp KWM, Penning ME et al. From glomerular endothelium to podocyte pathobiology in preeclampsia: a paradigm shift. Curr Hypertens Rep. 2015;17:54(8 pages).

Van Dinter MC. Ptyalism in pregnant women. J Obstet Gynecol Neonatal Nurs. 1990;20:206–9.

Van Lieshout LCEW, Koek GH, Spaanderman MA, et al. Placenta-derived factors involved in the pathogenesis of the liver in the syndrome of haemolysis, elevated liver enzymes and low platelets (HELLP). Pregnancy Hypertens. 2019;18:42–8.

Veenendaal MVE, Van Abeelen AFM, Painter RC, et al. Consequences of hyperemesis gravidarum for off-spring: a systematic review and meta-analysis. Br J Obstet Gynaecol. 2011;118:1302–13.

Vogel JP, Chawanpaiboon S, Moller A-B, et al. The global epidemiology of preterm birth. Best Pract Res Clin Obstet Gynecol. 2018;52:3–12.

Von Salmuth V, Van der Heiden Y, Bekkers I, et al. The role of hepatic sinusoidal obstruction in the pathogenesis of the hepatic involvement in HELLP syndrome: Exploring the literature. Pregnancy Hypertens. 2020;19:37–43.

Wadhwa PD, Entringer S, Buss C, et al. The contribution of maternal stress to preterm birth: Issues and considerations. Clin Perinatol. 2011;38:351–84.

Walters C, West S, Nippita TA. Pelvic gridle pain. Aust J Gen Pract. 2018;47:439–43.

Westbrook RH, Dusheiko G, Williamson C. Pregnancy and liver disease. J Hepatol. 2016;64:933–45.

Wortham M, Sander M. Mechanisms of β-cell functional adaptation to changes in workload. Diabetes Obes Metab. 2016;18(suppl. 1):78–86.

Wu P, Haththotuwa R, Kwok CS, et al. Preeclampsia and future cardiovascuar health. A systemic review and meta-analysis. Circ Cardiovasc Qual Outcomes. 2017;10:e003497.

Zhang J, Merialdi M, Platt LD, Kramer MS. Defining normal and abnormal fetal growth: promises and challenges. Am J Obstet Gynecol. 2010:522–528.

Zhang C, Rawal S, Seng Chong Y. Risk factors for gestational diabetes: is prevention possible? Diabetologia. 2016;59:1385–90.

Zhang H, Dou R, Yang H, et al. Maternal and neonatal outcomes of placenta increta and percreta from a multicenter study in China. J Mat Fetal Neonatal Med. 2019;32:2622–7.

Preexistent chronic disorders, often directly affecting pregnancy

Abstract

The first two chapters describe the strategy in mammalian pregnancy in general and human pregnancy in particular, how to secure the survival of the species without compromising maternal health. The first chapter discusses the specific adaptive strategy that a pregnant woman utilizes to achieve this goal. She temporarily accommodates an immunologically different human being within her body and by supplying this new life with sufficient O_2, nutrients and disposing of its metabolic waste products, enables it to grow and mature, in line with its genetic potential. She does this in a setting, that allows her to shield the infant from external stress factors, such as excessive heat, – cold and – physical forces and, last but not least, she provides the infant with the means to safely exit the maternal body to the outer world at a suitable time. Yet, even seemingly-healthy women may develop common pregnancy complications, such as early pregnancy loss, placental syndromes, preterm birth and gestational diabetes. These complications are often superimposed on a preexistent, often latent defect in the maternal cardiovascular system (▶ sect. 3.1), renal function (▶ sect. 3.2), metabolism (▶ sect. 3.3), certain liver functions (▶ sect. 3.4), or the immune – (▶ sect. 3.5) and clotting systems (▶ sect. 3.6). Such a defect limits a woman's capacity to adapt to pregnancy and therefore, predisposes her to one of these pregnancy complications. This chapter describes the course and outcome of pregnancy in women with a chronic disorder affecting one of these six maternal functions and also, whether pregnancy will alter the course of her underlying chronic disorder.

L. L. H. Peeters et al., *Pathophysiology of pregnancy complications*,
https://doi.org/10.1007/978-90-368-2571-9_3

3

> **Highlights**
>
> 1. Pregnancy requires sufficient functional reserve capacity of the heart/vascular bed, and the volume regulatory- and immune systems. Women affected by a chronic disorder that reduces the reserve capacity of the related organs or systems, are at higher risk of developing placental syndromes in the second half of pregnancy;
> 2. Pregnant women with a chronic metabolic disorder or certain chronic liver diseases are at higher risk of abnormal fetal growth, fetal death (*diabetes mellitus*) or a placental syndrome;
> 3. Pregnancy may alleviate (*autoimmune diseases*), worsen (*thrombophilia*) or have little impact (*ulcerative colitis*) on the clinical presentation of a preexistent chronic disorder.

3.1 Cardiovascular diseases

3.1.1 Introduction

Under normal circumstances, pregnancy induces a series of adaptations in the maternal cardiovascular system, most of them being triggered and coordinated by hormones produced by the corpus luteum and placenta (detailed in ▶ Chap. 1). The cardiovascular functional reserve capacity determines a woman's ability to properly institute the adaptive changes required for a normal pregnancy. Many preexistent cardiovascular disorders are characterized by a reduced circulatory reserve capacity, predisposing affected women during pregnancy to complications, such as early pregnancy loss, preterm birth and a placental syndrome. In the sections below, we discuss the impact of various common preexistent cardiovascular disorders on pregnancy and conversely, whether and if so, how pregnancy may alter the course of these disorders. The clinical management during pregnancy has been summarized elsewhere (Emmanuel and Thorne 2015).

3.1.2 Systemic arterial hypertension

Systemic arterial hypertension affects about 15 % of the human population worldwide (Rossier et al. 2017), rendering it the most critical and expensive public health problem. Even though genetic and environmental factors are involved in its development, an unhealthy lifestyle is an important contributor. Although hypertension may have developed in response to other abnormalities such as, for instance, a renal artery stenosis or an aldosterone-producing adenoma, in most patients with high blood pressure there is no apparent cause and therefore, referred to as 'primary' or 'essential' hypertension. In hemodynamic terms, blood pressure is determined by cardiac output and vascular resistance, so hypertension must be due to a rise in either one or both of these two variables. Current theories on the pathogenesis of the disorder emphasize the primary role of an increased systemic vascular resistance in all forms of hypertension, even in cases where cardiac output is elevated. However, it remains obscure, as to what causes the rise in resistance. Histological specimens show a reduced lumen-to-media ratio, even in the very early stages of hypertension, which results from medial hypertrophy.

Once hypertension has developed, chronic exposure of the arterial wall to the enhanced mechanical strain associated with the raised pressure, amplifies this process of medial hypertrophy. This phenomenon, known as inward eutrophic remodeling (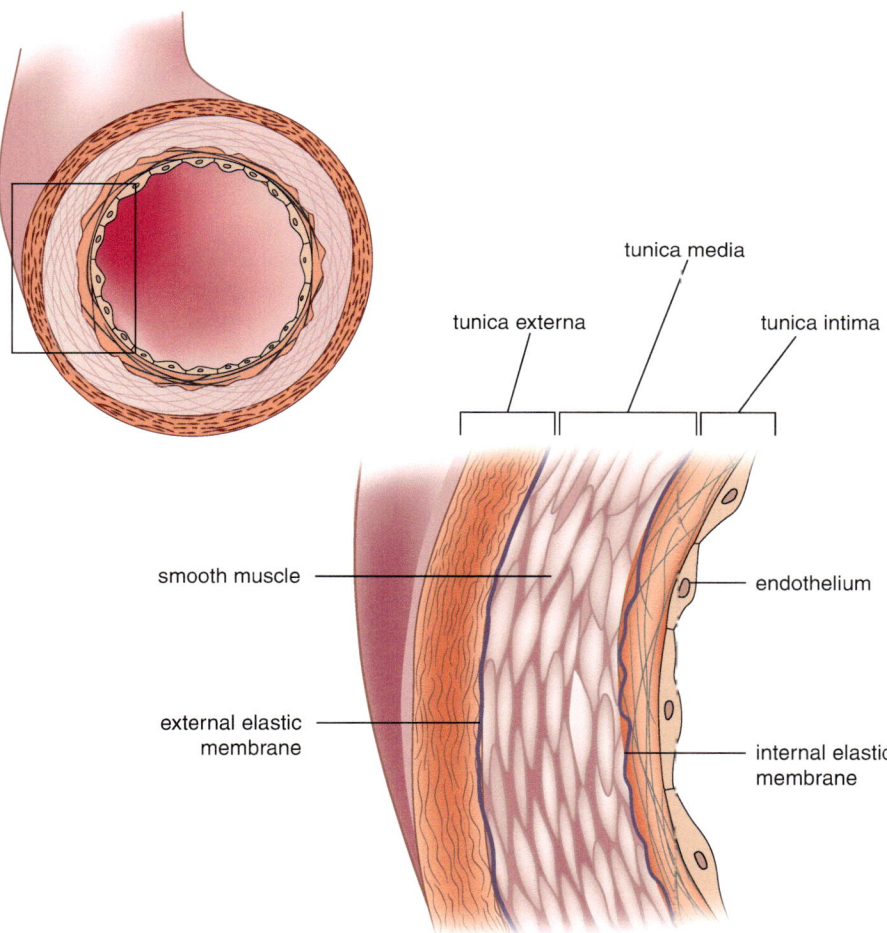 fig. 3.1) reduces wall stress at the expense of a higher resistance to flow. This development is clinically relevant as indicated by the higher incidence of cardiovascular events (e.g. myocardial infarction and stroke) in hypertensive, symptom-free subjects identified with reduced small vessels' lumen-to-media ratio, relative to their counterparts without this abnormality (Mathiassen et al. 2007).

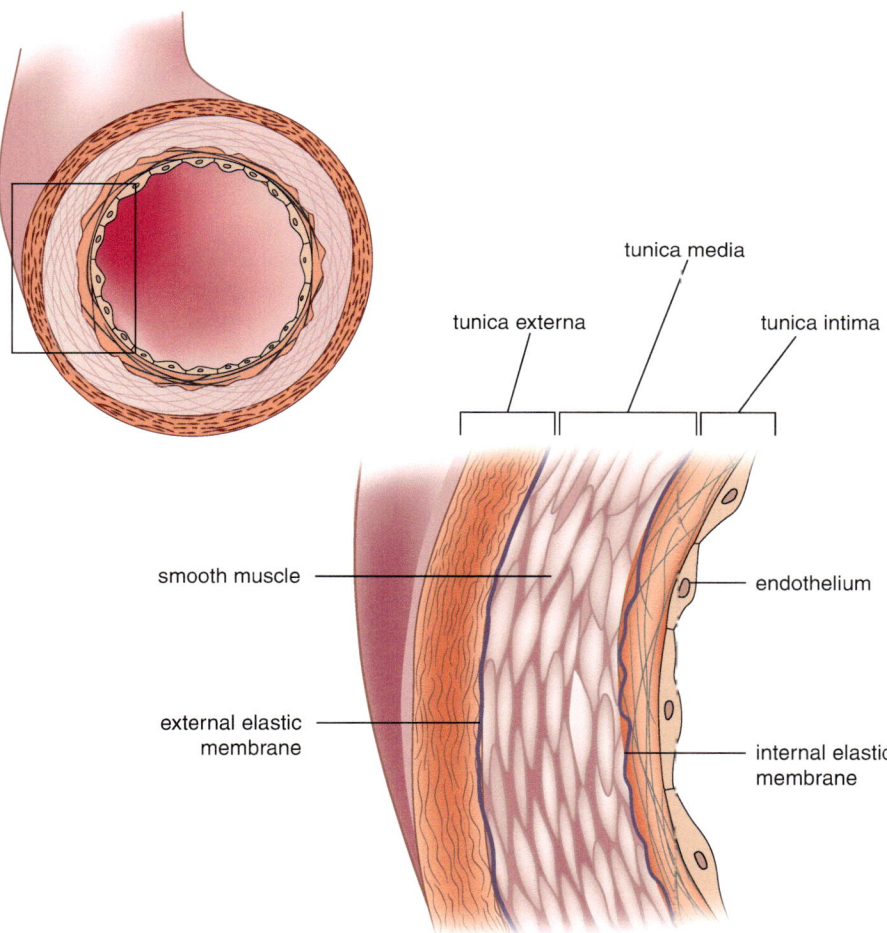

Figure 3.1   Chronic arterial hypertension with inward eutrophic remodeling of small arteries, an effect that leads to a lower lumen-to-media ratio (Mulvany 2012), because (1) the *tunica intima* (endothelium) has less capacity to release NO in response to shear stress; (2) the *tunica media* (smooth muscle cells) is stiffer due to collagen deposition and elastin degradation; (3) the *tunica externa* (adventitia) is less compliant because of more collagen deposition and accumulation of fibroblasts

3

Effect of systemic arterial hypertension on pregnancy

Since a hyperdynamic circulation that develops in response to a fall in systemic vascular resistance (SVR) is an important adaptive response in the early phase of a normal pregnancy, the maternal blood vessels should be able to dilate. Therefore, it is plausible that women with hypertension and inwardly remodeled, stiffer, small arteries are less capable of dilating their vasculature in response to pregnancy. This concept is supported by indirect evidence, such as a smaller rise in plasma volume (Spaanderman et al. 2001) and a lack of decline in arterial pressure in early pregnancy (McDonald-Wallis et al. 2012). Interestingly, formerly preeclamptic women show a clearly smaller adaptive circulatory and volume response to their next pregnancy than their counterparts, who had a normal pregnancy course and outcome (Lopez van Balen et al. 2013). This finding suggests a relation between the magnitude of the vasodilator response and the risk of developing a placental syndrome. In hypertensive women, the reduced capacity of the arterial bed to dilate, hinders the institution of a hyperdynamic circulation. It is conceivable that this defective response limits the maternal capacity to develop enough 'redundant shunt flow' by midpregnancy. Moreover, the lower arterial dilatory capacity applies to the entire systemic cardiovascular system, including the uterine vasculature, where spiral-artery remodeling is key in creating a sufficiently large uteroplacental vascular bed. Both subnormal reserve flow and poorly remodeled uterine spiral arteries predispose to placental dysfunction, usually clinically emerging in the second half of pregnancy.

Impact of pregnancy on the systemic arterial hypertension

Although the pathophysiological mechanisms are still only partly understood, it is clear that a pregnancy complicated by a placental syndrome predisposes to cardiovascular disease later in life. This is in line with the concept that vasoconstriction or inability to dilate the vasculature not only underlies hypertensive disorders of pregnancy. It is also associated with ischemic cardiovascular complications a few decades later. Moreover, also normotensive women that developed a placental syndrome in their pregnancy are at higher risk of developing a cardiovascular disorder later in life. It follows that pregnancy appears to be a physiologic stress test for the cardiovascular system, identifying not only hypertensive-, but also normotensive women at risk of cardiovascular disorders later in life. Besides, a placental syndrome does not seem to alter the course of systemic arterial hypertension, suggesting that pregnancy does not seem to accelerate the loss of already limited cardiovascular reserves, at least in the subgroup of hypertensive women.

3.1.3 Pulmonary arterial hypertension (PAH)

Pulmonary arterial hypertension (PAH) is defined as a (resting) mean pulmonary arterial pressure (mPAP) – assessed by right heart catheterization – of more than 25 mmHg, a figure, well above the upper limit of 20 mmHg for a normal resting mPAP (14 ± 3 mmHg). The etiology of PAH varies widely and, according to a recent definition by the WHO, includes left ventricular failure, chronic obstructive lung disease, other pulmonary disorders and pulmonary embolism. Most women with PAH can be classified in WHO group 1, consisting of individuals with idiopathic PAH and PAH being either heritable or secondary to a connective tissue disorder (Banerjee and Ventetuolo 2017). WHO group-1 PAH results from an abnormal proliferation of endothelial and smooth muscle cells in the wall of pulmonary arterioles. Eventually, PAH affects right-ventricular functional capacity. The disorder occurs several-fold more often in women than in men, with pregnancy being a condition prone to clinical deterioration. Still, pregnancies affected by PAH are rare with an incidence of 1.1/100,000 women (Obican and Cleary 2014). In a large proportion of pregnant PAH-affected women, the condition results from preexistent left heart disease, often a residual effect of congenital heart disease (CHD). PAH in pregnancy is idiopathic in 25–50 % of the cases (Franco et al. 2019).

The first clinical signs of PAH are fatigue and stress dyspnea, aspecific symptoms that do neither immediately alert the patient nor the physician. As a consequence, over 20 % of PAH patients are only diagnosed after having been symptomatic for over 2 years. The early signs are caused by right ventricular insufficiency, that limits the ability to properly raise cardiac output during exercise. As PAH progresses, symptoms worsen with eventually signs of overt right ventricular failure (e.g. stress-induced chest pain, syncope and development of peripheral edema, pleural effusion, sometimes even ascites). Nocturnal hypoxemia and sleep apnoea are common.

Lung volumes in PAH patients are often mildly to moderately reduced. Transthoracic cardiac ultrasound is key in diagnosing PAH as it provides both an image of the cardiac effects of PAH and enables estimation of mPAP from the continuous wave Doppler measurements.

Women with PAH who are already pregnant, should be offered the option of therapeutic abortion (Franco et al. 2019). Pregnant women with PAH who choose to continue their pregnancy, should be followed-up regularly in a specialized PAH center, which is to include regular cardiac ultrasound along with monitoring fetal growth. They should also be informed about the increased risk of deteriorating PAH, particularly during labor and postpartum. Pregnancy activates the coagulation system. Although there are no studies indicating an increased risk of thromboembolism in PAH patients, postmortem histopathology suggests a high incidence of thromboembolic events in PAH-affected women. This finding and the nonspecific risk factors for thrombosis, such as heart failure and immobility, provide a rationale for anticoagulation prophylaxis in pregnant PAH patients.

Impact of PAH on pregnancy

The risk of PAH-affected pregnant women to develop a hypertensive pregnancy disorder, preterm birth, fetal growth restriction and fetal mortality, is clearly higher than that in a large control group of pregnant women without PAH (Thomas et al. 2017).

Impact of pregnancy on PAH

An important adaptive response to pregnancy is the about 30 % fall in total peripheral vascular resistance (SVR) triggering the circulatory compensations detailed in ► Chap. 1. These include falls in colloid-osmotic pressure and plasma osmolality, along with hemodilution. In PAH, the pulmonary vascular resistance fails to decline in concert with the SVR in order to accommodate these effects (Lane and Trow 2011). This increases the strain exerted upon the right ventricle and with it, further reduces its already marginal compensatory capacity (◘ fig. 3.2). In women with PAH, the risk of right ventricular failure is particularly high during labor and postpartum, due to labor-related stress, pain, and extra metabolic demands. The postpartum period is characterized by large volume

3

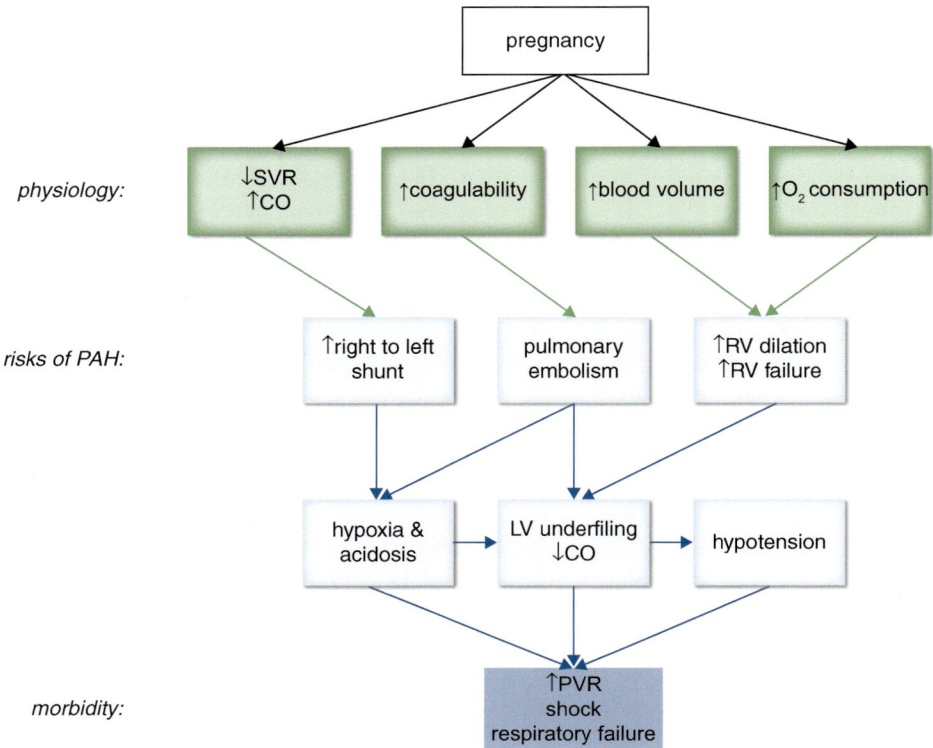

physiology:

risks of PAH:

morbidity:

☐ **Figure 3.2**   Pregnancy induces various adaptations in the maternal cardiovascular system that are associated with extra risks for pulmonary arterial hypertension (PAH) patients, as indicated by the grey boxes. The development of one of these complications in turn, may initiate a vicious circle that ends in maternal mortality. *Abbreviations*: CO, cardiac output; PAH-CHD, PAH associated with congenital heart disease; LV, left ventricle; RV, right ventricle; PVR, pulmonary vascular resistance; SVR, systemic vascular resistance (Olsson and Channick 2016)

shifts from the maternal interstitium to the intravascular compartment, which increases the vascular filling state and with it, puts extra strain upon the limited cardiac capacity to raise cardiac output.

Details about management of women with PAH have been elaborated in a recent guideline (Galiè et al. 2016; Olsson and Channick 2016). Yet, even nowadays the maternal mortality – mostly occurring postpartum – is at 16 % still high in spite of optimal treatment (Meng et al. 2017). The prognosis is particularly poor in women with PAH superimposed on cardiomyopathy or a valvular heart disease (Thomas et al. 2017).

3.1.4 Maternal arrhythmias

Maternal arrhythmias have become more prevalent over the last decades, as women with repaired congenital heart disease survive more often until their reproductive years, the maternal age of reproduction has also increased, and cardiac arrhythmias are age-dependent (Knotts and Garan 2014). Life-threatening arrhythmias in women of

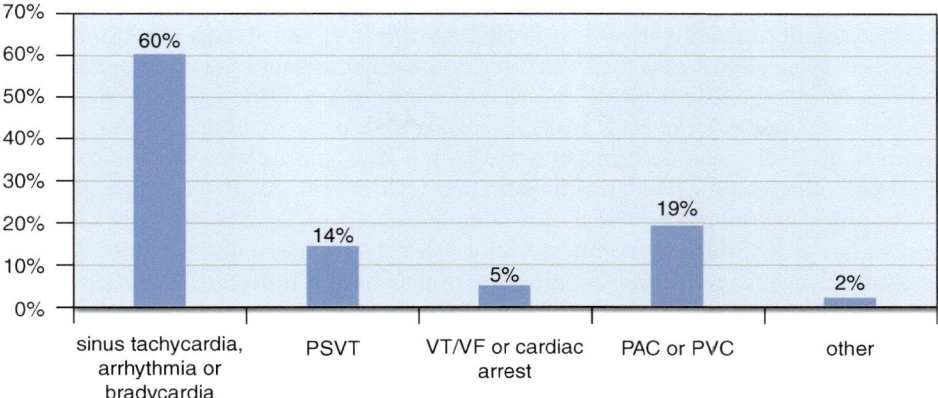

□ Figure 3.3 Diagnostic outcome among 218 pregnant women admitted to hospital because of cardiac arrhythmia. VT/VF: ventricular tachycardia/fibrillation; PSVT: paroxysmal supraventricular tachycardia; PAC or PVC: premature atrial complex or ventricular complex (*adapted from* Li et al. 2008)

childbearing age are rare. Also, in most cases of hospital admission for 'arrhythmia' during pregnancy, no true arrhythmia is found, but rather benign sinus tachycardia (heart rate > 100 bpm) or bradycardia (heart rate < 60 bpm) (□ fig. 3.3).

During pregnancy, cardiac output increases by a rise in both stroke volume and heart rate. Whereas the early-pregnancy rise in cardiac output mostly results from an increase in stroke volume, a higher heart rate becomes more important to sustain the elevated cardiac output in advanced pregnancy. The latter results from a rise in resting sinus node rate. Near term, the heart rate has usually increased by about 20 bpm, but rarely exceeds 100 bpm.

At any rate, the physiologic changes that boost cardiac filling can be expected to facilitate the development of arrhythmias by raising end-diastolic volume as well as myocardial stretch. Animal experiments suggest that – in addition to these mechanical factors – also the elevated circulating levels of catecholamines, estrogens and hCG may play a role as they may lower the threshold to develop arrhythmias in pregnancy. However, only arrhythmias causing unstable hemodynamic responses or debilitating maternal symptoms, are relevant. A hemodynamically significant arrhythmia is a major concern, as it may interfere with cardiovascular function and with it, threaten maternal health, and thus also fetal well-being. In this regard, it is pivotal to consider carefully the risk-benefit ratio of any (chronic) treatment, because there are often conflicting interests of mother and infant, particularly when maternal cardiovascular function is still stable. Indeed, on the one hand anti-arrhythmic drugs may be fetotoxic, whereas on the other hand, a too generous application of electrical cardioversion and radiofrequency ablation may be hazardous for the fetus. The latter emphasizes the importance of a comprehensive diagnostic work-up in each pregnant woman diagnosed with arrhythmia. If an electrocardiogram (ECG) at rest shows a sinus rhythm of over 100 bpm and external causes such as severe anemia, hyperthyroidism (prevalence 1 in 200 pregnancies) and drug abuse (e.g. cocaine, caffeine) have been excluded, the sinus tachycardia is probably physiologic in origin and does not need further treatment. Similarly, sinus bradycardia can be accepted after ruling out hypothyroidism and the use of medication, such as e.g. betablockers.

Premature atrial – (PACs) and ventricular contractions (PVCs) are also common arrhythmias, occurring in about half of all pregnancies. In the absence of organic heart disease, they are almost always benign. The same applies to paroxysmal supraventricular tachycardias. Diagnostic work-up and clinical management of these patients have been detailed elsewhere (Moore et al. 2012). Even though most arrhythmias in women with no previous cardiac disease turn out to be benign at diagnostic work-up, these women are at risk of developing fetal growth restriction (Henry et al. 2016). Obviously, arrhythmia in pregnancy should be managed by a multidisciplinary team particularly when the woman has arrhythmias superimposed on a preexistent organic heart condition. Management of pregnancy in women with arrhythmias has been detailed elsewhere (Metz and Khanna 2016).

3.1.5 Valvular heart disease (VHD)

Valvular heart disease (VHD) is the most common form of cardiovascular disease in pregnancy in developed countries. The condition is usually part of congenital heart disease (CHD), but it may also be a sequel of a previous endocarditis or of an immunological process, such as in rheumatic heart disease. Even though the prevalence of valvular disease as a complication of acute rheumatic fever has declined substantially in Western countries, it is still common in less affluent societies (Carapetis et al. 2016; Goldstein and Ward, 2017). Due to earlier intervention and better survival, the number of women, who had their – often congenital – valvular disease surgically corrected in childhood, has risen markedly.

Functionally, the affected valve may become stenotic or insufficient (or both) with aortic stenosis and mitral regurgitation as the most frequent manifestations. The risk of a valvular lesion complicating pregnancy depends on both type and severity of the lesion, and on the maternal pre-pregnancy left-ventricular systolic functional capacity (Roeder et al. 2011), as detailed in ◘ tab. 3.1.

In general, pregnant women tolerate regurgitant lesions better than stenotic ones (Campos et al. 1993). This can be explained by the physiological fall in systemic and pulmonary resistances, that leads to a fall in cardiac afterload. Consequently, the pressure drop across the valve will favor forward flow and with it, reduce the impact of an incompetent valve. On the other hand, when there is a stenotic lesion, an adaptive rise in cardiac output can be severely hindered. The most common and clinically relevant valve lesions and their impact on pregnancy and vice versa, are discussed in more detail below. Clinical management aspects, have been detailed elsewhere (Nishimura et al. 2014, 2017; Lau and Defaria Yeh 2019).

Mitral valve lesions

Mitral valve lesions (◘ fig. 3.4) are far more common than aortic valve disorders (Shi-Min Yuan and Song-Li Yan 2016) with *mitral stenosis* (MS) being the most frequently encountered serious valvular lesion during pregnancy. Although the incidence of MS secondary to acute rheumatic fever has declined markedly in developed countries, it continues to be a problem in developing areas. Moreover, due to the influx of female immigrants with a history of rheumatic fever in their childhood, MS is also still prevalent in developed countries (Nanna and Stergiopoulos 2014). Women with mild MS are

□ **Table 3.1**   Factors that determine the risk of pregnancy complications in women with a preexistent cardiac valvular lesion

low maternal and fetal risks	high maternal and fetal risks	high maternal risk
asympt. aortic stenosis, low mean outflow gradient (< 50 mmHg); normal LV function	severe aortic stenosis, irrespective of symptoms	ejection fraction < 40 %
aortic regurgitation, NYHA class I/II; normal LV function	aortic regurgitation, NYHA class III/IV	previous heart failure
mitral regurgitation, NYHA class I/II; normal LV function	mitral stenosis, NYHA class II/ III/IV	previous stroke or transient ischemic attack
mitral valve prolapse with none-to-moderate mitral regurgitation, normal LV function	mitral regurgitation, NYHA class III/IV	
mild to moderate mitral stenosis without pulmonary hypertension	aortic or mitral valve disease with pulmonary hypertension	
mild to moderate pulmonary valve stenosis	aortic or mitral valve disease with LV dysfunction	
	maternal cyanosis	
	reduced funct. status, NYHA class III/IV	

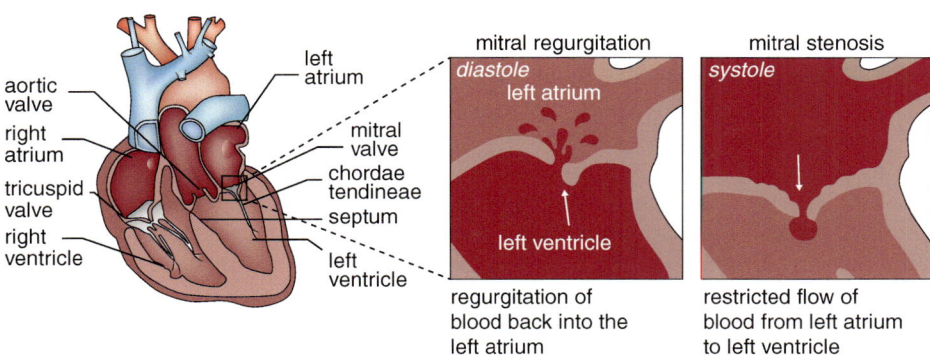

□ **Figure 3.4**   Display of mitral valve lesions. *Left panel*: anatomic location of mitral valve; *Right panel*: The two types of mitral valve pathology, mitral regurgitation and stenosis (*adopted from* Carapetis et al. 2016)

often asymptomatic, but during pregnancy they may develop extreme fatigue, dyspnea, orthopnea and resting tachycardia. This particular valve lesion compromises left-ventricular filling, and with it, limits the rise in cardiac output needed to compensate for the pregnancy-induced fall in systemic vascular resistance (Sliwa et al. 2015). The latter raises cardiovascular sympathetic activity, leading to a rise in heart rate and with it, shortening of the diastolic filling time. Consequently, the left atrium will accumulate

3

more fluid during diastole which will lead to atrial stretching, arrhythmias and loss of contractility. It will also hamper pulmonary drainage, which increases the risk of developing secondary pulmonary edema, pulmonary hypertension and even right-ventricular failure. Therefore, MS is probably the most serious VHD, with pregnancy imposing an extra risk for tipping the fragile cardiovascular balance of the patient. Obviously, the risk of perinatal complications in these women is also high (Sliwa et al. 2015).

Mitral valve insufficiency

Mitral valve insufficiency (MI) is not uncommon in pregnancy, as about one-third of women develop some degree of functional MI during pregnancy without clinically relevant hemodynamic consequences. The most common cause of MI in pregnancy is *mitral valve prolapse*, which is usually a benign mitral valve disorder affecting about 0.6 % of women of childbearing age. Although the prolapse may sometimes cause mild to moderate mitral regurgitation, most women with this lesion have a normal pregnancy course. In rare cases the hemodynamic changes may have a more serious adverse effect on the circulation, particularly, when the chordae tendineae (◘ fig. 3.4) have ruptured. Women with preexisting MI often tolerate pregnancy well, presumably because the fall in left ventricular afterload tends to ameliorate MI symptoms. However, this will no longer be the case, when MI is complicated by left-ventricular dysfunction, pulmonary edema or hypertension (Tsiaras and Poppas 2009, Dal-Bianco et al. 2014).

Aortic valve lesions

About a quarter of pregnant women with severe VHD have *aortic stenosis* (AS), ranking this lesion second in prevalence after mitral valve stenosis. A congenital bicuspid valve is the most common cause of aortic stenosis in young women. Because patients with symptomatic AS will usually be treated early in life, AS that is first detected during pregnancy is often mild. Nevertheless, in pathophysiological terms the pregnancy-related afterload reduction will intensify the functional impact of the stenosis and with it, enhance clinical symptoms. If the AS worsens, left ventricular systolic pressure and wall stress will rise, inducing compensatory left-ventricular hypertrophy with potential backlash, diastolic dysfunction, fibrosis, diminished coronary flow reserve and late systolic failure as sequelae. The extra strain upon the left ventricle further activates the sympathetic system resulting in an increase in both heart rate and myocardial contractility. However, due to the higher heart rate, diastolic filling time is reduced and this will further lower stroke volume. At the same time, enhanced sympathetic activity causes a redistribution of cardiac output in favor of brain and heart, but at the cost of skeletal muscles, skin, gastrointestinal tract, kidneys, and also the uteroplacental vascular bed. Therefore, pregnant women with aortic valve stenosis are at increased risk of both maternal and fetal complications, which currently are clinically well manageable (Orwat et al. 2016). Mild aortic stenosis may lead to fatigue, dyspnea and (pre-)syncope. Since these symptoms mimic commonly occurring pregnancy complaints, they do not always alarm the patient or the care provider. When the stenosis is more severe and the left ventricle is increasingly unable to eject a sufficient amount of blood during systole, life-threatening complications, such as therapy-resistant arrhythmias and cardiac failure may ensue. The reduced uteroplacental blood flow may ultimately lead to fetal growth restriction and preterm birth. *Aortic insufficiency* (AI) is also most often an after-effect of a bicuspid valve. It is characterized by partial backflow of the ejected stroke volume into the left ventricle during diastole. It lowers diastolic flow and pressure, thus leading to a higher pulse pressure and a diastolic pressure that sometimes falls to zero. AI leads to left-ventricular volume overload, which induces a gradual compensatory left-ventricular dilatation. Clinical symptoms resemble those of aortic valve stenosis: dyspnea, chest pain and syncope. Exercise-intolerance, frequently emerging through exertion-induced dyspnea, may be a sign of AI decompensation. Women with AI usually tolerate pregnancy well, as long as they succeed in maintaining their cardiac output. Accordingly, AI usually does not pose a serious risk for pregnancy and conversely, a preexistent AI rarely deteriorates during pregnancy. However, in severe cases, left ventricular dysfunction may ensue with arrhythmias and heart failure as the ultimate consequences. In advanced pregnancy, when the impact of pregnancy on maternal hemodynamics is greatest, women with AI may require medication to reduce cardiac afterload and volume overload. In general, bicuspid valves may be associated with accelerated dilation of the aortic root during pregnancy and an increased risk of dissection. The latter may also occur in women with a heritable connective tissue disorder (e.g. Marfan syndrome, Ehlers-Danlos syndrome and Loeys-Dietz syndrome), in particularly during the peripartum period, when there is increased lysis of collagen (Smok 2014).

Pulmonary valve lesions

Almost all cases of *pulmonary stenosis* (PS) and *pulmonary insufficiency* (PI) are congenital in origin and therefore, usually already diagnosed and treated in childhood. PI is seen most often after repair of tetralogy of Fallot and sometimes after valvuloplasty for PS. After surgery, cardiac function is usually normal, except in patients with residual PI as an after-effect of prolonged pre-surgical exposure to excess mechanical strain. Cardiac complications as a result of PS are extremely rare in pregnancy, even when PS is severe. On the other hand, the pregnancy-induced rise in cardiac output in women with PI may precipitate right-ventricular failure, in particular, when the right ventricular function was already impaired before pregnancy. Common symptoms include exertion-induced fatigue, dyspnea, atypical chest pain and syncope.

Tricuspid valve lesions

Tricuspid stenosis and insufficiency are extremely rare and almost always congenital in origin. The most common tricuspid valve lesion in this respect is tricuspid regurgitation, almost always developing as a sequel of another cardiac anomaly (Crousillat and Wood 2019). For more details about the impact of tricuspid regurgitation on pregnancy, the interested reader is referred to the related cardiology specialty literature.

Prosthetic heart valves

The rate of adverse pregnancy outcome in women with prosthetic heart valves is still high, as indicated by increased rates of pregnancy loss and perinatal mortality. Also, maternal mortality due to hemorrhagic or thromboembolic events is still relatively high, even though the risk of these complications has declined in the last decade (Arya 2019). The perinatal risks relate to intrauterine growth restriction, preterm birth and congenital malformations, mostly consisting of congenital heart disease or those related to intrauterine exposure to warfarin. Anticoagulant prophylaxis in these women during pregnancy is still challenging (Castellano et al. 2012; Yanagawa et al. 2016). Details about the clinical management of these patients has been reported elsewhere (Bhagra et al. 2017).

3.1.6 **Congenital heart disease (CHD)**

CHD refers to a series of cardiac disorders that in most cases require surgical repair in childhood. A symptom-free woman with a history of such a repair and adequate ventricular function has excellent chances of having a normal pregnancy. On the other hand, former CHD patients with (post-repair) pulmonary hypertension or a (pre-replacement) dilated aortic root, are at high risk of having a poor pregnancy outcome. The most frequently (repaired) CHDs observed in women of childbearing age are atrial septal defect (ASD), ventricular septal defect (VSD), patent foramen ovale (PFO), obstructive and leaky-valve lesions, and coarctation of the aorta (Head and Thorne 2005). ASD and PFO are associated with a left-to-right shunt, but it is rare that small shunts have a negative impact on pregnancy. Still, pregnancy may increase the preexistent tendency to atrial arrhythmias, because of more atrial stretch secondary to the higher cardiac preload. The risk of pregnancy complications in women with a small VSD or PFO and normal right-sided pressures is not higher than in their non-affected counterparts. On the other hand, pregnancy in (cyanotic) women with a right-to-left shunt can be considered life-threatening! The clinical management of these patients during pregnancy, has been discussed elsewhere (Canobbio et al. 2017).

In about half of the women with a repaired aortic coarctation, pregnancy will be uneventful. The other half is at increased risk of complications due to having developed an aneurysm at the repair site, or a post-repair pressure gradient over the coarctation of greater than 20 mmHg. They should be counseled preconceptionally as they will often have developed chronic hypertension requiring tailored management (Head and Thorne 2005). Detailed information on the consequences of pregnancy for women with complex CHDs, like Marfan's syndrome, tetralogy of Fallot and transposition of the great arteries, can be retrieved from the cardiology literature on this topic.

3.1.7 **Heart failure (HF)**

Heart failure (HF) is a complex clinical syndrome associated with a reduced or preserved ejection fraction, although the criterion for differentiating between these two entities varies among studies. Heart failure ensues when a primary cardiac event (e.g. myocardial infarction, myocarditis, valvular dysfunction) results in, usually left ventricular dysfunction. Initially, impaired ventricular filling or impaired ejection of blood may be asymptomatic, but symptoms, such as fatigue and dyspnea, will gradually develop. Without specific treatment, HF is almost always progressive. For clinical reasons and to facilitate development of measures to delay or even prevent HF from progressing, HF has been classified as follows (Yancy et al. 2013):

- stage A refers to an asymptomatic condition at high risk to progress to HF (e.g. in primary hypertension), but without structural heart disease;
- stage B refers to structural heart disease, but without symptoms or signs of HF;
- stage C refers to symptomatic structural heart disease with no, mild or severe limitation of physical abilities;
- stage D refers to refractory HF requiring specialized interventions.

HF often begins with reduced systolic function, e.g. a compromised ejection fraction (EF) (< about 40 %) with compensatory left ventricular dilation. However, HF may also begin with (asymptomatic) diastolic dysfunction with preserved ejection fraction and

▣ **Table 3.2**　Functional and structural causes of heart failure (HF) in pregnancy. Often, HF in pregnancy results from a combined structural/functional defect (*adopted from* Dennis 2015)		
functional causes of heart disease	**structural causes of heart disease**	
preload ↑ (*subnorm. contractility or lusitropy problem*)	**congenital**	**acquired**
either abnormal rate or rhythm, or afterload problem (*due to physiol. conditions or drugs (tocolytics, analgesia, i.v. fluids, drug overdose, illicit drug use.)*	uncorrected or corrected	*vascular → small vessels (e.g. coronary art.) → large vessels (e.g. aorta, pulm. art.)*
		pericardial → secondary to inflammation, edema
		myocardial → secondary to cardiomyopathy, edema, infection, hypertrophy, fibrosis, idiopathic
		valvular → stenotic or regurgitant lesions, secondary to inflammation/infection

without ventricular dilatation. Cardiac conditions that may lead to HF in pregnancy are summarized in ▣ tab. 3.2. So-called high output HF may occur in patients with severe anemia, hyperthyroidism, arteriovenous shunting (e.g. in beriberi). Isolated right ventricular failure usually results from severe pulmonary disease or pulmonary embolism.

Women with a preexistent cardiovascular risk condition (e.g. hypertension) or a cardiac disorder (e.g. CHD and VHD) with residual structural defect(s), are at increased risk to develop HF in pregnancy. As the normal hemodynamic adaptation to pregnancy includes a rise in cardiac work and blood volume, it is not surprising that in women at risk, cardiac reserves may be insufficient to meet the 30–40 % higher cardiovascular demands. When cardiac reserves are exhausted, the cardiovascular system responds with activation of the sympathetic nervous system in order to preserve blood supply to vital tissues at the cost of – among others – the uterus. When the mismatch between cardiac output and peripheral flow demands develops more abruptly, the 'normal' stress response will be inadequate to prevent adverse circulatory effects. It is plausible that the latter can trigger the development of a placental syndrome, with rises in blood pressure and heart rate, and compromised blood supply to the kidneys, splanchnic organs, skeletal muscles and skin and obviously also, the uteroplacental bed.

3.1.8　Peripartum cardiomyopathy (PPCM)

Interestingly, some seemingly healthy women develop PPCM, an often-lethal form of HF stage-D, characterized by severe systolic dysfunction developing in the final month of pregnancy or in the first five months postpartum. Typically, PPCM affects 1 of 1,000-4,000 live births in the US, the wide variation being related to large differences between the populations studied (Arany and Elkayam 2016). Maternal mortality in untreated PPCM patients may be as high as 50 %, with cardiac function in half of the survivors being persistently reduced. Insight into the etiology of PPCM is still incomplete, but possible contributors are myocarditis, raised myocyte apoptosis, abnormal immune response to pregnancy and genetic predisposition. The latter is supported by case-clustering in geographic regions. Recent evidence suggests that the pathophysiology of PPCM, is characterized by unbalanced peripartum/postpartum oxidative stress that triggers the proteolytic cleavage of prolactin into highly potent anti-angiogenic, pro-apoptotic, pro-inflammatory and cardiotoxic 16kDa sub-fragments that destroy the myocardial microcirculation, eventually resulting in ventricular dilation and systolic dysfunction (Hilfiker-Kleiner and Sliwa 2014). Overlap of PPCM with hypertensive pregnancy disorders provides evidence for the role of oxidative stress as an instigator of abnormal prolactin cleavage in genetically susceptible women (Parikh and Blauwet 2018). Actually, in hypertensive pregnancy disorders, such as preeclampsia, the dysfunctional placenta releases large amounts of Flt-1, that can be expected to facilitate abnormal prolactin cleavage. On the other hand, the source of the oxidative stress in women that develop PPMC some months postpartum, is still obscure. At any rate, prolactin inhibition by adding bromocriptine to standard cardiac support therapy improves left ventricular function in severely ill patients (Hilfiker-Kleiner et al. 2017), which provides additional evidence for abnormal prolactin-cleavage being key in the development of PPCM. The clinical management of PPCM has been reported in detail elsewhere (Arany and Elkayam 2016; Cunningham et al. 2019).

3.2 Renal disease

3.2.1 Introduction

Chronic kidney disease (CKD) has a huge impact on pregnancy, because of the central role of the kidneys in preserving hemodynamic homeostasis. Women with preexistent CKD encounter various challenges in pregnancy, as also indicated by the high rate of pregnancy complications they experience (listed in ◘ tab. 3.3). The incidence of these complications increases with the severity of the underlying CKD (◘ tab. 3.4). Another aspect with respect to pregnancy in these women is the need to critically evaluate the medication used to control CKD – preferably before pregnancy – in order to avert exposure of the embryo/fetus to their potential teratogenicity.

Characteristics and pathophysiology

The prevalence of CKD in women of childbearing age is about 4 % (Fischer 2007) and involves both primary renal diseases and renal disorders secondary to systemic illness. Pregnancy can trigger not only an exacerbation of the preexistent CKD, but also unmask a latent nephropathy. For instance, when renal reserve capacity (RRC), i.e. the ability of the kidney to raise GFR in response to certain stimuli, are already maximally utilized, the kidney cannot additionally increase its function during pregnancy. Such a situation may occur in women with diabetes and/or obesity (Chagnac et al. 2019), or in women with reduced nephron mass due to underlying subclinical renal disease (Jefferson and Shankland 2014). Below, the most often observed glomerular abnormalities are discussed.

Table 3.3 Adverse perinatal outcome in women with chronic kidney disease (CKD). (*based on data reported by* Gonzalez-Suarez et al. 2019)

maternal adverse events	fetal adverse events
worsening of kidney function	early pregnancy loss
flare of underlying disease	stillbirth
hypertensive complications	fetal asphyxia
medication-related effects	fetal growth restriction
preterm birth	low birthweight

Table 3.4 Stages of Chronic Kidney Disease (CKD). The risk of pregnancy complications increases with CKD stage. Women in CKD stage 4 and 5 are unable to respond to pregnancy with a rise in glomerular filtration rate (GFR) (*adopted from* Vellanki 2013)

stage	description renal functional damage	GFR (mL/min/m^2)
1.	Kidney damage, normal or raised GFR	> 90
2.	Kidney damage, mildly reduced GFR	60–89
3.	Moderately reduced GFR	30–59
4.	Severely reduced GFR	15–29
5.	Kidney failure	< 15 or dialysis

3.2.2 Focal segmental glomerulosclerosis (FSGS)

Focal segmental glomerulosclerosis (FSGS) is the most common glomerular disorder causing CKD, often progressing to end-stage renal disease (ESRD) (Smyth et al. 2013). It usually presents as (sub)acute nephrotic syndrome (without renal insufficiency) resulting from podocyte injury of varying etiology (◘ tab. 3.5 and ◘ fig. 3.6) (Jefferson and Shankland 2014) with circa 80 % being primary FSGS. The podocytes play a key role in the kidney's filter function. The cause of podocyte injury is both complex and multifactorial as summarized in ◘ tab. 3.5 and in the ◘ figures 3.5 and 3.6.

IgA nephropathy, vasculitis, lupus nephritis, viral infection, drugs or toxins may all lead to secondary FSGS (Fogo 2015). Clinically, FSGS may mimic the onset of preeclampsia. Therefore, it is crucial to correctly diagnose FSGS before starting treatment. If non-invasive evaluation is inconclusive, renal biopsy should be considered (Smyth et al. 2013). ◘ Figure 3.7 illustrates the actual damage within the glomerulus.

Impact of pregnancy on FSGS

The normal rise in GFR during pregnancy can be expected to worsen FSGS-related proteinuria. After ruling out secondary causes of FSGS that require specific therapy, control of blood pressure combined with a low-salt diet, are the cornerstones of FSGS-management.

| | **Table 3.5** | Classification by cause of focal segmental glomerulosclerosis (FSGS) |
classification	etiology	cause
primary	circulating permeabil-ity factor	unknown
secondary	glomerular hyperfil-tration	reduced nephron mass; – congenital (low birthweight, kidney dysplasia); – acquired nephron loss (reflux and diabetic nephropathy); adaptive response (e.g. obesity, sickle cell disease); viral infections (HIV, parvovirus B19, cytomegaly); drugs, toxins (heroin, lithium, steroids).
familial	podocyte gene dis-orders	nephrin, podocin, IFN2, α-actinin-4, phospholipase Cε1.

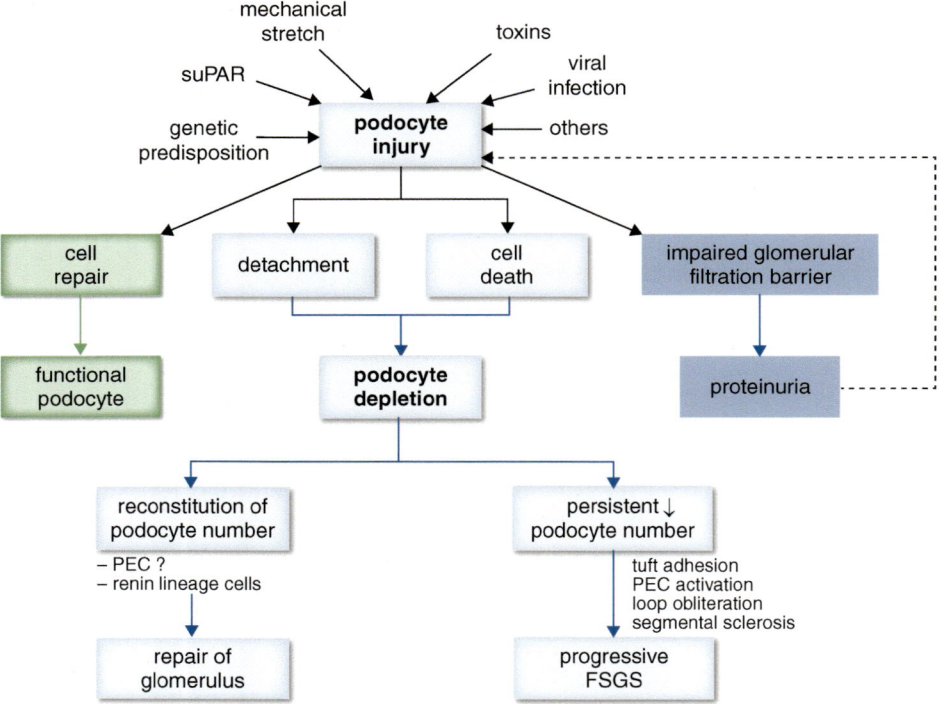

Figure 3.5 Focal segmental glomerulosclerosis (FSGS) is the result of ongoing podocyte depletion, that affects the glomerular filtration barrier. This leads to proteinuria and ongoing podocyte injury eventually resulting in end-stage renal disease. Yet, the reconstitution of podocyte number may be possible, enabling recovery of glomerular architecture and function. *Abbreviations*: *FSGS*, focal segmental glomerulosclerosis; *suPAR*, circulating (soluble) urokinase-type plasminogen-activator receptor fragments; *PEC*, parietal epithelial cells. (*for more details, see article by* Jefferson and Shankland 2014)

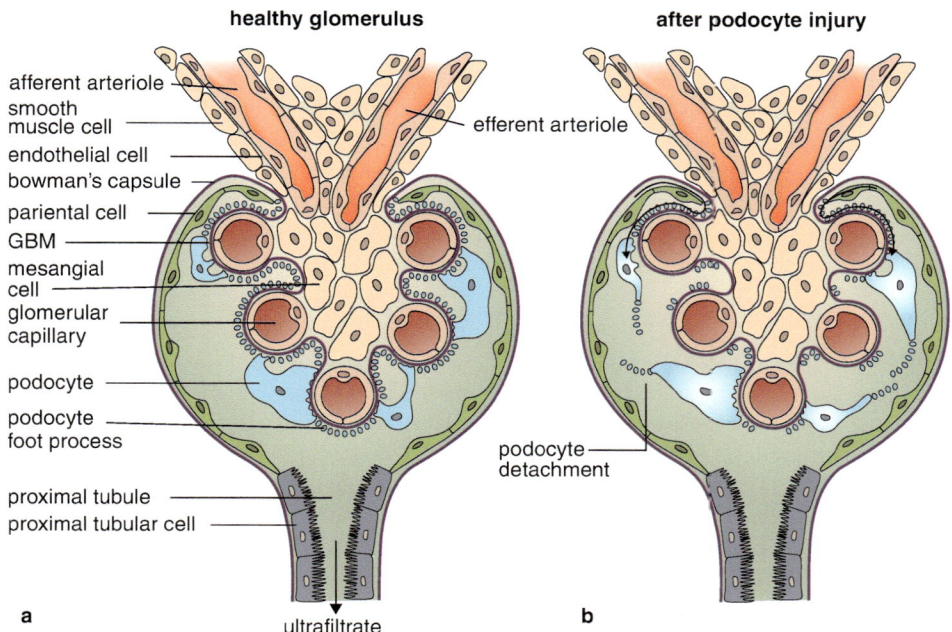

healthy glomerulus   **after podocyte injury**

afferent arteriole
smooth muscle cell
efferent arteriole
endothelial cell
bowman's capsule
pariental cell
GBM
mesangial cell
glomerular capillary
podocyte
podocyte foot process
podocyte detachment

proximal tubule
proximal tubular cell

a
ultrafiltrate
b

◼ Figure 3.6   Development of podocyte injury in focal segmental glomerulcsclerosis (FSGS). (**a**) Healthy glomerulus showing glomerular tuft, surrounded by Bowman's capsule, lined by parietal epithelial cells. The highly-specialized podocytes cover the glomerular capillary tuft and are key in preserving glomerular structure and permeability function. They have limited proliferative capacity. (**b**) Podocytes may be damaged by various factors (see text and ◼ fig. 3.5). Their injury leads to their detachment causing the migration of parietal epithelial cells (PECs) along Bowman's capsule to the areas of injury. These PECs may either be reparative or promote sclerosis, depending on the local micro-environment Abbreviation: GBM, glomerular basement membrane (*adopted from* Fogo 2011)

Impact of FSGS on pregnancy

Pregnant women with FSGS are at increased risk of the complications listed in ◼ tab. 3.3. The risk of developing these complications increase with more severe CKD (◼ tab. 3.4).

3.2.3 Lupus nephritis (LN)

Systemic lupus erythematosus (SLE) is the result of an interplay between genetic, epigenetic and environmental factors resulting in the loss of self-tolerance and with it, the life-long persistence of antinuclear antibodies (ANAs) and auto-active T- and B-cell clones (Anders and Rovin 2016). A subset of patients develops clinical signs in response to either viral infections or endocrine triggers with about 75 % of SLE patients developing LN, more often women than men. LN is amongst the most variable and dangerous renal diseases that can affect pregnant women.

Impact of pregnancy on LN

Pregnancy-induced changes in the immune function and endocrine environment may increase the rate of LN flares, that affect one out of four LN pregnancies (Vellanki 2013; Smyth et al. 2013). Flares may mimic preeclampsia, but can be identified by a targeted blood test (e.g. rising levels of anti-DNA-antibodies, hypocomplementemia) combined with a urine sediment ("active" urine sediment vs. isolated proteinuria) (Moroni and Ponticelli 2018). Renal functional deterioration during pregnancy occurs in about 5 % of all cases with mild renal dysfunction at the time of conception (◘ tab. 3.3: stage 1 and 2), and around 30 % of all cases with, at conception, more severe renal dysfunction (stage 3 and 4) (Fischer 2007).

Impact of LN on pregnancy

A woman with LN who intends to conceive, should be informed about pregnancy being safest after a period of at least six months remission, with blood pressure well-controlled, serum creatinine level below 130 µmol/L and daily dose of prednisone less than 10 mg (Vellanki 2013). During pregnancy, anticoagulant prophylaxis is required. With these optimal conditions at conception, her risk of a flare during pregnancy is about 30 % (Fischer 2007), which is half the risk of flares in case of less favorable conditions at conception. Flares impact pregnancy adversely. Without flares, pregnancy outcome is favorable for both mother and child in spite of an increased risk of the complications listed in ◘ tab. 3.3. Last but not least, the child is at increased risk of acquiring a congenital heart block as a result of exposure to maternal circulating anti-SSA antibodies (Vellanki 2013).

3.2.4 Minimal change disease (MCD)

MCD is a renal lesion mostly observed in children. Yet it accounts for 10–15 % of the cases of primary Nephrotic Syndrome (NS, proteinuria > 3.5 g/day) in adults (Smyth et al. 2013). MCD is a renal disorder that combines massive proteinuria with minimal morphological lesions (normal glomeruli at light microscopy and only foot-process effacement at electron microscopy). In most cases, long-term prognosis of MCD is favorable with no progression to higher stages of CKD. Insight in the pathogenesis is still incomplete. MCD is thought to result from a combination of immunologic dysregulation and changes in the podocytes that disrupts the integrity of the glomerular basement membrane (GBM). This enables albumin and other serum proteins to escape to the urinary tubules resulting in NS and secondary hypoalbuminemia, salt retention, hyperlipidemia, hemoconcentration, hypovolemia and hemostatic disorders (Vivarelli et al. 2017). Most patients respond favorably to standard prednisone therapy, although the rate of relapse is high. A subset of patients needs second-line steroid-sparing immunosuppression. Some steroid-unresponsive forms of MCD may deteriorate into FSGS.

Impact of pregnancy on MCD

Pregnancy is likely to increase preexistent MCD-related NS, but there are no reports suggesting that pregnancy alters the long-term natural course of MCD (O'Shaughnessy et al. 2017).

Impact of MCD on pregnancy

Although pregnancy may worsen the preexistent MCD-related NS, the few reported cases on pregnancy in MCD-affected women indicate that, in spite of preterm birth in most patients, the outcome for both mother and infant is favorable (O'Shaughnessy et al. 2017).

3.2.5 Membranous nephropathy (MN)

MN, another potential cause of NS, is histopathologically defined by the presence of immune complexes on the extra-capillary side of the GBM. Despite its annual incidence of only 1 in 100,000, it accounts for about 20 % of non-diabetic cases of NS in adults. The disease may affect anyone, irrespective of age, ethnic and racial background, men twice as often as women. The pathophysiology begins with normal glomeruli gradually developing homogeneous thickening of the capillary wall and formation/incorporation of typical spike-like deposits of immune complexes in the GBM. The active process ends with the development of tubulointerstitial fibrosis (Ronco and Debiec 2015). Experimental evidence supports the concept that circulating antibodies bind to integral membrane proteins of the podocyte (acting as auto-antigens) or exogenous antigens planted in the GBM, forming immune complexes (■ fig. 3.7). Deposits of these immune complexes activate the complement system and induce the formation of C5b-9 attack complexes,

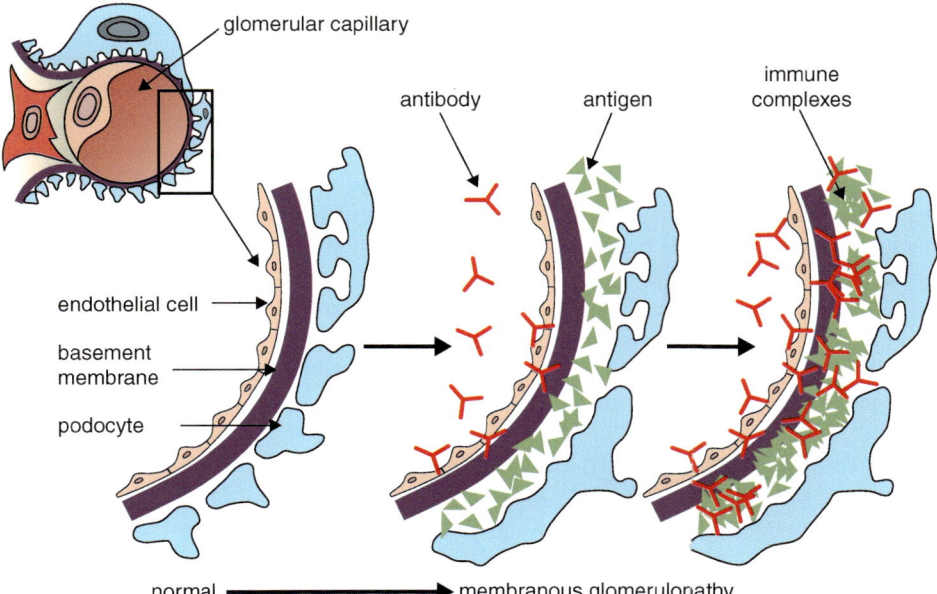

■ Figure 3.7 Pathogenesis of immune-mediated podocyte injury in membranous nephropathy (MN). Circulating antibodies bind to either *endogenous* integral membrane proteins of the podocyte that act as auto-antigens, or to *exogenous* antigens planted in the glomerular basement membrane, thus forming immune complexes. Deposits of these immune complexes activate the complement system and induce the formation of C5b-9 *attack complexes*, that in turn, damage podocytes leading to proteinuria. (*for details see article by Ronco and Debiec 2015*)

that damage the podocytes and with it, leads to proteinuria, as detailed elsewhere (Ronco and Debiec 2015). Three of every four cases are idiopathic, with the remaining one developing after various clinical conditions, such as infections (e.g. hepatitis B), autoimmune diseases (e.g. SLE), malignancy and drug intoxication.

Impact of pregnancy on MN

Only case reports have been published and these suggest that pregnancy does not affect the natural course of MN. Nevertheless, pregnancy may increase the proteinuria.

Impact of MN on pregnancy

The increased risk of the usual complications (■ tab. 3.3) also applies to pregnant MN-affected women. Exacerbations of NS during pregnancy usually respond well to corticosteroid (pulse) therapy. The limited information from case reports on this topic supports a favorable pregnancy outcome for both mother and infant (Malik et al. 2002; Ope-Adenuga et al. 2015).

3.2.6 IgA nephropathy

IgA nephropathy is the most common primary glomerulonephritis worldwide. Most cases will progress to ESRD. The incidence peaks in young adults of 20–30 years and thus, for affected women that intend to conceive, is a major concern.

The production of galactose-deficient IgA1 represents the first hit (Hit-1) in the pathogenesis of IgA nephropathy (■ fig. 3.8). Hit 2 consists of the formation of autoantibodies that recognize galactose-deficient IgA1. The subsequent hit 3 represents the formation of pathogenic immune complexes. However, key in the pathogenesis of IgA nephropathy is hit 4: the deposition of specific immune complexes in the glomeruli close to the mesangial cells. As also decribed above for MN, this hit 4 activates the complement system (Novak et al. 2018), but in contrast to the events in MN, it does not damage podocytes, but triggers the proliferation of resident mesangial cells, triggering the production of extracellular matrix proteins and inflammatory cytokines. These cytokines damage the filtration barrier resulting in hematuria and proteinuria. They also damage the mesangial cells, inducing their apoptosis via mesangium-podocyte-tubular crosstalk. This process eventually results in tubulosclerosis (Wu et al. 2018). The rate of renal function loss depends on features, such as mesangial hypercellularity, segmental glomerulosclerosis, tubular atrophy and interstitial fibrosis (Soares and Roberts 2017).

Impact of pregnancy on IgA nephropathy

The results of a recent meta-analysis suggest no accelerated loss of renal function during pregnancy in women with IgA nephropathy, who still have a partially preserved kidney function (Liu et al. 2016). The number, quality and comparability of the studies included in the analysis, though, were limited and no differentiation was made between mild and advanced stages of CKD. Therefore, it is conceivable that particularly women with stage 4 or 5 renal dysfunction (■ tab. 3.4) are at risk of accelerated pregnancy-related loss of renal function.

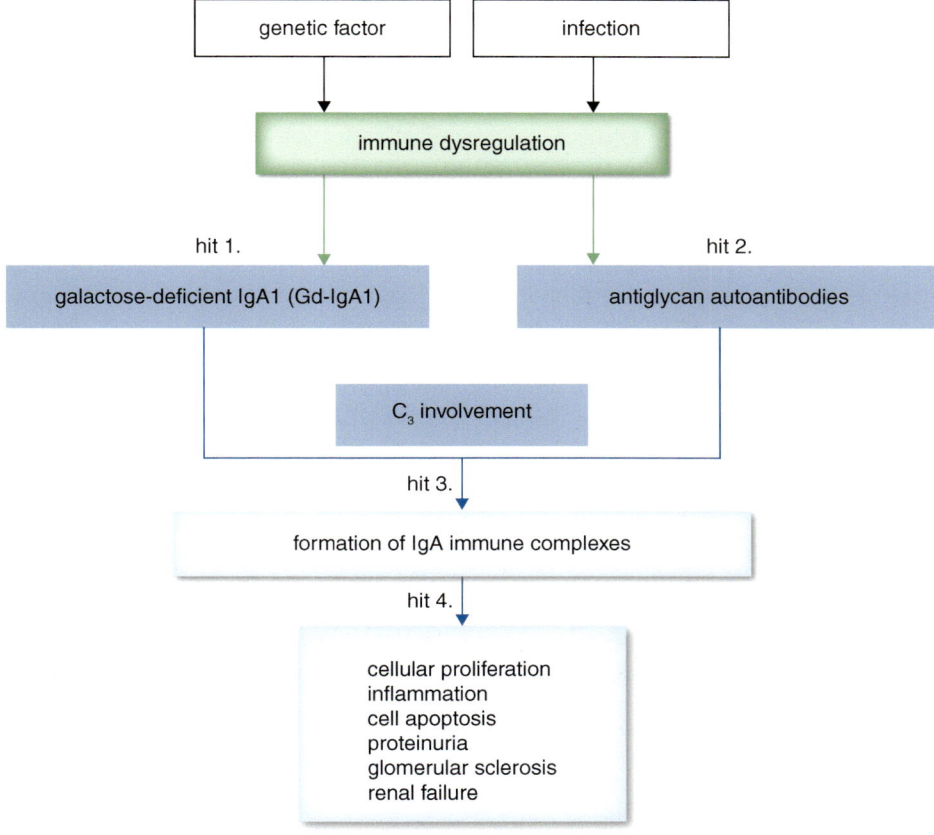

□ Figure 3.8   A generally accepted hypothesis about the pathogenesis of IgA nephropathy postu-
lates that immune complexes are formed in the circulation and then deposited in the mesangium as
described in the text. These deposits activate the complement system, which leads to local oxidative
stress along with an inflammatory response, that damages mesangial cells inducing their apoptosis,
eventually resulting in tubulosclerosis (*adopted from* Wu et al. 2018)

Impact of IgA nephropathy on pregnancy

Women with IgA nephropathy are at increased risk of the pregnancy disorders listed in
□ tab. 3.3.

3.2.7 Thin basement membrane nephropathy

This is a glomerular disorder with IgA nephropathy-like features that may lead to hematuria. The available data suggest no adverse impact of this rare disorder on pregnancy
course and outcome (Packham 2005).

Several other forms of glomerular damage, such as amyloid deposits or anti-GBM
disease (Goodpasture syndrome) may also occur in pregnancy but are extremely rare.
Nevertheless, the latter may be associated with significant maternal and fetal morbidity
(Huser et al. 2015).

3

3.2.8 Diabetic nephropathy (DN)

Diabetes mellitus (DM) complicates roughly 1 in 250 pregnancies in the UK, with an about 50 % rise in type-2 DM in the last decades, closely following the rising prevalence in obesity (Bramham 2017). DN is an important microvascular complication of DM and is characterized by albuminuria (urine albumin/creatinine ratio > 30 mg/g). Initially, DN is accompanied by glomerular hyperfiltration (Helal et al. 2012), but with reversal to hypofiltration (GFR below 60 ml/min/1.73 m²) and a fall in all other renal functions, in the following 15 to 20 years. In spite of optimal management, DN is still the leading cause of ESRD and a major contributor to morbidity and mortality in diabetic patients worldwide. Hyperglycemia initiates a cascade eventually resulting in renal damage mediated by oxidative stress, inflammation and hypertension (◘ fig. 3.9). The structural changes in the kidneys consist of excessive accumulation of extracellular matrix, causing expansion of the mesangial matrix, thickening of the GBM and tubulointerstitial fibrosis (◘ fig. 3.10).

Impact of pregnancy on DN

In most patients, pregnancy does not worsen preexistent DN. This applies in particular to patients with a tightly controlled glycemic status and normal blood pressure (with or without antihypertensive medication). However, some studies indicate that the risk of DN worsening is increased in patients with pre-pregnancy GFR below 60 mL/min/1.73 m² and/or proteinuria over 3 g/24h (Spotti 2019).

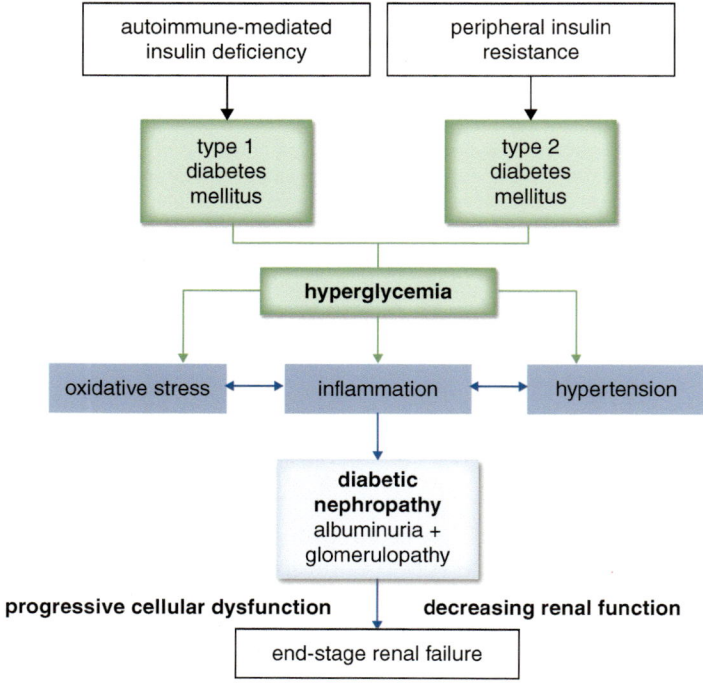

◘ **Figure 3.9** The central role of hyperglycemia in triggering the development and progression of diabetic nephropathy (*adopted from* Magee et al. 2017)

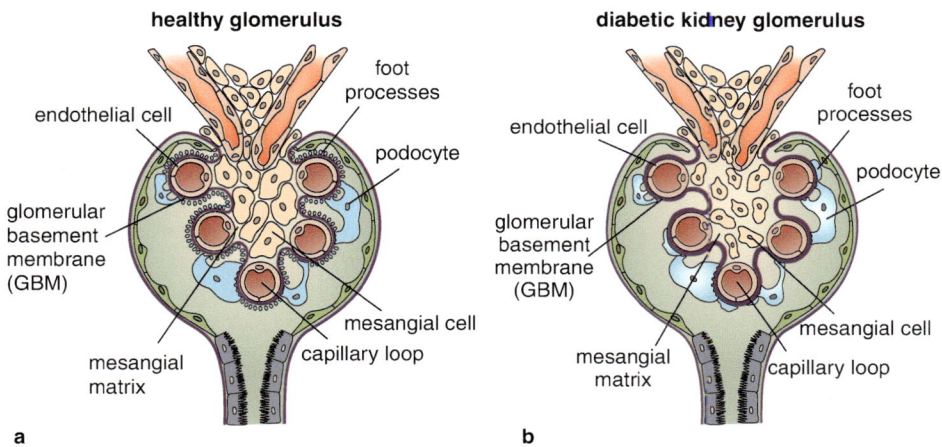

Figure 3.10 This figures illustrates the healthy glomerulus (**a**) and the structural changes in the glomerulus in *diabetic nephropathy* (**b**). Note the thickening of the glomerular basement membrane (GBM), fusion of the foot processes, the loss of podocytes with denuding of the GBM along with mesangial matrix expansion. The latter can even lead to complete blockage of the filtering function (*adopted from* Alicic et al. 2017)

Impact of DN on pregnancy

The outcome of pregnancy in women with DN is far worse than expected based on their stage of CKD. It is conceivable that the higher than expected rates of maternal and perinatal complications (■ tab. 3.3) are caused by the diabetes itself, resulting from the often lower cardiovascular reserve capacity, developing secondary to the endothelial dysfunction, the lower cardiovascular compliance and chronic hypertension. These diabetes-induced complications alone already increase the risk of developing a hypertensive pregnancy complication. Meanwhile, the fetus has to cope with a variable degree of placental insufficiency often accompanied by exposure to fluctuations in the transplacental glucose supply. Episodes of excessive transplacental glucose transfer accelerate fetal metabolism and cause concomitant episodes of fetal hypoxia, that occasionally may deteriorate to fetal asphyxic death. Postpartum, the (often premature) infant is at extra risk of a wide range of metabolic and prematurity-related complications, which may also raise perinatal mortality rate. Obviously, the incidence of these specific causes of perinatal morbidity and mortality declines with better quality of maternal glycemic control during pregnancy.

3.2.9 Pregnancy-Hemolytic Uremic Syndrome (P-HUS)

Hemolytic uremic syndrome (HUS) is defined by the classical triad of microangiopathic hemolytic anemia, thrombocytopenia and acute organ injury with the kidney being the primary target. The sub-classification of HUS is based on triggering factors, with P-HUS being a pregnancy-related thrombotic microangiopathy (TMA), that mostly develops postpartum. It is a rare disorder with an estimated incidence of 1 in 25,000 pregnancies, though, with high perinatal and maternal morbidity and mortality (Fakhouri et al. 2010).

3

P-HUS is an atypical HUS (aHUS) defined as a TMA, mediated by the chronic uncontrolled activity of the complement pathway causing endothelial damage followed by platelet activation. aHUS may develop at any age, with about half of the adults progressing to ESRD after the first aHUS episode (Fremeaux-Bacchi et al. 2013). The clinical presentation of P-HUS resembles that of other TMAs that may occur in pregnancy, such as Thrombotic Thrombocytopenic Purpura (TTP), Disseminated Intravascular Coagulation (DIC) and the HELLP (Hemolysis, Elevated Liver enzymes and Low Platelets) syndrome, but differs by being mediated by dysregulation of the complement pathway. The renal outcome in P-HUS is similar to that in aHUS, namely 76 % of the cases progressing to ESRD. In most cases P-HUS is diagnosed by ruling out all other possible causes of TMA. Timely diagnosis is key for successful clinical management, particularly to optimize the chance for renal functional rescue.

Impact of pregnancy on P-HUS

P-HUS is triggered by pregnancy (Fakhouri 2016) and has a similar clinical course as aHUS in the nonpregnant state.

Impact of P-HUS on pregnancy

P-HUS differs from other TMAs complicating pregnancy by having its onset in 80 % of the cases postpartum (Fakhouri 2016). Early diagnosis and prompt optimal clinical management is key to minimize the risk of permanent renal injury.

3.2.10 End-stage renal disease (ESRD)

Pregnancy outcome in women with ESRD has improved markedly over the past two decades and differs between women managed by permanent dialysis and kidney-donor-recipients.

ESRD managed by dialysis

In the last two decades, the previously observed low fertility rate in women with ESRD managed by dialysis has improved markedly, because of better and intensified dialysis regimens, increased use of erythropoietin and probably also more realistic counseling practices (Tangren et al. 2018). In general, hemodialysis results in more favorable pregnancy outcome than peritoneal dialysis. The use of more intensified hemodialysis protocols (e.g. more weekly hours/days dialysis) in a setting with optimal collaboration between nephrology and high-risk obstetrical teams, has increased life birth rates in these women from 37 % in the 1980s to over 80 % in the last decade (Tangren et al. 2018). This illustrates that pregnancy for these women has become more feasible and safer. Yet, these pregnancies still are at increased risk for maternal and perinatal complications. In a large meta-analysis, preterm birth rate was still surprisingly high (> 70 %) with more than half of the cases caused by interventions for obstetric reasons, such as fetal distress or growth restriction (Yang et al. 2010). Part of the remaining cases are dialysis-related, e.g. due to post-procedure dips in circulating progesterone levels and the partial take-over of the renal role in the regulation of blood volume and blood pressure. A common problem in pregnant women requiring dialysis is the difficulty of differentiating between hypertension as a symptom of a superimposed hypertensive disorder or being dialysis-related. Most of these women are anuric or have a renal disorder with chronic proteinuria. This feature eliminates the option of using *de-novo* proteinuria as a differentiating diagnostic criterion. Therefore, the clinician has to rely on other measures, such as the evolution of clinical signs, liver enzymes and platelet count. Fortunately, the reported rate of *de-novo* hypertensive disorders in these women is not higher than in healthy (nulliparous) controls (about 8.5 %, Yang et al. 2010). An unexpected complication observed in as many as 1 in 3 patients was the development of polyhydramnios, possibly resulting from fetal polyuria in response to increased urea and creatinine levels. The rate of this complication tends to fall with more intense hemodialysis. Details about clinical management of pregnant women on dialysis have been reported previously (Alkhunaizi et al. 2015).

Kidney transplant recipients

For women with ESRD and wishing to become a mother, kidney transplantation offers the best chance to have their own child. However, pregnancy in these women remains challenging, because of the side effects of immunosuppressive medication, the risk of both deteriorating allograft function and complications related to placental insufficiency/dysfunction, leading to placental syndromes, poor fetal growth, preterm birth and low birthweight (Majak et al. 2016). The risk of a complicated pregnancy increases inversely with the function of the renal graft, the presence of proteinuria and/or preexistent hypertension (Shah and Prasoon 2016; Bramham 2017).

3.2.11 Acute kidney injury (AKI) during pregnancy

Nowadays, maternal and fetal morbidity rarely results from pregnancy-related AKI (◘ tab. 3.6), particularly in the more developed countries. Since the 1980s, the incidence of AKI has declined worldwide, mostly due to a lower rate of sepsis in conjunction with abortion and childbirth and to better obstetrical care reflected in improved management of postpartum bleeding and placental abruption. A recently reported figure for the incidence of AKI was 1 in 15,000 pregnancies, though, with wide interregional variation, partly resulting from a lack of uniform criteria for AKI (Jim and Garovic 2017).

◘ **Table 3.6** Causes of acute kidney injury during pregnancy (*adopted from* Van Hook 2014)

prerenal	intrarenal (intrinsic)	postrenal
hypotension due to: – shock/sepsis – heart failure	*renal ischemia*: – acute tubular necrosis – acute cortical necrosis	uterine *compression* causing hydronephrosis.
hypovolemia due to: – hemorrhage – diarrhea/vomiting – shock/sepsis	*pregnancy-induced*: – acute fatty liver – PE/HELLP/eclampsia – microangiopathy	obstruction ureters or bladder outlet due to stones or tumor.

severe hypoxemia due to:
– amniotic fluid
  embolism
– pulmonary embolism
	(Auto)immune and other:
	– TTP/aHUS
	– lupus nephritis
	– toxicity (medication,
	  drugs)
		injury ureters or bladder during cesarean section.

3

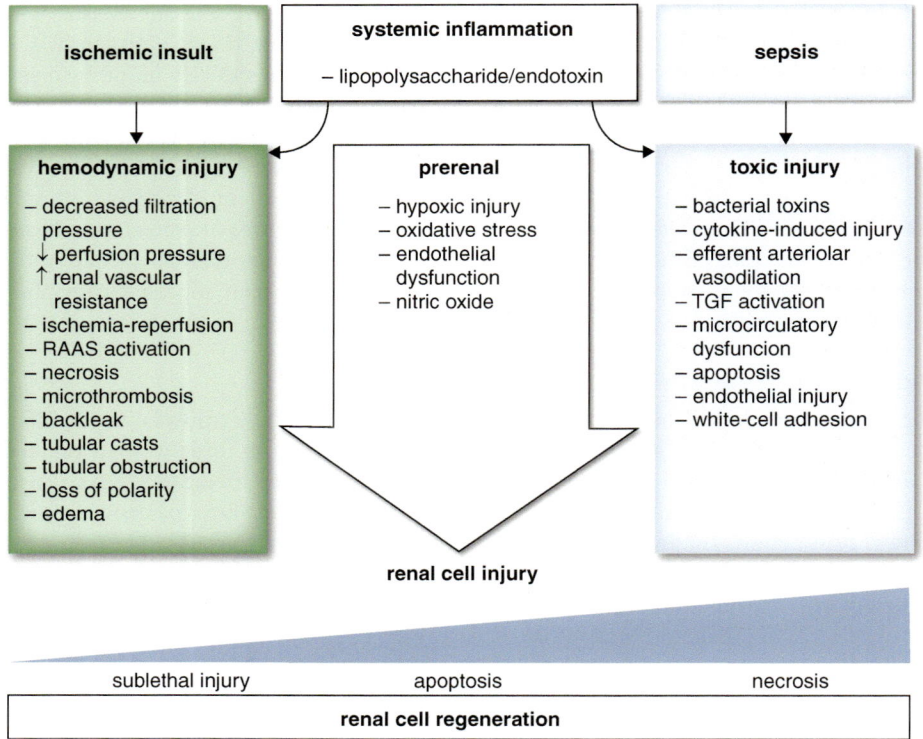

□ **Figure 3.11**   Potential pathways implicated in the *pathogenesis* of *acute kidney injury* due to ischemia or sepsis. Timing of activation of each pathway, their interaction, and hierarchy of these pathways remain unknown. *Abbreviations: RAAS*: Renin-Angiotensin-Aldosterone System. *TGF*: tubuloglomerular feedback (*adopted from* Belomo and Kellum 2012)

Probably the most common causes of AKI in pregnancy are ischemic events due to severe bleeding, septic shock (□ fig. 3.11) or an acute fall in intravascular filling. AKI secondary to glomerulonephritis or acute non-pregnancy-related renal disease may also occur in pregnancy. Etiologies include primary glomerular disease, such as membranoproliferative- or poststreptococcal glomerulonephritis, and all the causes described earlier in this chapter. Yet, the etiological heterogeneity of AKI in pregnancy is high, implicating that management must be tailored to the underlying condition as detailed elsewhere (Acharya 2016).

3.2.12 General discussion

The preceding section provides an overview of the potential impact of CKD on pregnancy. The kidneys play a key role in early pregnancy to preserve cardiovascular function after the pregnancy-related induction of systemic vascular relaxation. Absence of compensatory rises in vascular tone and circulating volume would lead to a fall in cardiovascular filling state and with it, a fall in cardiac pre- and afterload and blood pressure.

This emphasizes the importance of the kidneys. If the kidneys fail to generate these adaptations, the mother activates her autonomic nervous system to generate the so-called 'survival' response, which consists of rises in cardiovascular sympathetic tone and adrenal output of catecholamines in order to preserve blood flow at sufficient pressure to brain and heart. This survival response redirects cardiac output at the cost of non-vital organs, such as the GI-tract, kidneys, skeletal tissue and also the uterus, in early pregnancy resulting in miscarriage. However, if the renal response is defective, the survival response may be activated to such an extend, that pregnancy continues to beyond the first trimester, though, at the cost of the pregnancy complications listed in ◘ tab. 3.3. The pathophysiology of the various types of CKD also shows some interesting overlaps. CKD may be the endpoint of various (often combined) insults on the glomeruli that can be classified as follows. (1) abnormal intraglomerular pressure (e.g. FSGS), (2) clogging of the glomerular filter by e.g. large circulating immune complexes, e.g. in lupus-, membranous- and IgA nephropathies, (3) glomerular microcirculatory damage by oxidative stress/inflammation (diabetic nephropathy), and (4) direct damage of podocytes by toxins/ischemia (e.g. certain drugs/medications, TMA, P-HUS, prolonged severe hypotension).

3.3 Metabolic disorders

3.3.1 Introduction

Glucose is by far the most important metabolic substrate to fuel the oxidative metabolism, in pregnancy as well as in the non-pregnant state. Therefore, it is not surprising that glucose supply and uptake are tightly controlled. In the non-pregnant state, glucose uptake is insulin-dependent in all tissues, except for the brain, where glucose uptake depends on the blood glucose level. This difference implies that cerebral glucose uptake can be prioritized at the cost of that of other organs. This feature is particularly important, when either the glucose pool is too small to meet total peripheral demands (fasting state) or has become less accessible for non-cerebral organs due to insulin deficiency. In the non-pregnant state, this mechanism enables preferential supply of a relatively larger portion of the available glucose pool to the brain, which obliges other tissues to switch to alternative substrates, such as non-esterized fatty acids, glycerol, acetate and amino acids, in order to fuel their oxidative metabolism (shown in ◘ fig. 3.12). However, in pregnancy, the preferential glucose availability does no longer exclusively apply to the brain, but also to the uteroplacental bed.

In the first half of pregnancy, the overnight fast induces a larger fall in glucose and amino acids, and a larger rise in free fatty acids than in the pre-pregnant state ('accelerated starvation'). This response results from hepatic insulin resistance and obliges the mother to fuel her oxidative metabolism with non-carbohydrate substrates. At the same time, high circulating estrogen levels increase peripheral insulin sensitivity, which accelerates the maternal accretion of circulating carbohydrates in energy stores (so-called "facilitated anabolism"), an effect, further enhanced by the higher maternal appetite in early pregnancy. It follows that in this period of pregnancy, the focus of the maternal metabolism is to accumulate sufficiently large energy stores that can be mobilized in the second half of pregnancy, when fetal demands increase rapidly.

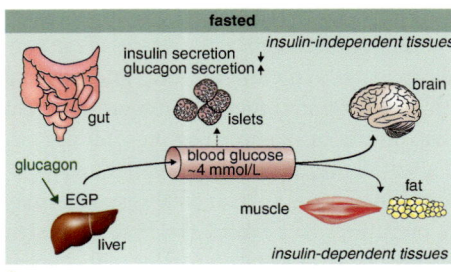
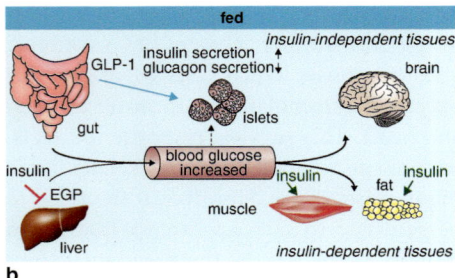

◻ Figure 3.12   Overview of normal glucose homeostasis: *Fasting state* (**a**). The blood glucose level determines the balance between endogenous glucose production (EGP) and glucose uptake by insulin-independent tissues (brain). Insulin-dependent tissues use non-glucose nutrients in response to a low insulin-to-glucagon ratio, thus preventing hypoglycemia to develop. *Fed state* (**b**). Carbohydrates absorbed in the gut stimulate insulin output and inhibit glucagon output, thus raising the insulin-to-glucagon ratio. The latter suppresses EGP and adipose tissue lipolysis, enabling insulin-dependent tissues to utilize glucose again. This state promotes anabolism. *Abbreviation*: GLP-1: glucagon-like peptide 1 (raises insulin output and inhibits glucagon output in response to glucose) (*adopted from* Nolan et al. 2011)

In more advanced pregnancy, the mother develops insulin resistance, which enables a larger fraction of the total glucose pool to be preferentially distributed to the brain *and* the uteroplacental bed. This is reflected by longer postprandial episodes of elevated maternal blood glucose levels, an effect that is beneficial for fetal growth, as it is associated with transient boosts in transplacental glucose uptake. The insulin resistance in advanced pregnancy reinforces this effect by further constraining glucose utilization by non-uterine organs. The relative or absolute insulin deficiency in diabetic pregnancy, can be expected to affect these carefully orchestrated metabolic adjustments and with it, adversely impact pregnancy course and outcome. In the following section, these metabolic disorders will be discussed.

3.3.2 Carbohydrate disorders

Carbohydrate disorders consist of metabolic syndrome (MetS) and diabetes mellitus (DM) type 1 and 2 and represent the most common metabolic disorders that may complicate pregnancy. When pregnancy-induced insulin resistance causes relative insulin deficiency in women affected with one of these disorders, mean circulating glucose level together with transplacental glucose uptake rise. This accelerates fetal growth, often resulting in macrosomia. It also increases the risk of fetal asphyxia, as the accelerated glucose uptake is not matched by (flow-dependent) extra oxygen uptake required to either metabolize or store the extra glucose in glycogen or fat. This mismatch is generally thought to be responsible for the development of fetal hypoxia, which in severe cases may result in fetal demise.

MetS is a complex metabolic disorder characterized by (1) overweight/obesity, (2) reduced insulin sensitivity, (3) reduced glucose tolerance, (4) abnormal circulating levels of lipid-derived metabolic substrates, and (5) elevated resting blood pressure. MetS and type-2-DM develop as an aftereffect of an adverse response of ß-cells and adipose tissue to chronic excess fuel, that leads to so-called nutrient spill-over, insulin resistance and metabolic stress, with the latter being potentially damaging for many organs

(Nolan et al. 2011). Therefore, it is conceivable that insulin resistance is a defense mechanism to prevent nutrient-related toxic effects. The diagnosis of MetS is based on clinical criteria (elevated circulating levels of fasting glucose and triglycerides, along with a raised blood pressure and waist circumference), as specified elsewhere (Kassi et al. 2011). Its prevalence in high-income countries ranges from 25 % to 34 % (Kassi et al. 2011). People diagnosed with MetS preserve normoglycemia by chronically raising their circulating insulin levels (Gerich 2003). Yet, their insulin-generating capacity not only declines with age, but also with deteriorating basic features of MetS. It follows that MetS patients are at risk of developing type-2-DM. They are also highly likely to benefit from measures that mitigate the contributing basic features to at least delay the progression of MetS to type-2-DM.

DM is a metabolic disorder that affects about 8% of adults worldwide, men and women equally, with around 10 % of cases being *type-1-DM* (Balsells et al. 2009; Tao et al. 2015). About 80 % of type-1-DM cases develop as a sequel of a virus-induced, progressive, autoimmune-mediated, apoptotic loss of pancreatic β-cells in susceptible individuals (Op de Beeck and Elzirik 2016). It reduces partly or completely the pancreatic insulin secreting capacity. The resulting insulin deficiency alters the metabolism and is accompanied by hyperglycemia and insulin resistance (◘ fig. 3.13).

Type-2-DM is characterized by a state of insulin resistance, with compensatory hyperinsulinemia, though insufficient to preserve normoglycemia. In these patients, the

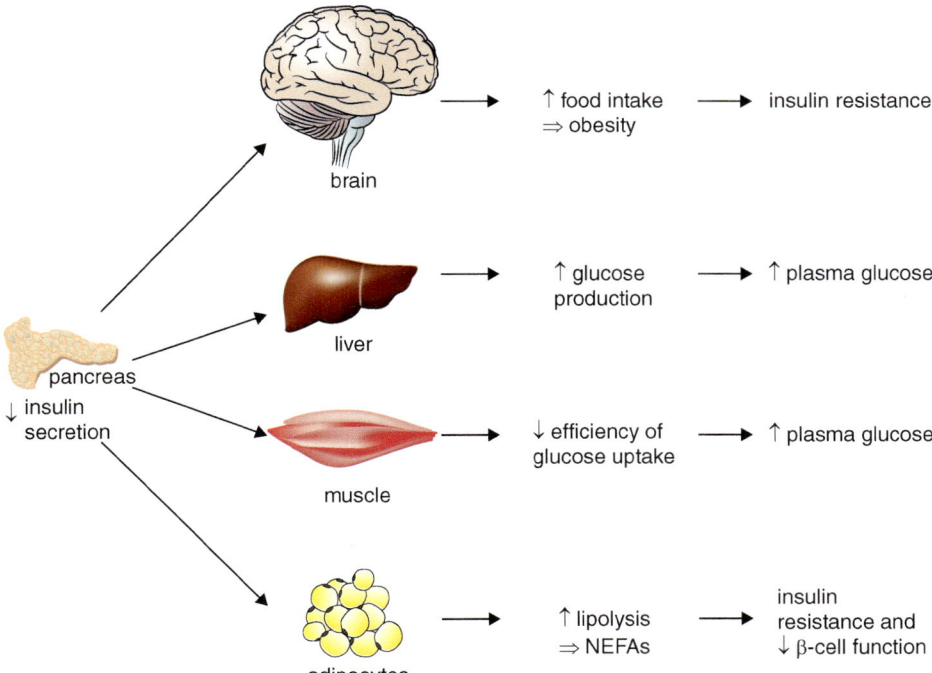

◘ **Figure 3.13**   Insulin deficiency leads to more food intake and with it, weight gain. It also diminishes hepatic glucose production and glucose uptake by non-cerebral tissues, like muscle. This effect in turn, triggers lipolysis to generate alternative substrates to fuel the oxidative metabolism of these non-cerebral tissues. Meanwhile, lipolysis raises circulating levels of non-esterized fatty acids (NEFAs) and together with the developing obesity, increase insulin resistance, thus starting a viscious circle (*adopted from* Kahn et al. 2006)

3

insulin secreting capacity is usually reduced. In the pathogenesis of type-2-DM, genetic susceptibility and environmental risk factors, such as unhealthy food habits, obesity, sedentary lifestyle and poor stress management, also contribute (Gerich 2003; Chatterjee et al. 2017). However, in type-2-DM, β-cells are dysfunctional rather than destroyed, which suggests that the abnormality is at least partially reversible (Fujioka 2007). This β-cells dysfunction already develops in pre-diabetes and is associated with a fall in insulin secretory capacity, while concomitant insulin demands may be raised, due to the above-mentioned insulin-resistance promoting factors. When the insulin secretory capacity becomes insufficient to preserve normoglycemia, pre-diabetes has evolved to overt type-2-DM. Over the past decades, the worldwide prevalence of type-2-DM has increased steadily in concert with the obesity epidemic (Balsells et al. 2009).

Gestational diabetes (GDM) overlaps with type-2-DM with overt disease being triggered by pregnancy. As GDM is a quite common pregnancy-induced disorder, it has been discussed in ▶ Chap. 2.

Impact of preexistent DM on pregnancy

The risk of early complications does not differ between women with type-1 and type 2-DM pregnancies and – until about 8 to 10 weeks of amenorrhea – depends almost entirely on the quality of glucose control during organogenesis. Even in the best centers, the incidence of congenital malformation and mortality is 2 to 5 times higher than in the background population (◘ fig. 3.14) (McCance 2015). This suggests that preventive measures, most importantly tight regulation of normoglycemia already before conception (Wender-Ozegowska et al. 2005), is only partly effective. The most common early-pregnancy complications of DM are miscarriage and congenital malformations, such as cardiac anomalies, diaphragmatic hernias and neural tube defects (Rosenn et al. 1994).

In advanced pregnancy, diabetic patients is at increased risk of complications due to either poor glycemic control (e.g. macrosomia, unexplained late fetal demise, preterm birth and neonatal hypoglycemia) (HAPO-study 2008), or preexistent DM-induced micro- and macroangiopathy (fetal growth restriction, placental syndromes). These two sets of complications develop along different, but also interrelated pathophysiological pathways (Paneni et al. 2014). This aspect supports the concept that ideally, clinical management should begin several months prior to conception and also requires a multidisciplinary approach.

Impact of pregnancy on preexistent DM

Impact of pregnancy on preexistent DM consists of the effect on insulin requirements. Early in pregnancy, this may lead to hypoglycemic episodes due to the temporarily increased insulin sensitivity, altered eating patterns and occasional morning sickness. In contrast, when pregnancy advances into the second half, insulin demands rise by about 40 % (Paneni et al. 2014), although individual changes may vary from no change to a threefold rise. The rise in insulin levels is primarily caused by increased levels of insulin-resistance promoting hormones, such as progesterone, prolactin, placental lactogen and cortisol. Pre existent retinopathy may deteriorate, particularly, when glucose control is suddenly tightened (Paneni et al. 2014). Women with diabetic nephropathy and increased circulating creatinine levels at conception, are at increased risk to respond to pregnancy with a permanent loss of renal function (Paneni et al. 2014). Finally, a relevant aspect of diabetic pregnancy is its long-term impact on the offspring (Fraser and Lawlor 2014; Ma et al. 2015), as summarized in ◘ fig. 3.15.

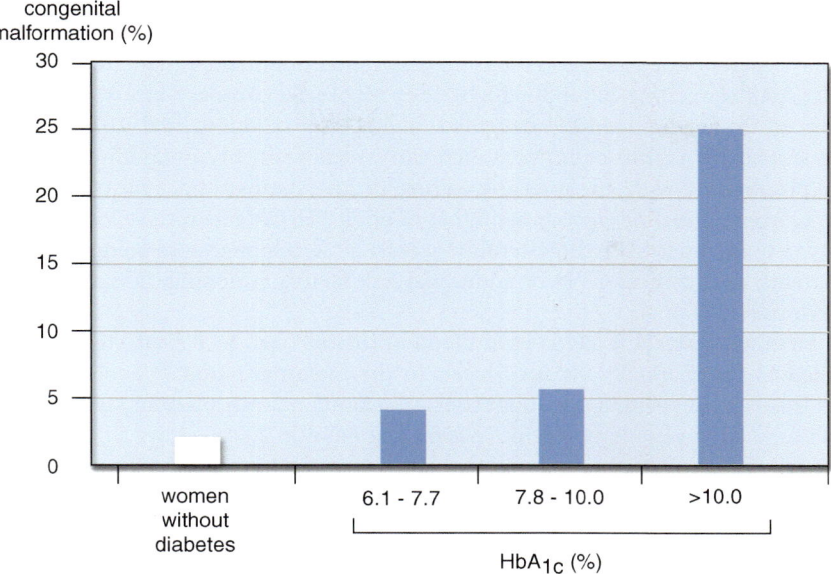

○ **Figure 3.14**   Risk of congenital malformations in pregnant women with diabetes mellitus is raised above the background population rate of 2 %, even in women with normal HbA1c levels. The risk increases sharply with increasingly poor blood glucose control in early pregnancy (*adopted from* Rosenn et al. 1994)

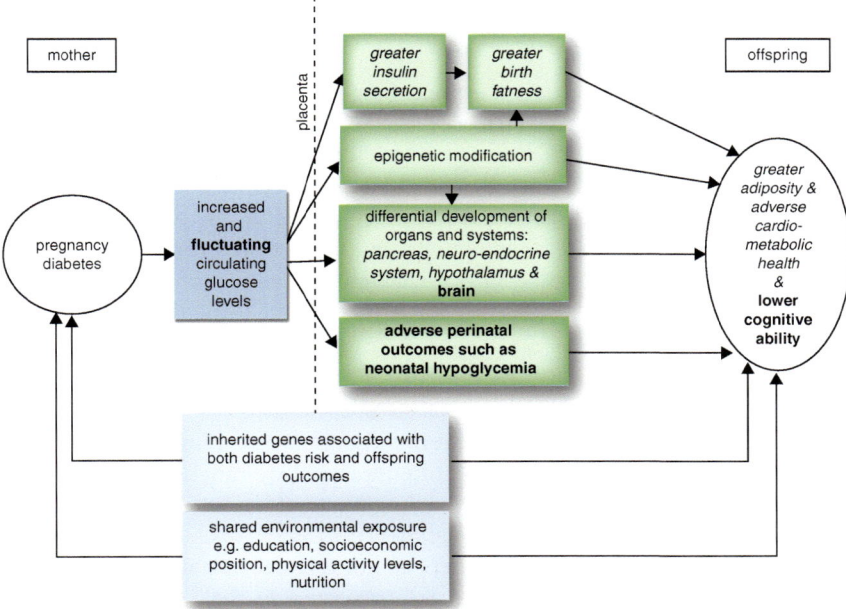

○ **Figure 3.15**   Simplified presentation of potential pathways linking gestational diabetes mellitus with long-term offspring greater adiposity, adverse cardiometabolic health and lower cognitive ability. Pathways specific to offspring adiposity and cardiometabolic health are shown in *italics* and pathways specific to cognitive ability in **bold**, with common pathways in standard font (*adopted from* Fraser and Lawlor 2014)

3.3.3 Familiar hypercholesterolemia (FH)

Familiar hypercholesterolemia (FH) is an autosomal dominant genetic disorder with a prevalence of about 1 in 200 individuals. The risk of fatal coronary-artery disease before 60 years of age in untreated FH patients is about 30 % (Gidding et al. 2015). Therefore, FH-patients benefit from being identified early, ideally already in childhood, to enable timely prophylaxis with cholesterol-lowering drugs (statins) and adjustments in food intake. Current guidelines recommend that all adult FH-patients receive long-term statin therapy to lower their LDL-cholesterol by at least 50 %, a higher dose being perscribed in FH-patients with clinical CVD or additional risk factors (smoking, DM, family history of early-onset CVD).

At birth, cholesterol levels in cord blood of infants born to FH-affected mothers are unrelated to the markedly elevated levels in the maternal blood (Napoli and Palinski 2001). This is in line with a previous report indicating no transplacental transfer of large cholesterol-carrying apolipoproteins (Napoli and Palinski 2001). However, fatty streaks – precursors of advanced atherosclerotic lesions – are fairly common in the near-term fetal aorta of infants of women with FH. Presumably, these fatty streaks are already formed early in pregnancy, when the placenta is still permeable for large cholesterol-carrying apolipoproteins (Napoli et al. 1997). With pregnancy advancing into the third trimester, fetal plasma levels of these compounds decline steadily, while maternal plasma levels remain high, probably reflecting the declining placental permeability for these compounds. There is evidence suggesting that onset of the atherogenic process in early fetal life leads to more rapid progression of atherosclerotic lesions in childhood and adolescence (Napoli and Palinski 2001).

Impact of pregnancy on FH

Reducing circulating cholesterol levels in (non-pregnant) FH women by cholesterol-lowering drugs (statins) reduces the increased cardiovascular risk (CVR) (Gidding et al. 2015). However, most guidelines recommend pre-conceptional discontinuation of statins to avert the potential risk of statin-related birth defects, although the evidence for the latter is still inconclusive (Kusters et al. 2012). Presumably, the potential rise in long-term cardiovascular risk due to the temporary cessation of statin treatment is small. As soon as newer statin-based drugs become available with a solid record of being safe with respect to birth defects, it is probably preferable to continue using this preventive medication during pregnancy.

Impact of FH on pregnancy

FH pregnancies do not differ appreciably from those in matched healthy controls (Eapen et al. 2012), in spite of the increased risk of endothelial dysfunction (◻ fig. 3.16), activated clotting system, and the tendency of LDL-cholesterol levels to rise after discontinuation of the statin prophylaxis (Rahman et al. 2017).

Nevertheless, autopsies on fetuses after an unexplained intrauterine demise often show a higher density of aortic fatty streaks compared to their normally developing counterparts. In addition, 6–13-year-old children born after in-utero exposure to high maternal circulating LDL-cholesterol levels have markedly higher LDL-cholesterol levels than their counterparts not having experienced this exposure (Christensen et al. 2016). Although this could be due to a common genetic background, it has also been suggested

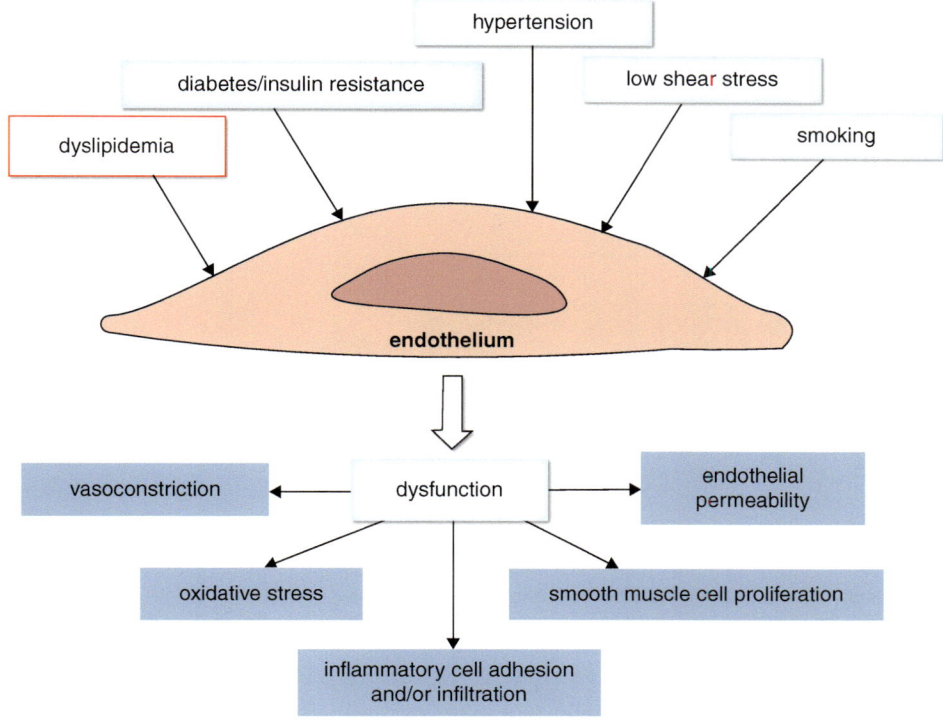

□ Figure 3.16   Induction of endothelial dysfunction by common cardiovascular risk factors

that fetal exposure to raised maternal LDL-cholesterol levels induces adverse epigenetic imprinting presumably increasing the risk of premature CVD later in life. Most guidelines recommend replacement in the pre-conceptional period of statins by bile acids sequestrants (e.g. cholestyramine), as they lower maternal LDL-cholesterol levels without reaching the maternal blood. However, their efficacy to reduce LDL-cholesterol is modest relative to that of statins, whereas their use is often accompanied by uncomfortable intestinal side effects (Scaldaferri et al. 2013).

3.3.4 Hyperhomocysteinemia (HHC)

The amino acid homocysteine is formed by the transmethylation of methionine (□ fig. 3.17) and is involved in various key metabolic processes. The serum homocysteine level is determined by (1) dietary factors such as the intake of folic acid and vitamin B_{12}, (2) physiologic changes, e.g. renal impairment, and (3) variation in the activity of enzymes in various pathways.

HHC is usually defined by a fasting level in excess of 15 μmol/L (Aubard et al. 2000) with the methionine loading test only providing relevant extra discrimination in selected subgroups (Van der Griend et al. 2000; Smulders 2000). The prevalence of HHC is 5–10 % among healthy controls. Epidemiological data indicate that HHC is an

3

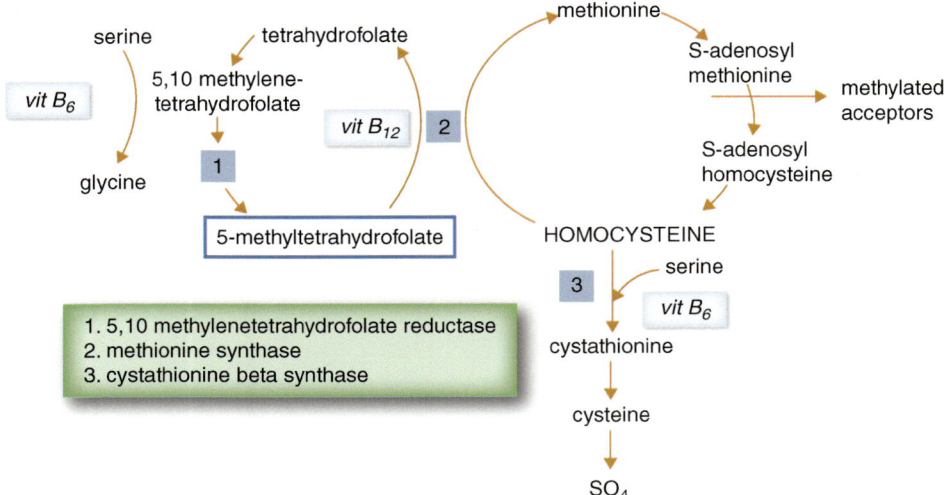

Figure 3.17   Schematic display of the metabolic pathways of homocysteine. Hyperhomocysteinemia usually results from a point mutation of the gene, that encodes for methylene tetrahydrofolate reductase as shown in the diagram (*adopted from* Hague 2003)

independent, graded risk factor for cardiovascular disease (CVD). However, the risk of CVD in patients with the most important inherited cause of HHC – a point mutation in the methylene tetrahydrofolate reductase gene – is not increased. This feature together with a lack of insight in the underlying pathophysiology linking HHC to CVD explains why it is still unclear, whether HHC is cause or effect of CVD (Van der Griend et al. 2000). In-vitro and animal studies suggest that HHC induces endothelial dysfunction, a key early event in the atherosclerotic process leading to both impaired endothelial anti-coagulant properties and vasomotor dysregulation. Nevertheless, the outcome of various intervention studies in CVD-patients with HHC managed with homocysteine-lowering supplementation of vitamins B_6, B_{12} and folic acid, was disappointing as this intervention did not reduce the risk of CV events (Marti-Carvajal et al. 2013).

Impact of pregnancy on HHC

Circulating homocysteine levels fall during pregnancy, presumably because of the pregnancy-induced hemodilution and increased glomerular filtration rate.

Impact of HHC on pregnancy

Abnormal homocysteine metabolism in early pregnancy has been associated with neural tube defects (Steegers-Theunissen et al. 1994) and recurrent miscarriages (Eichholzer et al. 2006). Therefore, there is consensus to recommend a daily use of 0.4 mg folic acid during the peri-conceptional period, so as to reduce the risk of neural tube defects (Hague 2003). Several studies suggest that HHC and folic acid deficiency predispose to placental syndromes. However, experimental evidence in support of this concept is still lacking and the available information points more towards an association rather than a causal relationship of elevated homocysteine levels with the raised incidence of placental syndromes (Mignini et al. 2005). On the other hand, a large meta-analysis showed a marginally higher rate of low-birthweight infants born from HHC pregnancies (Hogeveen et al. 2012), a rate that was lower in women who had continued folic acid supplementation throughout their pregnancy (Lassi et al. 2013).

3.4 Selected hepatic disorders

3.4.1 Introduction

Only disruption of some liver functions has a direct adverse impact on pregnancy. The following three hepatic functions are important for the maternal metabolism during pregnancy; (1) main storage site for glycogen and with it, (2) securing gluconeogenesis and with it, the uteroplacental glucose supply in the starved state, and (3) the metabolization of the large amounts of steroid hormones produced by the placenta. The liver is also important for the digestion of fat-based nutrients and is involved in various immune functions. Finally, in pregnancy, the liver may become a target for *vascular* complications because of its unique microcirculation, as e.g. observed in the HELLP syndrome (detailed in ► Chap. 2).

In this section, only hepatic disorders will be discussed, that may directly interfere with pregnancy. Other hepatic disorders without clear direct adverse effect on pregnancy, such as infectious disorders, primary sclerosing cholangitis, hepatic cirrhosis with portal hypertension, Wilson's disease and hepatocellular adenoma, are described in ► Chap. 4.

Pregnancy doesn't alter the blood flow or the function tests of the liver, except for those directly related to the breakdown of placental products (alkaline phosphatase, α-fetoprotein). Nearly 3 % of pregnancies are complicated by some form of liver disease that is potentially fatal for mother and child (Mikolasevic et al. 2018). Therefore, all pregnant women, including those without complaints, should undergo standard work-up at intake to identify the ones with abnormal liver tests in order to rule out asymptomatic chronic hepatitis or biliary pathology. It is plausible that the pregnancy-induced change in the intestinal microbiome also affects gut-liver signaling. However, the underlying mechanism is still unknown (Dixon and Williamson 2016). The smooth-muscle relaxation induced during early pregnancy, not only results in the institution of a high-flow/low-resistance circulation, but also affects the tone of the gall bladder and biliary system.

3.4.2 Intrahepatic Cholestasis of Pregnancy (ICP)

Cholestasis indicates impeded bile flow in the biliary system between the liver and duodenum. ICP in this context refers to the abnormal, pregnancy-specific metabolic form of cholestasis resulting from abnormal bile formation (◘ fig. 3.18). The prevalence of ICP ranges from 0.3 to 5.6 % and is the most common liver disorder in pregnancy (Geenes and Williamson 2009). Clinically, ICP is characterized by generalized pruritus accompanied by elevated circulating levels of aminotransferase and bile acids, but without other liver disease. One out of eight ICP patients also develops jaundice. The disorder usually develops after the 30th week of pregnancy and resolves again within 48 hours postpartum. The pruritis is most severe on the hand palms and feet soles. Pruritus affects one in four pregnant women. However, only a small fraction of these women has ICP.

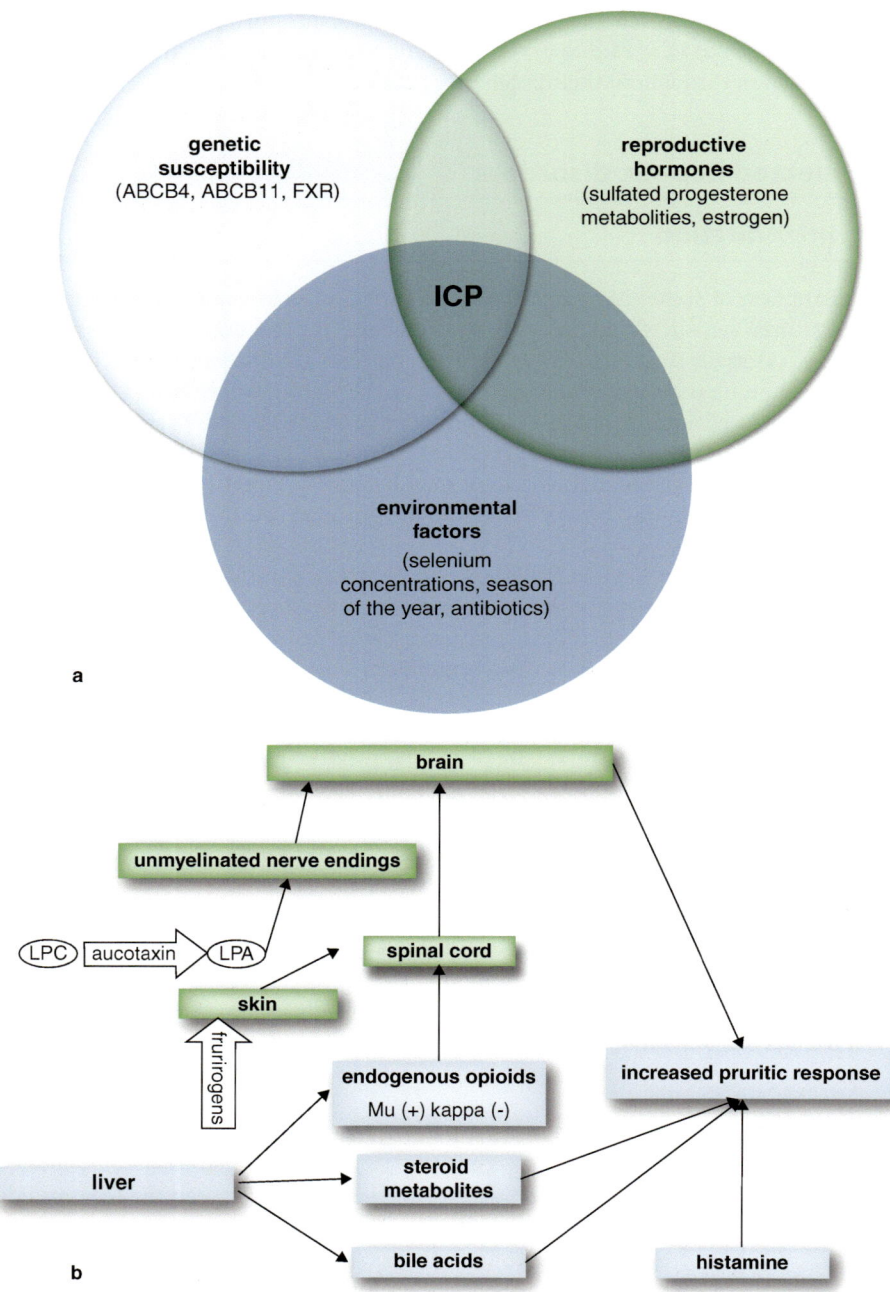

■ **Figure 3.18**   (**a**) Pathogenesis of intrahepatic cholestatic of pregnancy (ICP) starts with genetic susceptibility, that coincides with the presence of steroid metabolites and environmental factors. Most relevant steroid metabolites are sulphate metabolites of progesterone. Mutations in certain genes (e.g. ABCB4, ABCB11, FRX) encoding for bile transporter proteins cause genetic susceptibility. (**b**) Mechanism responsible for the development of the typical complaint of itch in ICP-affected women. *Abbreviations*: *LPC*: lysophosphatidylcholine; *LPA*: lysophosphatidic acid, (Dixon and Williamson 2016)

Ultrasound is safe and is the preferred technique to determine, whether or not abnormal liver tests result from a biliary tract disorder. On ultrasound, biliary ducts are *not* dilated, and the hepatic parenchyma has a normal appearance.

Insight into the etiology of ICP is still incomplete due to its complex multifactorial pathogenesis with input related to genetic susceptibility (mutations in genes encoding for hepatobiliary transporters), placental hormones (e.g. estrogens, progesterone, growth factors) and environmental factors (e.g. advanced maternal age, antibiotic use, selenium and/or vitamin-D deficiencies) (Dixon and Williamson 2016; de Vloo and Nevens 2019). Women with a history of cholestasis during oral contraceptive use or after having suffered from ICP in a previous pregnancy, are at risk of recurrent ICP. The fact that women with ICP are asymptomatic in the nonpregnant state, suggests that the elevated levels of reproductive hormones unmask their genetic susceptibility to develop ICP.

Impact of pregnancy on the intrahepatic bile draining system

Pregnancy induces various changes that may trigger ICP in susceptible women. (1) large amounts of placenta-derived steroid hormones need to be metabolized by the liver and therefore, may exceed the hepatic capacity to produce and transfer assembled gall components to the biliary system (endocrine factor). (2) pregnancy-induced lower motility of both the biliary system and GI-tract reduces the gall bladder's ability to eject most of its content during digestion, a condition that facilitates gall stasis in the biliary system and with it, thickening of gall, which increases its viscosity and thus further impedes biliary gall flux (mechanical factor). (3) pregnancy-induced changes in the composition of the intestinal microbiome are likely to affect the bile-acid pool, thus reducing the liver's capacity to metabolize fat-containing compounds (intestinal factor). (Dixon and Williamson 2016; Zakharia et al. 2018).

Impact of ICP on pregnancy

ICP is associated with an increased rate of adverse pregnancy outcomes, such as spontaneous preterm birth, meconium-stained amniotic fluid, fetal asphyxia and fetal mortality. The rate of fetal complications seems to increase as a function of maternal bile acid levels, particularly when levels exceed 40 µmol/L. It has been suggested that fetal asphyxia develops secondary to fetal arrhythmias, which seem to be a side-effect of high fetal bile acid levels. There is also evidence for direct cardiac and placental toxicity of elevated bile acid levels giving rise to left-ventricular dysfunction (Sanhal et al. 2017; Vasavan et al. 2018) and placental dysfunction, respectively (Dixon and Williamson 2016).

ICP does not seem to adversely affect maternal health during pregnancy, other than causing discomfort due to itch. Early delivery at 37 weeks is encouraged, because of the elevated risk of fetal death, that rarely occurs before 37 weeks. Earlier preterm birth carries an increased risk of respiratory distress in the neonate as bile acids have been found to adversely impact pulmonary surfactant production. Details about management of ICP are reported elsewhere (Imam et al. 2012; Ovadia and Williamson 2016). Even though the symptoms of ICP resolve rapidly postpartum, indirect evidence suggests that former ICP-patients are at increased risk of developing other hepatic disorders later in life, such as chronic hepatitis, gallstone disease, liver fibrosis/cirrhosis, cholangitis and hepatobiliary cancer (Wikström-Shemer et al. 2015).

3.4.3 Acute fatty liver of pregnancy (AFLP)

Acute fatty liver of pregnancy (AFLP) is a rare obstetric emergency disorder of mito-chondria β-oxidation causing hepatic microvesicular steatosis. AFLP affects between 5–30 of every 100,000 pregnant women (Morton and Laurie 2018) and usually develops in the third trimester of pregnancy, at a median gestation age of 36 weeks. Most women present with a 1 to 2 weeks history of anorexia, nausea, vomiting, mid-epigastric- or right-upper-quadrant abdominal pain, headache and occasionally jaundice. The clinical condition may rapidly deteriorate to hepatic failure and even encephalopathy. At presentation, AFLP may resemble severe preeclampsia (PE), HELLP syndrome and ICP. By applying the so-called 'Swansea criteria', which refers to a set of clinical and laboratory variables (Liu et al. 2017), it is possible that most cases of AFLP can successfully be differentiated from these three pregnancy disorders, which limits the need of performing a liver biopsy in suspected patients and with it the risk, as these patients often (relatively), also have a coagulopathy (Morton and Laurie 2018). Typical for AFLP is the development of acute hepatic failure due to fatty infiltration of the liver, a condition that may further deteriorate secondary to the (disseminated intravascular) coagulopathy, impaired renal function, electrolyte abnormalities, hypoglycemia, in fulminant cases advancing to multi-organ failure. Data from the 1980s suggested maternal mortality rates of more than 70 %, but more recent estimates are much lower, namely only circa 2 % (Liu et al. 2017). This dramatic fall in mortality is probably a result of a combination of more awareness of AFLP, and with it, earlier recognition, intervention and delivery (Dekker et al. 2011), together with aggressive management of complications. Recent data on perinatal mortality in AFLP-affected pregnancies ranges from 10 to 20 % (Liu et al. 2017) with most cases caused by intrauterine fetal death or as a sequel of severe fetal acidosis or prematurity. For some reason, the severity of the maternal illness does not correlate with incidence and severity of fetal complications. Risk factors of AFLP include nulliparity, multiple pregnancy, male fetus and most importantly, a *fetal* fatty-acid-oxidation disorder. There is some data suggesting an increased risk in women with a body mass index (BMI) below 20 kg/m^2 (Naoum et al. 2019).

Key in the pathophysiology of AFLP is a defect in the free fatty acid (FFA) metabolism (◻ fig. 3.19). In about one of five AFPL cases, the fetus is homozygous for long-chain acyl-coenzyme-A dehydrogenase (LCHAD) deficiency indicating that the mother is almost always heterozygous for LCHAD deficiency. The combination of a homozygous fetal defect and a heterozygous maternal defect result in an approximate 80 % maternal chance of developing AFLP, more so, since pregnancy-induced endocrine changes also reduce the oxidation rate of long- and medium-chain fatty acids. At any rate, the fetus is forced to discard large amounts of non-oxidized long- and medium-chain FFA metabolites into the maternal blood, where they accumulate and eventually become hepatotoxic to the mother. Other enzyme deficiencies of fetoplacental mitochondrial oxidation have also been associated with the development of AFLP (Naoum et al. 2019). A hallmark finding in patients with AFLP is multi-organ fatty infiltration.

Widespread micro-vesicular fatty hepatic steatosis disrupts the hepatic production of cholesterol, fibrinogen and coagulation factors and also impairs the hepatic capacity to conjugate hydrophobic metabolites, a defect that compromises the clearance of e.g. bilirubin. AFLP-induced liver and kidney dysfunctions recover completely in most patients in the first 6 months postpartum (Xiong et al. 2015). In contrast, circulating

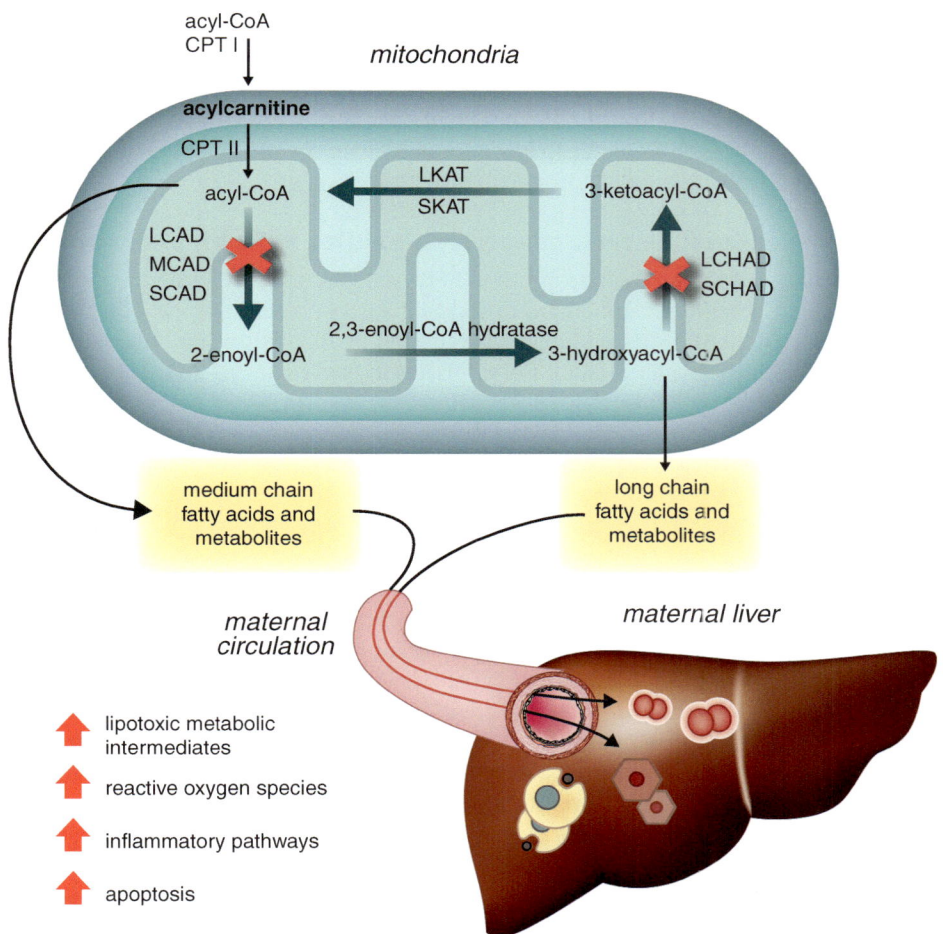

Figure 3.19   Pathophysiology of acute fatty liver of pregnancy (AFLP). It has been postulated that AFLP develops in pregnancies with a fetus that is affected by impaired mitochondrial β-oxidation of fatty acids because of a homozygous enzyme deficiency. This deficiency leads to elevated circulating levels of FFA metabolites in the fetus that cross over to the maternal blood. Pregnant women, who are heterozygous for fatty-acid-oxidation enzyme defects, may be more susceptible to the pregnancy-related higher metabolic demands and with it, more susceptible to liver injury caused by e.g. lipotoxic metabolic intermediates (*adopted from* Naoum et al. 2019). *Abbreviations*: *LCAD, MCAD, SCAD*: long-, medium- and short-chain acyl-coenzyme-A dehydrogenase; *LCHAD, SCHAD*: long-, short-chain 3-hydroxyacyl-coenzyme A dehydrogenase; *LKAT, SKAT*: long-, short-chain 3 ketoacyl coenzyme-S thiolase; *CPT*, carnitine palmitoyltransferase

FFAs increase mildly with advancing normal pregnancy. Their transplacental uptake is gradient-dependent. For the fetus, FFAs are important building stones for growth and development.

Impact of pregnancy on maternal hepatic FFA oxidation

Pregnancy hormones reduce the maternal hepatic capacity to oxidize FFAs (Naoum et al. 2019). Pregnant women, heterozygous for a defect of the LCHAD enzyme *and* carrying an infant that is homozygous for this particular enzyme defect, have a major metabolic issue. During pregnancy, these women will be challenged with a large amount of fetal non-oxidized FFAs that needs metabolization in their liver. However, the capacity to oxidize these molecules is limited because of their heterozygosity for the LCHAD enzyme. As a consequence, these non-oxidized FFAs accumulate in the maternal blood to hepatotoxic levels eventually causing AFLP.

Impact of maternal hepatic capacity to oxidize FFAs on pregnancy

Pregnancy hormones lower the rate of hepatic FFA oxidation. In the second half of pregnancy, maternal fat stores are mobilized to secure the transplacental supply of fat precursors, such as cholesterol, FFAs and glycerol, required by the fetus as building stones for fetal tissue accretion in general, and for brain tissue, in particular.

3.4.4 Auto-immune hepatitis

Autoimmune hepatitis (AIH) is an autoimmune liver disorder defined by a progressive hepatocellular inflammation unrelated to excessive alcohol consumption, viral infection, exposure to hepatotoxic drugs or a genetic disorder (Braga et al. 2016). It occurs at all ages with prevalence ranging from 11 to 25 cases per 100,000, often affecting young women of childbearing age. The clinical presentation of AIH varies widely from no symptoms in most patients to fulminant hepatic failure in one-third of affected subjects (Lohse and Mieli-Vergani 2011). AIH patients may present themselves with nonspecific symptoms, such as generalized fatigue or arthralgias (without arthritis), complaints that may trigger systematic diagnostic work-up. AIH is often diagnosed in subjects with abnormal liver function during routine medical testing. At least one-third of AIH patients has already cirrhosis at presentation indicating a considerable period of subclinical disease before the diagnosis is made.

AIH is a multifactorial, polygenic disorder resulting from autoreactivity against liver autoantigens (LAGs) (Heneghan et al. 2013). The phenotype of AIH is heterogeneous and fluctuating. The trigger that sparks the development of AIH is still unknown (Floreani et al. 2018). Damage is likely to be orchestrated by CD4 T-lymphocytes that recognize an autoantigenic liver enzyme, as detailed elsewhere (Manns et al. 2015; Theocharidou and Heneghan 2018). AIH seems to develop in a genetically susceptible host, when the yet-unknown trigger leads to a T-cell-mediated immune response that targets liver autoantigens. The diagnosis of AIH is based on the raised of immunoglobulin G/ hypergammaglobulinemia, detection of both typical autoantibodies and a typical pattern on liver histology. The induced cascade of events results in liver damage due to necro-inflammatory and fibrotic processes. Raised circulating liver transaminase levels reflect the degree of inflammatory activity. The so-called 'interface hepatitis' on histology is typical and is often paralleled by bridging necrosis and multi-lobular necrosis. The clinical aspects and follow-up of patients have been detailed elsewhere (Heneghan et al. 2013; Manns et al. 2015).

Impact of pregnancy on AIH

The response of AIH to pregnancy is mixed: In about 10 % of AIH patients, AIH signs improve, whereas in another 20 %, the rate of exacerbations rises (Braga et al. 2016;

Llovet et al. 2019). Postpartum, there is a transient rise in the rate of AIH flare-ups (to 25–30 %). The latter are defined by a transient rise in the circulating levels of liver enzymes and total IgG (asymptomatic) that require medication to be modified. These flares may be related to the sharp postpartum fall in blood estrogen levels.

Impact of AIH on pregnancy course and outcome

Reports on the rate of spontaneous first-trimester abortions in women with AIH varies from no rise (Grønbæk et al. 2018), to one-third of all pregnancies (Braga et al. 2016). AIH patients with an ongoing pregnancy are at increased risk to deliver preterm (Braga et al. 2016) and to give birth to a growth-restricted infant (Grønbæk et al. 2018). The rate of congenital malformations and that of serious maternal complications does not differ from that in a healthy control population (Grønbæk et al. 2018). Nevertheless, these data support the view that women with AIH should seek preconceptional counseling, that should include evaluation of liver function (with also assessment of presence/absence of cirrhosis and portal hypertension) and quality of the immunosuppressive therapy. During pregnancy, these women should continue their treatment with corticosteroids and/or azathioprine. The use of azathioprine in pregnancy is considered safe, as it has not been found to increase the risk of birth defects. Clinical management of these patients during pregnancy has been detailed elsewhere (Tran et al. 2016).

3.4.5 Primary sclerosing cholangitis (PSC)

PSC is a chronic, progressive cholangiopathy, often associated with inflammatory bowel syndrome (IBS), has male predominance (2:1), occurs at a median age of 41 years, and has an overall incidence rate of 1 patient per 100,000 inhabitants (Molodecky et al. 2011). Although the cause of PSC is still obscure, there is consensus about PSC only developing in genetically susceptible individuals secondary to an immune-mediated liver disease triggered by environmental factors (Horsley-Silva et al. 2016) and with a highly disease-specific antimitochondrial antibody identified in about 95 % of patients. Typical for PSC is the interplay between inflammation, fibrosis and cholestasis in the biliary ductal system (◘ fig. 3.20) that eventually leads to the formation of multifocal bile duct strictures and obstructions, in most patients sooner or later leading to liver cirrhosis, portal hypertension and liver failure (Chapman et al. 2010; Karlsen et al. 2017; Dyson et al. 2018).

Symptoms of PSC include fatigue, jaundice, pruritus and steatorrhea. Management involves assessment of comorbid IBD and the exclusion of other related cholangiopathic disorders. The prognosis of PSC is poor, not only because of the high risk of progression to liver cirrhosis, but also because of an increased risk of hepatobiliary and colorectal cancer. The serum of PSC patients contains a wide range of autoantibodies, consistent with an altered state of immune regulation.

The diagnosis of PSC in patients with a cholestatic biochemical profile is made by cholangiography (e.g. magnetic resonance cholangiography, endoscopic retrograde cholangiography, percutaneous transhepatic cholangiography), which will show typical bile duct changes with multifocal strictures and segmental dilations, but also after having excluded other disorders known to be accompanied by secondary sclerosing cholangitis. Patients with clinical, biochemical and histological features of PSC, but normal cholangiogram will be classified as small-duct PSC (Chapman et al. 2010).

3

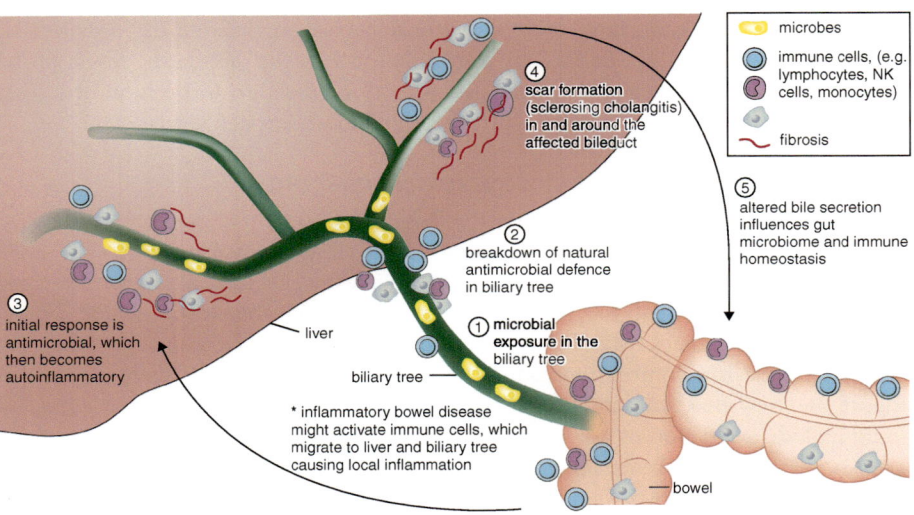

□ Figure 3.20   Presumed sequence of events (1 to 5) in the pathogenesis of primary sclerotic cholangitis (PSC). Environmental factors (e.g. certain eating habits) may trigger the development of PSC in
genetically susceptible individuals. *: Alternative hypothesis for the onset of the peribiliary inflammatory process. NK= natural killer (*adopted from* Dyson et al. 2018)

Impact of pregnancy on PSC

Fertility in women with PSC (without portal hypertension) appears to be normal.
Reports on the impact of pregnancy on PSC are limited. No serious deterioration of liver
function during or after pregnancy has been reported. Pregnancy leads to a rise in liver
enzymes and pruritus of 20 % and 40 % of PSC women, respectively, but does not trigger
more flares (Wellge et al. 2011).

Impact of PSC on pregnancy course and outcome

Preterm birth rate is 3 to 4 times higher in women with PSC than in healthy controls
(Ludvigsson et al. 2014), the highest risk being observed in women with concomitant
IBD (Zakharia et al. 2018). The rate of other pregnancy disorders, and the maternal and
perinatal outcomes are similar is as in healthy controls (Wellge et al. 2011). Early diagnosis and the use of ursodeoxycholic acid, usually controls pruritus and also has a favorable effect on pregnancy outcome. Persistent and severe, therapy-resistant pruritus may
necessitate earlier induction of labor. More details about the management of pregnancy
in women with PSC, has been reported elsewhere (Chapman et al. 2010).

3.4.6 Hepatic cirrhosis and portal hypertension

Liver cirrhosis is defined as permanent liver scarring, that develops after irreversible tissue
damage secondary to chronic inflammation, because of either alcohol abuse or a cholestatic, metabolic or autoimmune disorder (□ fig. 3.21) (Tsochatzis et al. 2014). Typical histological features of post-inflammatory liver damage are regenerative nodules surrounded by
fibrous bands throughout the liver (Schuppan and Afdhal 2008). Liver scarring results from
accelerated collagen production, fibrosis and nodular regeneration. It distorts the hepatic

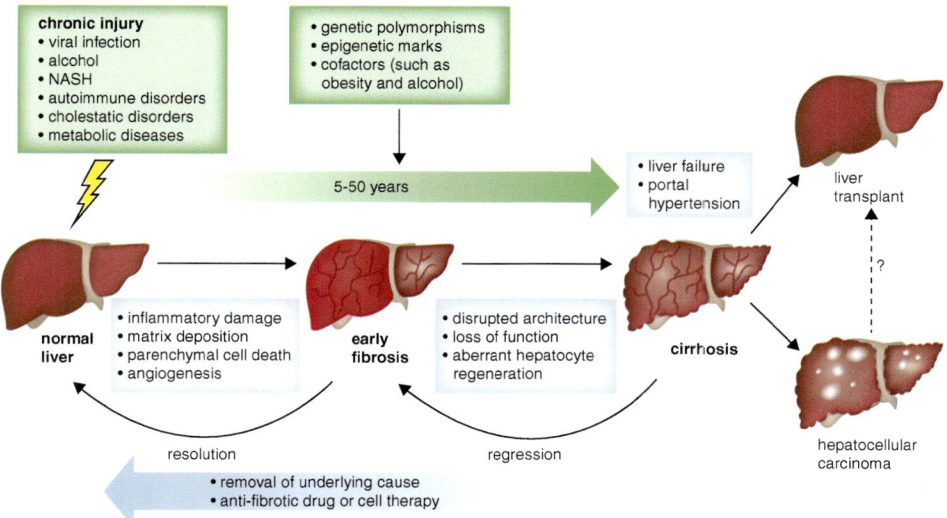

Figure 3.21   Liver fibrosis and repair: The natural course of chronic liver disease development. NASH: non-alcoholic steatohepatitis. *Abbreviations*: NASH: non-alcoholic steatohepatitis. (Source: Pellicoro et al. 2014)

microarchitecture by creating barriers between hepatocytes and sinusoids. These structural changes lead to: (1) Metabolic and endocrine liver dysfunction; (2) Increased portal resistance and pressure, (3) The development of portal shunts via extrahepatic collaterals, and (4) Splenomegaly. Also, the impaired hepatic metabolic functions lead to hepatic spillover into the blood of – sometimes toxic – substances that are normally cleared by the liver.

Initially, the symptoms of hepatic cirrhosis are often nonspecific (anorexia, weight loss, weakness and fatigue). Signs of decompensation are likely to develop with advancing disease. These include jaundice, pruritus, upper gastrointestinal bleeding from esophageal varices or peptic ulcer, ascites and confusion due to hepatic encephalopathy. Hepatic cirrhosis is often associated with abnormal findings on physical examination (e.g. jaundice, spider angiomas, gynecomastia, ascites, splenomegaly and palmar erythema) along with abnormal laboratory findings (increased serum levels of bilirubin, aminotransferases, alkaline phosphatase and γ-glutamyl transpeptidase). However, diagnosing and staging hepatic cirrhosis requires histologic confirmation by liver biopsy (Muir 2015). The prevalence of cirrhosis in the US is 0.3 %, a third being women, often after suffering from hepatitis B or C, or after chronic alcohol abuse (Giard and Terrault 2016). Several scoring systems have been developed to determine the prognosis of severe liver disorders (Tiniakos 2010; Causey et al. 2012), but these may also be valuable in preconceptional counseling of women with severe liver disease to assess the risk of maternal hepatic decompensation or variceal bleeding during pregnancy.

Idiopathic [non-cirrhotic] portal hypertension (IPH)

Idiopathic [non-cirrhotic] portal hypertension (IPH) refers to a set of disorders with common denominator impeded portal flow secondary to extra-hepatic causes. IPH is accompanied by splenomegaly, but a key difference to portal hypertension complicating liver cirrhosis is the preservation of liver function with patent hepatic and portal

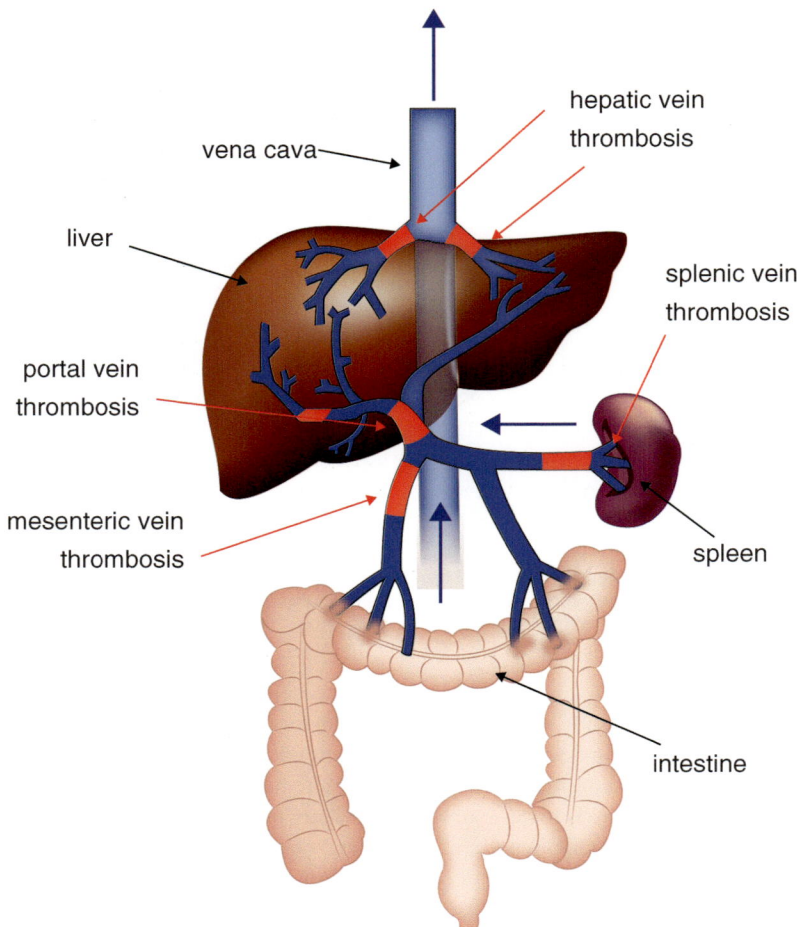

Figure 3.22 Budd-Chiari syndrome, resulting from a partial or complete obstruction of the hepatic venous drainage, usually resulting from the downstream formation of a thrombus

veins. The prevalence of this series of disorders is also low (Hernandez-Gea et al. 2018). Because of preserved liver functions, fertility is normal. IPH may be caused by either extrahepatic portal vein obstruction (EHPVO, e.g. by portal, mesenteric- or splenic-vein thrombosis) or by disorders that otherwise interfere with portal drainage, such as the *Budd-Chiari Syndrome* (BCS) that refers to an obstruction of the hepatic vein by a clot or granulomatous phlebitis in the hepatic vein, just proximal to the outlet into the inferior vena cava (■ fig. 3.22). Importantly, hepatic outflow obstruction due to cardiac and pericardial disease, or the sinusoidal obstruction syndrome (SOS) are excluded from this definition, because of their different pathophysiology and clinical implications (Hernández-Gea et al. 2019). Another cause of IPH is schistosomiasis, an infectious disorder of the intestinal tract and liver causing periportal fibrosis impeding portal influx into the liver. The incidence of variceal bleeding in pregnant women with cirrhotic and non-cirrhotic IPH is comparable. Nevertheless, both pregnancy outcome and maternal prognosis are much better in the latter subgroup, probably because of their preserved liver function (Aggarwal et al. 2014). However, these non-cirrhotic IPH patients are still at high risk to develop a thrombotic complication during or after their pregnancy. Therefore, they can be expected to benefit from preconceptional counseling, in order to adopt strategies to minimize the risk of these complications, as specified in the guidelines on this topic (Rautou et al. 2009; Bissonnette et al. 2015).

Impact of pregnancy on cirrhotic liver disease with portal hypertension

Pregnancy in women affected with this disorder is rare due to the low prevalence of cirrhosis in women of reproductive age. Moreover, these women are often infertile due to frequent anovulatory cycles, because of endocrine dysfunction. Therefore, the rate of pregnancies with preexistent liver cirrhosis is still unclear (Russell and Craigo 1998; Puljic et al. 2016). Biosynthetic functions of the liver often deteriorate in pregnant women with hepatic cirrhosis, with 10 % of them even progressing to hepatic decompensation, as indicated by the development of ascites, variceal bleeding and encephalopathy. Maternal mortality in these women is 1.6 %, the primary cause being massive bleeding from esophageal varices (Westbrook et al. 2016). These bleedings mostly occur in midpregnancy, when total blood volume is highest and the growing uterus exerts an increasingly higher pressure upon the inferior vena cava. A higher caval pressure downstream of the inflow of the hepatic veins also raises the resistance to flow in the portal circulation and, hence, portal venous pressure. The latter also applies to the second stage of labor when active pushing hinders venous return (■ fig. 3.23). A patient with preexistent esophageal varices has a 1 in 4 risk of developing variceal bleeding during pregnancy. Obviously, this complication is associated with a high maternal mortality rate.

Impact on pregnancy in a woman with chronic cirrhotic liver disease and portal hypertension

Pregnancies in these patients are at increased risk of spontaneous early pregnancy loss, preterm birth, hypertensive pregnancy disorders, fetal growth restriction and postpartum hemorrhage (Puljic et al. 2016). The incidence of these complication increases with the severity of the liver dysfunction (Westbrook et al. 2016).

3.5 Autoimmune disorders

3.5.1 Introduction

The immune system provides essential protection against pathogenic microorganisms. However, it may also attack self-antigens located on its own cells. The presence of pro-inflammatory signals during the differentiation of the common precursor cell – the naïve CD4 T helper cell – determines, whether or not this key immune cell develops into a Th17- (pro-inflammation) or a Treg cell (anti-inflammation). Preferential differentiation of CD4 cells into Th17 cells may result in imbalance because of Th17 dominance.

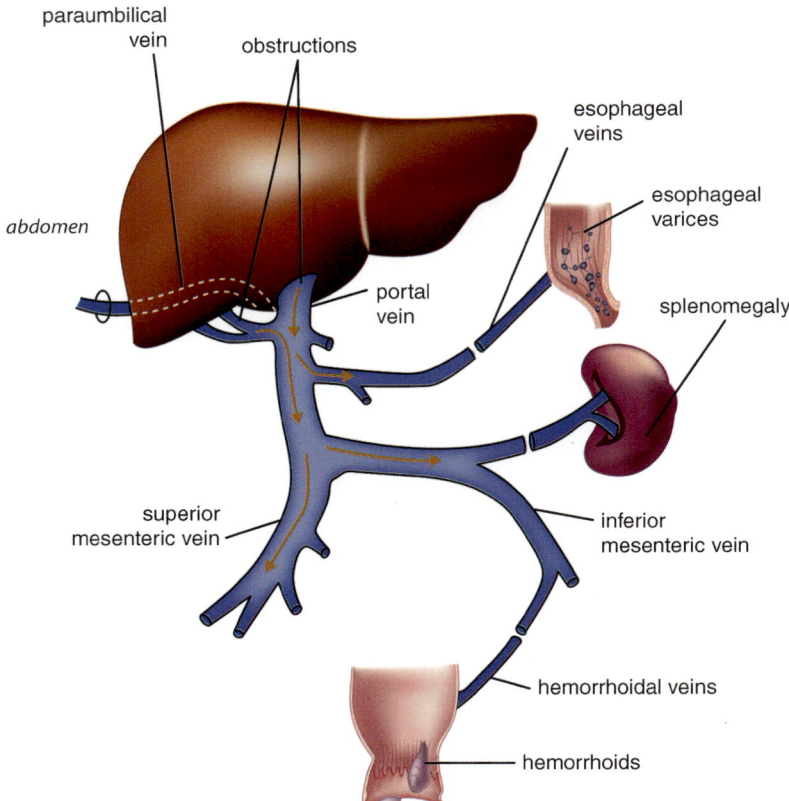

paraumbilical
vein

obstructions

esophageal
veins

esophageal
varices

abdomen

portal
vein

splenomegaly

superior
mesenteric vein

inferior
mesenteric vein

hemorrhoidal veins

hemorrhoids

◘ **Figure 3.23**   Redirection of portal venous flow, because of downstream obstruction with secondary portal hypertension: The drainage of the portal vein and that of the superior and inferior mesenteric veins reverses to be redirected to alternative draining sites as shown in the figure. This event may lead to esophageal varices, splenomegaly and hemorrhoids

This may happen, when differentiation pathways evolve in an environment dominated by pro-inflammatory signals (Lee 2018; Lee et al. 2015). Autoimmune disorders (AIDs) develop secondary to aberrant interactions between genetic and environmental factors (◘ fig. 3.24).

The most common site of these aberrant interactions is the human mucosa in gut and other mucosal cavities, where the commensal microbiome actively modulates the immune system. AIDs may develop in response to changes in composition and function of these microbiomes. Environmental factors, such as these microbiomes in concert with their metabolites, induce epigenetic changes and with it, alter gene expression of immune cells and the cytokines they release causing aberrant immune responses, which are typical for AIDs (Chen et al. 2017, ◘ fig. 3.25). AIDs may exist (active or latent) before pregnancy, but also flare, or develop de novo in pregnancy. In the sections below, we describe how various AIDs may interact with pregnancy.

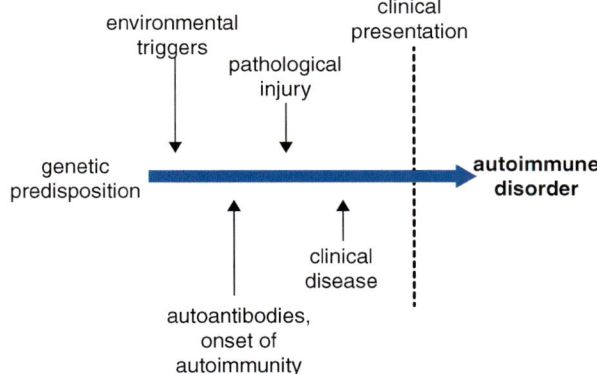

Figure 3.24   Pathogenic events prior to the development of symptoms in autoimmune disorders (*adopted from* Jonsson et al. 2011

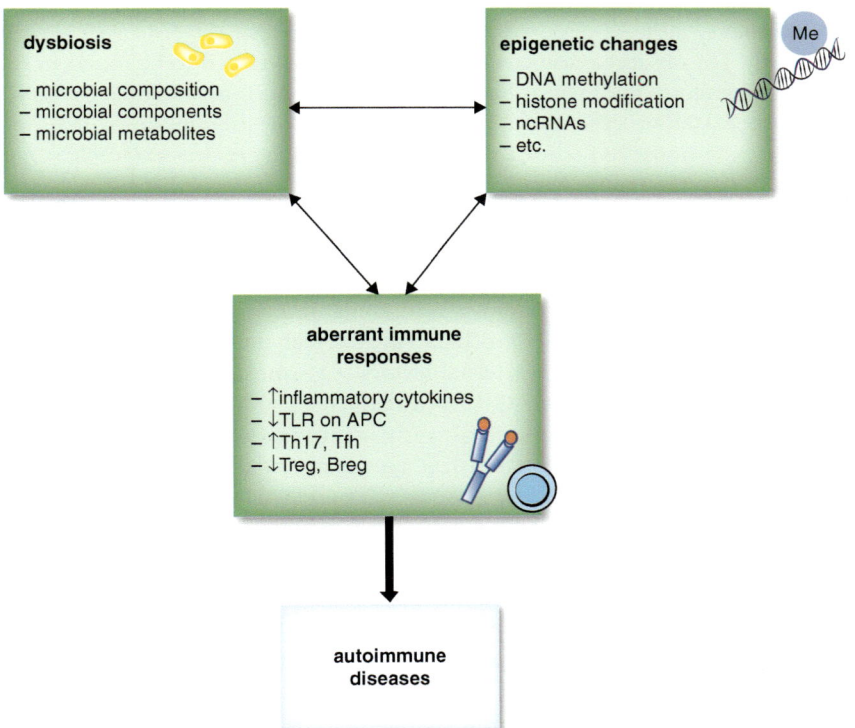

Figure 3.25   Presumed mechanism of how human dysbiosis and resulting epigenetic changes interact to trigger aberrant immune responses in autoimmune disorders (AIDs) by producing both pro-inflammatory cytokines and dysregulated immune cells. Of note is the reciprocity of immunological changes affecting the microbiome and human epigenome. Presumably, AIDs only develop in carriers of a particular set of susceptibility genes. *Abbreviations*: *ncRNA*, noncoding RNA; *Me*, abnormal methylation; *TLR*, toll-like receptors; *APC*, antigen-presenting cells; *Treg/Breg*, regulatory T/B cells (*for details: see review by* Chen et al. 2017)

3

3.5.2 Antiphospholipid syndrome (APS)

APS is an acquired, autoantibody-mediated disorder, characterized by the presence in the peripheral circulation of antiphospholipid antibodies (aPL), directed against negatively-charged phospholipids, a group of inner- and outer-cell membrane antigens. The 3 most important phospholipids are lupus anticoagulant (LA), β_2-glycoprotein-1 (β_2GP1) and anticardiolipin antibodies (aCL).

The pathogenesis of APS is still unknown, although it is widely accepted that APS involves endothelial cell and platelet activation resulting in a procoagulant phenotype (Arachchillage and Laffan 2017) (◘ fig. 3.26). Its clinical presentation in the nonpregnant state consists of multiple, often recurrent, vascular thromboses (TAPS) and in pregnancy, of recurrent pregnancy loss (OAPS). According to the 2006 revised consensus 'Sapporo' criteria, the APS is diagnosed on the basis of lab tests providing persistently positive functional LA assay and/or the presence of anti-β_2GP1 and/or aCL, plus a thrombotic event (Linnemann 2018). Frequently, patients with APS also have other clinical features, such as moderate thrombocytopenia, Coombs-positive hemolytic anemia, heart valve disease or renal microangiopathy. In half of the cases, APS coincides with other autoimmune disorders, often systemic lupus erythematosus (SLE). These cases are termed 'secondary APS' as opposed to 'primary APS', which refers to APS developing autonomously. For obscure reasons, circulating aPL levels may also be found in healthy individuals. Therefore, the mere presence of circulating aPL is not sufficient to trigger APS. This aspect supports the so-called 'second-hit hypothesis', implicating that APS can only develop in response to tissue damage (caused by oxidative stress, trauma, surgery or infection) and the subsequent removal of cellular debris, a process that seems to provoke the formation of immune complexes on the surface of endothelial cells (Antovic et al. 2018). The presumed mechanism of clearance of cellular debris by e.g. apoptosis, necrosis, necroptosis and autophagy proceeds abnormally, and with it, allows the immune system to identify previously-unknown own intracellular proteins, which may induce (auto) antibody production. Epidemiological data suggest that the development of APS not only requires exposure to certain external factors (e.g. smoking), but also the presence of susceptibility genes (Islam et al. 2018). In the general population, the prevalence of APS is 1–5 %. Various clinical conditions, such as infections, myocardial infarction and stroke, may be accompanied by the transient appearance of positive aPL titers. However, the prevalence of APS is highest among young and middle-aged adults and more often in women than in men, partly because of OAPS (Linnemann 2018).

Impact of pregnancy on APS

Pregnancy may not only induce a flare in preexistent APS, but also its *de-novo* development. Embryo implantation and placentation involves trophoblast invasion into the decidua and spiral arteries, a process accompanied by tissue damage. Pregnancy also induces the institution of a hyperdynamic circulation, which leads to more mechanical strain exerted upon blood cells and the endothelial lining of the vascular bed. It is plausible that these effects combined, act as a second-hit in symptom-free women with chronically raised circulating aPL levels. The exposure to raised aPL levels in combination with the higher shear stress may affect endothelial function (Velásquez et al. 2018), and with it, adversely impact the institution of a hyperdynamic circulation and early placental development. Presumably, in some women these effects eventually evolve into pregnancy

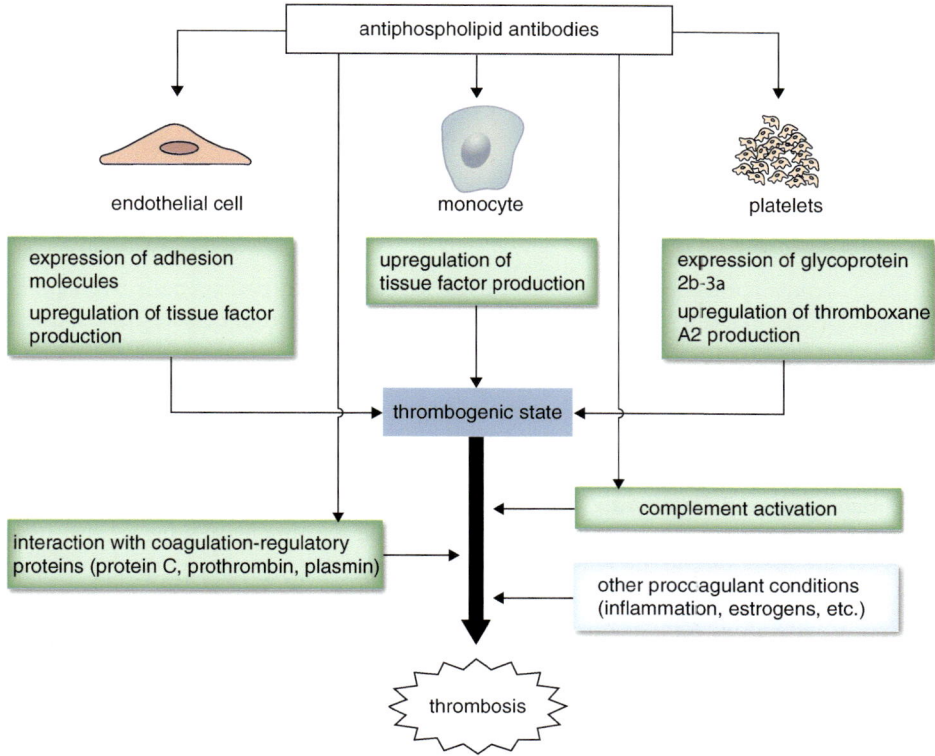

◻ Figure 3.26   Pathogenesis of thrombosis in the antiphospholipid syndrome (*adopted from* Ruiz-Iras-torza et al. 2010)

disorders, such as placental syndromes, fetal growth restriction and preterm birth. The endothelial dysfunction is also thrombogenic and with it, increases the thrombogenic effect of pregnancy itself.

A rare, serious form of OAPS is the so-called 'catastrophic APS' (CAPS), which is a highly variable and potentially lethal presentation of OAPS. It is characterized by multiple thromboses, usually affecting small vessels, eventually resulting in multi-organ failure. CAPS is defined by the simultaneously involvement of more than 2 organs (almost always including the kidneys) combined with positive aPL titers, with often positivity of all 3 aPLs. The diagnostic work-up can be complex, because of clinical overlap with other TMAs and hypertensive pregnancy disorders. The clinical management has been detailed elsewhere (Silver 2018).

Impact of APS on pregnancy

OAPS refers to the chronic presence of a positive aPL titer in women with a history of early recurrent pregnancy loss, stillbirth or preterm birth < 34 gestational weeks due to a placental syndrome and/or placental insufficiency. OAPS does not require a history of thromboembolism. A positive titer early in pregnancy, particularly for LA, predisposes to poor placentation (Antovic et al. 2018), an effect enhanced by the concomitant

3

activation of the complement system (Holers et al. 2002; Ruiz-Irastorza et al. 2010). The negative impact on pregnancy outcome is reflected in higher rates of miscarriage, hypertensive disorders, fetal growth restriction, preterm birth, perinatal mortality, and thromboembolic events (Liu and Sun 2019). Clinical management of OAPS consists of antithrombotic treatment as specified elsewhere (Antovic et al. 2018).

3.5.3 Systemic Lupus Erythematosus (SLE)

SLE is a chronic autoimmune connective tissue disorder with pathogenesis overlapping with that of APS regarding defects in clearance and elimination of cellular debris. These defects may lead to aberrant uptake of macrophages, which then present antigens to T and B cells, thus driving the autoimmune process. The pathogenesis also involves susceptibility genes that interact with environmental factors, which in SLE include ultraviolet light, various drugs, hormones (e.g. estrogens), infections and viruses. These interactions trigger the production of antibodies directed against double-stranded DNA (dsDNA) and small nuclear RNA-binding proteins. This, in turn, results in irreversible loss of immunologic self-tolerance with clinical symptoms usually only developing several years later (D'Cruz et al. 2007). The current understanding is that multiple leucocyte subsets, along with inflammatory cytokines, chemokines and regulatory mediators, normally involved in host protection against invading pathogens, contribute to the inflammatory events that lead to the deposition of autoantibodies and immune complexes, which cause tissue destruction and organ failure (Vilas-Boas et al. 2015). The extremely diverse spectrum of clinical symptoms is consistent with its multisystem involvement. Common targets are skin, kidneys, and the musculoskeletal and hematopoietic systems. This aspect complicates SLE classification and with it, risk prediction and tailored clinical management. This has led to the internationally accepted "SLICC-consensus" on diagnosing SLE using clinical combined with immunological criteria (Petri et al. 2012).

The prevalence of SLE in developed countries varies between 50 and 100 cases per 100,000 individuals with a female/male ratio of 7/1, mostly affecting women of reproductive age (Kuhn et al. 2016; Goulielmos et al. 2018). Also, more than half of SLE patients develop lupus nephritis (detailed in the previous section on kidney disease). Particularly lupus nephritis contributes to the raised risk of maternal/perinatal morbidity/mortality in SLE women.

Impact of pregnancy on SLE

Pregnancy may exacerbate SLE activity, particularly in patients that had active disease in the six months before conception. Their risk of a flare during pregnancy is over 60 %, which is 3 times higher than in their counterparts, who were in remission in the six months before conception. Nevertheless, even low-risk women have a 2 to 3 times higher rate of flares in pregnancy than before pregnancy (Singh and Chowdhary 2015). Some of the normal pregnancy-induced physiologic changes may mimic a lupus flare, such as fatigue, non-inflammatory joint pains, melasma, palmar erythema and some lab indices, such as anemia, thrombocytopenia, and an increased erythrocyte sedimentation rate. Therefore, disease activity during pregnancy is to be monitored regularly using standard 'SLE-activity-indices', to optimize early flare recognition (with kidneys and blood being primary targets in pregnancy), followed by prompt clinical management as detailed elsewhere (Singh and Chowdhary 2015). The incidence of SLE flares is highest in the third trimester of pregnancy.

Impact of SLE on pregnancy

The disrupted immunologic self-tolerance in SLE affects the normal maternal toler-ance to the conceptus. Therefore, SLE can be expected to affect implantation and pla-cental development, and therefore, to be associated with a high rate of pregnancy losses. Poor placental development in SLE women – particularly if kidneys are involved – implies that placental insufficiency is likely to jeopardize fetal wellbeing as indicated by increased rates of stillbirth, preterm birth, fetal asphyxia and fetal growth restric-tion. The rate of superimposed placental disorders, such as preeclampsia and the HELLP syndrome is also increased, particularly with renal involvement. Furthermore, circulat-ing antibodies against SSA/Ro and SSB/LA ribonucleoproteins in the maternal blood predispose the fetus to the development of a so-called 'neonatal lupus syndrome' with (irreversible) congenital heart block (CHB), which is clinically most relevant (Buyon et al. 1998). CHB is rare as it has been observed in the newborns of only 2 % of preg-nant women with an autoimmune connective tissue disorder and circulating anti-SSA/Ro antibodies (Brucato et al. 2001). The clinical management of pregnant women with SLE has been elaborated in various excellent reviews (Stojan and Baer 2012; Lateef and Petri 2017). Some of the drugs that serve to control SLE in the non-pregnant state may be teratogenic. Therefore, SLE patients who wish to conceive should be offered pre-conceptional counseling to discuss all aspects of pregnancy in women with SLE, opti-mize their preconceptional condition, critically evaluate their SLE medication, and secure the timely beginning of thromboprophylaxis.

3.5.4 Auto-immune nephropathy

Auto-immune nephropathy, such as some forms of focal segmental glomerulosclerosis (FSGS), lupus nephritis (LN), minimal-change disease (MCD), membranous nephrop-athy (MN) and IgA nephropathy, have been discussed in detail in ▶ sect. 3.2 on renal diseases.

3.5.5 Rheumatoid arthritis (RA)

RA is a polygenic, multifactorial, autoimmune disorder of still unknown cause, that leads to inflammation of the inner layer of the joint capsule and the synovial mem-brane, with the primary target being the joints of the fingers and knees. The symmet-rical inflammatory polyarthritis gradually damages the adjacent cartilage and bone, eventually resulting not only in deformities, but also in systemic features, such as car-diovascular, pulmonary, skeletal and psychological disorders (McInnes and Schett 2011; Nandakumar 2018). RA is a chronic disease with substantial physical and emotional impact on both patient and society. The personal burden results from musculoskeletal deficits gradually not only eroding physical function and quality of life, but also caus-ing cumulative comorbid risk. The socioeconomic burden relates to functional disabil-ity, reduced work capacity and reduced societal participation. Patients with more severe symptoms and joint damage show more often circulating autoantibodies, presumably due to the formation of immune complexes with citrulline-containing antigens, accom-panied by abundant complement activation (Smolen et al. 2016).

The overall prevalence of RA is about 1 % with 5–50 new cases per 100,000 persons annually. Geographically, the rate of RA declines going from North to South (in the northern hemisphere) and from urban to rural areas. A family history of the disease increases the risk of RA 3 to 5-fold. Increased concordance rates in twins indicate an important contribution of genetic factors to the pathogenesis, which is estimated to be about half for individuals that are positive for rheumatoid factor (RF), and below 20 % for those that are seronegative for RF (Smolen et al. 2016). RA is diagnosed based on the 2010 American College of Rheumatology/European League Against Rheumatism classification criteria for RA as detailed elsewhere (Zamanpoor 2019).

Impact of pregnancy on RA

Pregnancy ameliorates RA symptoms in many patients, particularly in the third trimester (De Man et al. 2008). Moreover, about two-thirds of pregnant women with RA reported less pain and swelling during pregnancy than before conception. Meanwhile, most postpartum patients reported more RA flares of RA activity, which also supports the concept that pregnancy tends to lower RA activity (Hazes et al. 2011; Ince-Ascan and Dolhain 2015).

Impact of RA on pregnancy

Women affected by RA have been reported to suffer more often from subfertility. Pregnancy course and outcome in women with well-controlled RA at conception does not differ appreciably from those in the background population (Smeele and Dolhain 2019). However, high RA activity at conception, is associated with more preterm birth and/or fetal growth restriction (Hazes et al. 2011; Ince-Ascan and Dolhain 2015). Some of the drugs prescribed to control RA (e.g. methotrexate) are teratogenic. Therefore, a woman with RA that wishes to conceive should be offered preconceptional counseling to optimize disease control with safe medication in order to maximize her chances of an uneventful pregnancy.

3.5.6 Auto-immune hypothyroidism

Autoimmune thyroid disorders (AITD) are the most common autoimmune disorders and consists of two clinically distinct and functionally opposing phenotypes, namely Graves' disease [GD] and Hashimoto's thyroiditis [HT]. They share a similar immune-mediated pathogenesis, driven by the interaction between susceptibility genes and environmental triggers, eventually resulting in the production of thyroid autoantibodies and lymphocytic infiltration in the thyroid (Lee et al. 2015). Known environmental risk factors are radiation, iodine, selenium, smoking, stress and drugs (Antonelli et al. 2015). Thyroid autoimmunity is associated with the presence in the blood of either thyroid-stimulating antibodies directed against the thyroid hormone receptor (TRAs) or thyroid-inhibiting antibodies directed against thyroglobulin or thyroperoxidase (De Leo and Pearce 2018). The estimated prevalence of AITD is about 5 % (Antonelli et al. 2015) with a strong female predominance as indicated by a female/male ratio of about 5–10 to 1 (Effraimidis and Wiersinga 2014). GD is the most common cause of *hyperthyroidism* in women of childbearing age and thought to be triggered by circulating TRAs. About 2 to 3 % of pregnant women have some form of thyroid dysfunction, whereas another

10 % have a subclinical autoimmune thyroid disease and thus, normal thyroid function (Negro and Mestman 2011). Therefore, awareness of this disorder is highly relevant for care-providers (De Leo and Pearce 2018). Finally, several studies have found thyroid autoimmunity and raised circulating TSH levels to be independent risk factors for thyroid malignancy.

Impact of pregnancy on AITD

The peak of human chorionic gonadotrophin (hCG) levels at between 8 to 11 weeks pregnancy may be accompanied by transient gestational thyrotoxicosis, as hCG also binds to the TSH-receptor, stimulating thyroxin production (Negro and Mestman 2011); Pearce 2015). Some indirect evidence suggests a rise in the chance of developing AITD with increasing parity (Van de Boogaard et al. 2011).

Impact of AITD on pregnancy

Pregnant women with thyroid-inhibiting antibodies directed against thyroperoxidase or thyroglobulin in their blood, are at increased risk of developing (sub)clinical *hypo-thyroidism*, and with it, pregnancy complications, such as miscarriage, preterm birth, preeclampsia, and postpartum HT, that usually progresses to permanent autoimmune hypothyroidism (Van de Boogaard et al. 2011; De Leo and Pearce 2018; Korevaar et al. 2019). Untreated maternal hypothyroidism also predisposes the unborn child to lower scores in neuropsychological tests for intelligence, attention, language, reading ability, school performance and visual motor performance at the age of 7–9 years (Negro and Mestman 2011). The risk of these adverse effects can be reduced effectively by substituting levothyroxine from early pregnancy onwards, using TSH levels as a reference (Negro and Mestman 2011). Conversely, TRAs readily cross the placenta, and from about 16 weeks pregnancy onward, may stimulate the fetal thyroid, potentially inducing fetal hyperthyroidism. Maternal hyperthyroidism is associated with an increased risk of hypertensive pregnancy disorders. More details on management of AIDT in pregnancy, have been provided elsewhere (Pearce 2015).

3.5.7 Multiple sclerosis (MS)

Multiple sclerosis (MS) is an inflammatory demyelinating disorder of the brain and spinal cord with polygenic and environmental factors involved. The pathogenesis of MS is still poorly understood (Lemus et al. 2019), partly because of its highly heterogenous clinical phenotype with sensory and visual nuisances, motor impairments, fatigue, pain and cognitive deficits. The disorder is characterized by a pattern of relapses interrupted by periods of relatively mild symptoms (◘ fig. 3.27).

The temporal and anatomical dispersion of the structural lesions within the central nervous system (CNS) and spinal cord – typical hallmarks of MS – are accompanied by variation in symptoms. These are caused by immune cell infiltration across the blood-brain barrier that promote inflammation, demyelination, gliosis and neuroaxonal degeneration, eventually affecting neuronal signaling. T-cells appear early in lesion formation and the disease is considered autoimmune, initiated by autoreactive lymphocytes leading to abnormal responses against CNS autoantigens, the precise nature of which, though, remains obscure. The onset of MS is on average at 30 years of age, about 3 times

3

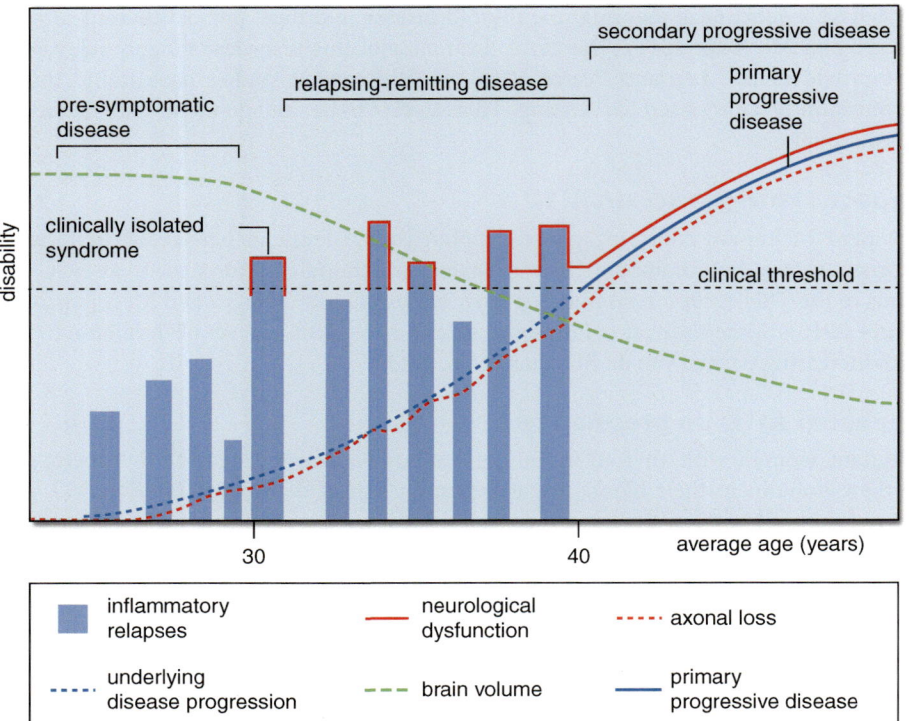

◻ **Figure 3.27**   Clinical course of the most common form of multiple sclerosis (MS), which is characterized by a relapsing and remitting disease pattern (red solid line in figure), affects about 85 % of the patients. The relapses coincide with focal CNS inflammation, demyelination and white matter lesions. Eventually, the only partial improvement after each relapse implies progression of the disability in 80 % of the cases, eventually resulting in the development of secondary progressive disease, characterized by progressive neurologic decline along with CNS atrophy (*adopted from* Dendrou et al. 2015)

more often in women than in men, with half of the patients being wheelchair-dependent within 25 years of diagnosis. MS is the most common cause of disability among young adults (Dendrou et al. 2015). The exact cause of MS is still obscure, although there is evidence for the disease only arising in genetically susceptible individuals and with ambiguous events and environmental factors influencing disease penetrance. Genetic variation accounts for about one-third of the overall disease risk. Despite the fact that nongenetic factors contribute proportionally about twice as much as genetic factors, progress in identifying these factors is slow (Dendrou et al. 2015).

Impact of pregnancy on MS

Pregnancy in MS-affected women is associated with a 70 % decline in relapse rate in the third trimester, a transient effect as indicated by the postpartum return to the pre-pregnant relapse rate within 2 years (Voskuhl and Momtazee 2017). In this respect, MS resembles other cell-mediated autoimmune disorders, such as psoriasis and rheumatoid arthritis, that also ameliorate during pregnancy. Unfortunately, the pregnancy-induced immunomodulation is complex as it involves placental hormones that alter the maternal metabolism, gut microbiome and volume homeostasis, which are accompanied by adjustments in the cardiovascular, renal and respiratory functions. Some follow-up studies have identified estrogen to be responsible for the beneficial effects on MS symptoms, particularly with respect to cognition. Even though the favorable effect of pregnancy on MS is only temporal, it may be reassuring for women with a family history of MS to learn that pregnancies do not increase the risk of developing MS, nor adversely impact the long-term course of MS, and may even delay the pace of worsening disability (Voskuhl and Momtazee 2017; Thöne et al. 2017).

Impact of MS on pregnancy

If possible, any woman with a chronic disease who considers to become pregnant should be counseled preconceptionally, thus allowing the best management strategy to be discussed beforehand. This is most important in women with an aggressive disease such as MS (Bove et al. 2014). In contrast to previously discussed auto-immune disorders, MS does predispose to adverse pregnancy outcome (Bove et al. 2014; Thöne et al. 2017). An important aspect of pregnancy in a woman with MS is, to what extent the various disease-modifying therapies to control MS are teratogenous and thus, whether they are safe to be continued in pregnancy. The risk of congenital malformations in the offspring of MS patients is about 5 %, almost twice the rate in the general population (Voskuhl and Momtazee 2017). Lack of consistency in type of congenital defects complicates the (preconceptional) choice for the most suitable drug regiment at lowest risk for the infant. This problem is a consequence of the low number of sufficiently powered studies addressing drug safety in pregnancy in MS patients.

3.5.8 Myasthenia gravis (MG)

MG is an autoimmune disorder characterized by the presence of (auto)antibodies directed against acetylcholine receptors or functionally-related molecules in the post-synaptic membrane at the neuromuscular junction (Gilhus 2016). To offer safe and optimal anesthesia to MG patients is therefore particularly challenging. Typical for the clinic phenotype of MG is generalized or localized weakness of skeletal muscles, mostly proximal and usually symmetric, though nearly always with asymmetric weakness of oculo-bulbar muscles causing (asymmetric) diplopia and ptosis. Non-motor symptoms, such as pain and headache, are also observed (Tong et al. 2018). Exercise worsens muscle weakness, as does repetitive muscle use (fatigue). In the morning, muscle strength is often normal, with weakness gradually developing over the course of the day, and fluctuating between days (Gilhus 2016). The prevalence of MG is 150–250 patients per million individuals, affecting twice as many women as men (Varner 2013). MG is diagnosed by identifying circulating titres of the autoantibodies mentioned above in individuals, who had developed the typical symptoms.

Impact of pregnancy on MG

The impact of pregnancy on MG is highly variable. In circa one-third of MG-affected women, the disorder deteriorates in early pregnancy to gradually ameliorate again in the remainder of pregnancy, with some women having a postpartum flare. In the other two-thirds of pregnant MG patients, clinical symptoms do not change appreciably, and may even ameliorate with advancing pregnancy, some women even reaching complete remission near term. During pregnancy, particularly intercurrent infections may trigger a MG exacerbation and therefore, should be treated without delay (Varner 2013; Hamel and Ciafaloni 2018). One of six infants born from MG-affected women develops transient neonatal MG, since the related autoantibodies easily cross the placenta. This complication is to be suspected, if a risk infant develops lethargy, a faint cry, difficulty sucking and breathing and generalized muscle weakness, within 4 days postnatally. The prognosis is favorable, provided that it is properly managed. Symptoms gradually fade within about 3 weeks.

Impact of MG on pregnancy

MG has no adverse impact on pregnancy. Nevertheless, a woman affected with MG and wishing to conceive is strongly advised to seek preconceptional counseling with her neurologist to optimize treatment with the best possible safety profile for her and her infant. MG treatment has been detailed elsewhere (Sanders et al. 2018; Hamel and Ciafaloni 2018). Although course and outcome of pregnancy does not differ from that in the general obstetric population, MG patients more often require assisted vaginal delivery (forceps or vacuum), because of fatigue (Varner 2013; Hassan and Yasawy 2017).

3.5.9 Autoimmune thrombocytopenia (ITP)

About 10 % of pregnancies are complicated by thrombocytopenia, defined by a platelet count below 100,000/μL. Over 75 % of these cases are caused by benign gestational (self-limiting) thrombocytopenia (GTP) and only 3 % by ITP. ITP is an acquired autoimmune disorder, characterized by antibody-mediated platelet destruction and variably impaired platelet production. The cause of ITP may also be a combination of genetic predisposition, immune dysregulation and environmental insults (such as infection and post-vaccination) resulting in an abnormal T cell response in the spleen. ITP is a disorder with thrombocytopenia being the common outcome of different pathophysiological pathways that lead to peripheral platelet destruction by the immune system and/or subnormal platelet production in the bone marrow. The effect of accelerated platelet destruction may be amplified by an immune response against megakaryocytes combined with insufficient stimulation by thrombopoietin (Cines et al. 2014; Audia et al. 2016, 2017; Li et al. 2018).

GTP – as opposed to ITP – is mostly observed in the third trimester. However, spontaneous bleedings, particularly in skin and mucosa, are usually a feature of ITP as they occur in two-thirds of ITP patients (Audia et al. 2017). The prevalence of ITP in pregnancy ranges from 0.1 to 1 case per 1,000 women. ITP is often a diagnostic and management challenge, frequently only diagnosed by exclusion (Fogerty 2018). Steroids are useful, both as a diagnostic test and as the first line of treatment, since they may induce (transient) remission in more than 80 % of affected women. If a pregnant ITP patient has severe thrombocytopenia (< 70,000/μL platelets) or thrombocytopenic bleedings in the third trimester, unresponsive to steroids, intravenous immunoglobulin is an appropriate first-line alternative. Additional clinical aspects and management of ITP have been detailed previously (Provan et al. 2010; Sankaran and Robinson 2011; Audia et al. 2016).

Impact of pregnancy on ITP

There are no studies reporting an adverse impact of pregnancy on preexistent ITP.

Impact of ITP on pregnancy

The rate of fetal growth restriction, fetal intracranial hemorrhage, intrauterine fetal death and preterm birth was clearly lower in ITP-affected women, that had undergone splenectomy prior to pregnancy (surgery group) as compared to a matched, conservatively-managed control group of ITP-affected women (Rezk et al. 2018). Also, the rate of bleeding episodes in the surgery group was lower than in the control group. This finding supports the view that ITP resembles other autoimmune disorders in adversely affecting pregnancy. Steroid treatment in the control group is likely to have contributed to the less favorable outcome of pregnancy in the control group, as indicated by higher rates of hypertensive disorders and diabetes. Besides, the autoantibodies that continue to circulate in the control group readily cross the placenta, potentially inducing thrombocytopenia in the infants, which may explain the postnatally detected signs of bleeding in 9–15 % of these infants (Fogerty 2018). Therefore, the infants of ITP-patients managed conservatively are at increased risk of bleedings, particularly during the second stage of labor, and therefore, ought to be managed as atraumatic as possible.

3.5.10 Hereditary angioedema (HAE)

Most cases of HAE are caused by any one of numerous genetic defects that lead to decreased functional levels of the C1 inhibitor, key in the regulation of several inflammatory pathways, resulting in failure to control local bradykinin production (Banerji and Riedl 2016). Affected individuals present with intermittent cutaneous (hands, feet, face, genitals) or mucosal (GI-tract) swellings, occurring in a frequency varying from once a week to less than once a year. These swellings typically develop in several hours and persist for a few days as detailed elsewhere (Longhurst and Cicardi 2012). About 2 % of swellings involve the larynx and can be fatal, if untreated. The prevalence is 1 in 50–100,000 persons of any ethnic group, many affected persons not being aware of the diagnosis. Therefore, awareness of the possibility of this disorder in pregnant women is critical for care providers dealing with high-risk pregnant women. Pregnant women may occasionally experience a higher frequency of attacks. Presumably, high estrogen levels as prevail during pregnancy, and oral contraceptive use, act as triggers for such attacks. Diagnostics and management have been detailed elsewhere (Banerji and Riedl 2016).

3.5.11 Immunodeficiency syndromes

Since the prevalence of primary immunodeficiency disorders and common variable immune deficiency is low, particularly in pregnant women, little is known about their impact on pregnancy. The limited data available on pregnancy in women affected by one of these disorders supports a benign pregnancy course and outcome (Gundlapalli et al. 2015).

3

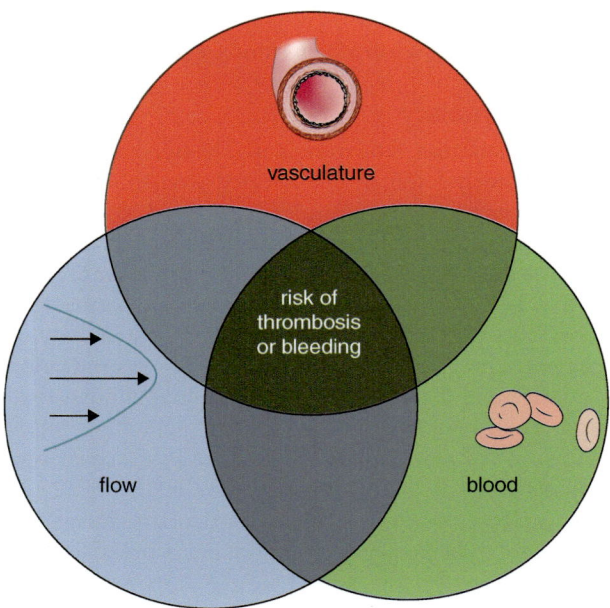

○ **Figure 3.28**   Diagram illustrating how an imbalance in vascular function, blood composition and blood flow dynamics (shear stress) contributes to risk of thrombosis or bleeding (*adopted from* Wolberg et al. 2012)

3.6   Clotting disorders

Normal hemostasis is the outcome of the interplay between (1) blood composition, (2) vessel wall and (3) blood flow rheology, the so-called Virchow's triad. An abnormality in one of these three components predisposes to thrombosis or bleeding (○ fig. 3.28).

The section below describes chronologically, the pathophysiology of thrombosis or bleeding, initiated (1) by abnormal circulating components, (2) by abnormal function of vessel wall ingredients, and (3) by abnormal blood flow properties. The human body produces and removes 10^{11} platelets daily to maintain normal steady-state platelet count. Platelet production must be tightly regulated to avert abnormal bleeding, blood vessel occlusion and organ damage, as detailed elsewhere (Grozovsky et al. 2015). Platelets are key in the pathophysiology of abnormal hemostasis, e.g. because of either abnormal platelet number (thrombocytosis, thrombopenia) or platelet function (thrombopathy).

3.6.1   Thrombocytosis

Thrombocytosis refers to the condition in adults with the number of circulating platelets exceeding the upper limit of the normal range (450×10^9/L) because of one of the following three pathophysiologic mechanisms. Firstly, *reactive thrombocytosis* (RT) is a usually transient condition that develops secondary to a specific acute event (trauma, surgery, acute blood loss) or as a side-effect of certain chronic disorders, such as inflammatory bowel disease, rheumatoid arthritis, iron deficiency, malignancy, hemolytic anemia or some drugs. RT accounts for over 80 % of thrombocytosis cases (Schafer 2001). It is usually characterized by a mild subclinical course without (thromboembolic) complications. It has been postulated that the primary disorder induces a rise in interleukin-6 (IL-6), which in turn upregulates thrombopoietin (TPO)-messenger-RNA expression in the liver (Schafer 2004). This suggests that IL-6 is key in triggering RT. The focus of management is treating the underlying disease. Secondly, *essential (or primary) thrombocytosis* (ET) is a myeloproliferative disorder, accounting for about 14 % of all cases of thrombocytosis and, in contrast to RT, predisposes to thrombosis, bleeding and conversion to acute leukemia. The incidence of thrombotic events is unrelated to platelet count in low-risk ET-patients. On the other hand, the risk of bleeding tends to be higher, when thrombocytosis is extreme (platelet count in excess of $1,000 \times 10^9$/L), presumably due to enhanced uptake of clotting factors by platelets. Thirdly, *familial thrombocytosis* is a rare autosomal dominant disorder, usually resulting from a mutation in the TPO-gene. It leads to deregulated gene translation and with it, overproduction of TPO. Affected family members have excessively high plasma TPO levels. Probably, the highly variable phenotype of familial thrombocytosis results from variation in the type of mutation as detailed previously (Schafer 2004).

Impact of pregnancy on thrombocytosis

Pregnancy does not seem to alter the course and severity of the various forms of preexistent thrombocytosis (Elliott 2003).

Impact of thrombocytosis on pregnancy

In women with RT, the risk of venous thromboembolism (VTE) in pregnancy is similar to that in healthy pregnant controls, unless the RT-patient is confronted with one of the events listed above (trauma, surgery including cesarean section, etc.) (Atalla et al. 2000). On the other hand, the risk of pregnant ET-patients to develop VTE is slightly higher than in healthy controls (Skeith et al. 2017). The most common pregnancy complication in ET-patients is first-trimester spontaneous abortion. If pregnancy in RT and ET patients has advanced to beyond the first trimester, the outcome of that pregnancy does not differ from that in healthy controls (Valera et al. 2011). Clinical management of the various forms of thrombocytosis in pregnancy has been detailed elsewhere (Harrison et al. 2010).

3.6.2 Acquired thrombocytopenia (aTP)

Acquired thrombocytopenia (aTP) refers to a condition in adults with blood platelet count below 100×10^9/L (Cooper and Ghanima 2019). Apart from some rare hereditary forms of aTP (Franchini et al. 2017), the disorder only develops in response to a specific trigger (◘ tab. 3.7), which emphasizes the importance of examining the blood for these triggers in patients with thrombocytopenia (after ruling out pseudo-thrombocytopenia or a EDTA-effect).

Signs of abnormal hemostasis, such as e.g. petechiae, only develop, when platelet count is below 60×10^9/L (George 2000). In this context, it is important to indicate that pregnancy is associated with around a 10 % decline in platelet count, probably due to the physiologic hemodilution. This fall is also seen in women with a preexistent condition

3

◘ Table 3.7   Etiology of acquired thrombocytopenia in adults

etiology	subgroups
pseudothrombocytopenia	in-vitro phenomenon, caused by platelet aggregation in a peripheral blood smear.
autoimmune	ITP; aplastic anemia.
infections	viral (e.g. influenza, zika, CMV, HCV, HIV, EBV); bacterial (e.g. tuberculosis, helicobacter pylori); parasitic (e.g. toxoplasmosis, malaria).
nutritional deficits	vitamin B_{12}, folic acid deficiency.
DIC	septicemia.
splenomegaly	portal hypertension, liver cirrhosis.
microangiopathy	TTP, HUS.
pregnancy-related	HELLP syndrome.
medications	heparin-induced, chemotherapy, radiotherapy.
neoplasms	myelodysplastic, neoplastic BM infiltration.

Abbreviations: *ITP*, Immune thrombocytopenic purpura; *DIC*, disseminated intravascular coagulation; *CMV*, cytomegaly virus; *HCV*, hepatitis C virus; *EBV*, Epstein-Barr virus; *TTP*, thrombotic thrombocytopenic purpura; *HUS*, hemolytic uremic syndrome; *HELLP*, syndrome of hemolysis, elevated liver enzymes and low platelets; *BM*, bone marrow.

accompanied by thrombocytopenia and in women that develop a pregnancy-related complication (see ◘ tab. 3.7 and ◘ fig. 3.29).

With respect to pregnancy, the most relevant (pregnancy-independent) triggers for aTP are hemolytic uremic syndrome (HUS), immune thrombocytopenic purpura (ITP), (non-immune) thrombotic thrombocytopenic purpura (TTP), and medication-induced aTP. HUS and ITP have been discussed in ▶ sect. 3.2 (renal diseases) and ▶ sect. 3.5 (autoimmune disorders) of this chapter, respectively. Therefore, only TTP and medication-induced thrombocytopenia, will be discussed below.

3.6.3 Thrombotic thrombocytopenic purpura (TTP)

TTP develops in concert with microangiopathic hemolytic anemia as part of the thrombotic microangiopathies (TMAs). It leads to microvascular thrombosis and consumption thrombocytopenia along with end-organ damage. Although TTP is characterized by aTP, its pathogenesis begins with abnormal cleavage of the Von Willebrand factor (VWF) at the endothelium due to a deficiency of the enzyme ADAMTS13. Normally, ADAMTS13 cleaves VWF into small peptide chains, but in the presence of subnormal (or absent) amounts of this enzyme, large VWF fragments will accumulate. In the microcirculation, the large multimers enable platelets to bind to them. This facilitates microthrombi formation and potential downstream organ damage. Preeclampsia and the HELLP syndrome are typical examples of pregnancy-induced TMAs.

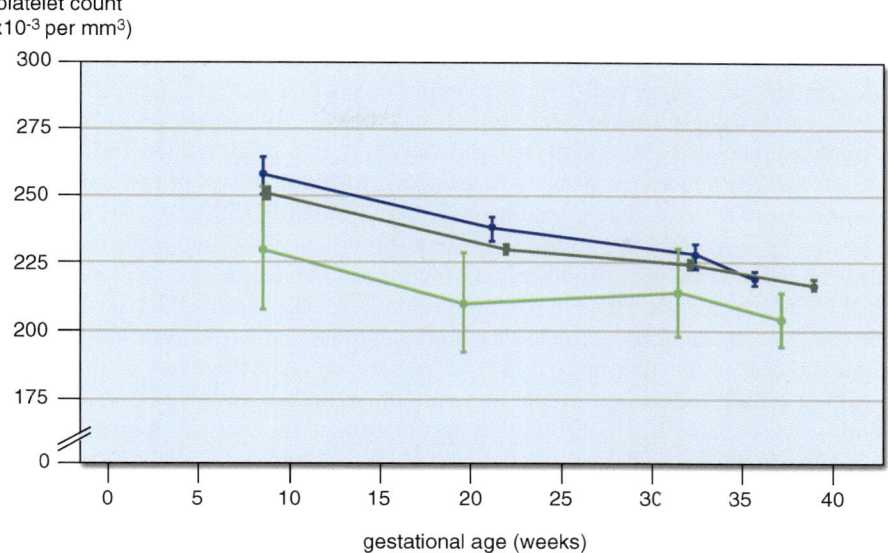

platelet count
(x10^{-3} per mm^3)

Figure 3.29   Mean platelet count in women with a pregnancy-related thrombocytopenia (blue line), a normal pregnancy (dark-green line) and a preexistent disorder accompanied by thrombocytopenia (light-green line). The platelet count of all 3 groups declines with advancing gestational age (*adopted from* Reese et al. 2018)

With a combined prevalence of 1 in 25,000 pregnancies, TTP and complement-mediated HUS are rare disorders in pregnancy (Neave and Scully 2018). This aspect and the clinical overlap with HELLP and preeclampsia, makes their diagnosis extra challenging during pregnancy. However, late diagnosis and delayed start of the appropriate management predisposes the patient and her pregnancy to serious sequels.

Impact of pregnancy on TTP

Preeclampsia and HELLP syndrome are pregnancy-specific TTPs. Apparently, the pregnancy-induced hemodynamic changes facilitate the development of TTP, superimposed on a hypertensive pregnancy complication. It is plausible that pregnancy can also trigger TTP in TMAs unrelated to pregnancy, because of the higher shear stress prevailing in certain organs. The kidneys are particularly prone to such an effect triggered by the renal hyperperfusion.

Impact of TTP on pregnancy

TTP preferentially develops in late pregnancy or postpartum but can also develop early in pregnancy. The rate of fetal loss in untreated TTP is markedly increased. Conversely, timely and appropriate treatment normalizes the prognosis of pregnancy (Neave and Scully 2018).

3.6.4 Medication-induced thrombocytopenia

Several drugs, such as certain antibiotics and chemotherapeutics are known to elicit aTP in susceptible patients. A well-known example of such an iatrogenic disorder is *heparin-induced thrombocytopenia (HIT)* type-I and type-II. HIT-type-I refers to a benign nonimmune-mediated response to heparins resulting in a mild, transient aTP, affecting up to 10 % of patients on heparin. aTP develops within 2–3 days of the start of heparin administration with platelet count returning to baseline within 4 days, irrespective of ongoing heparin administration. It only requires watchful waiting, while continuously evaluating the possibility of mistakenly having missed the diagnosis of HIT-type-II. This is highly relevant, since HIT-type-II may initially overlap with HIT-type-I, but with immense clinical implications including limb gangrene and even death. HIT-type-II is a clinical problem affecting up to 1–5 % of all patients receiving heparin, the variation depending on the indication for the heparin administration and type of heparin used (Donovan et al. 2010). Early recognition and treatment are crucial, given the universal use of heparin products. ◘ Figure 3.30 displays the pathophysiology of HIT-type-II. The clinical management of HIT-type-II has been detailed elsewhere (Donovan et al. 2010).

Impact of pregnancy on HIT

There are no reports showing that pregnancy alters the likelihood or severity of HIT that develops during pregnancy. Pregnancy by itself increases the risk of thromboembolic events, mostly related to the pregnancy-specific endocrine environment. It is unknown whether this modulates the development of HIT. A case report on HIT-type-II that developed after a cesarean birth emphasizes the importance of alertness for this complication to develop in pregnant or postpartum patients (Riess et al. 2005).

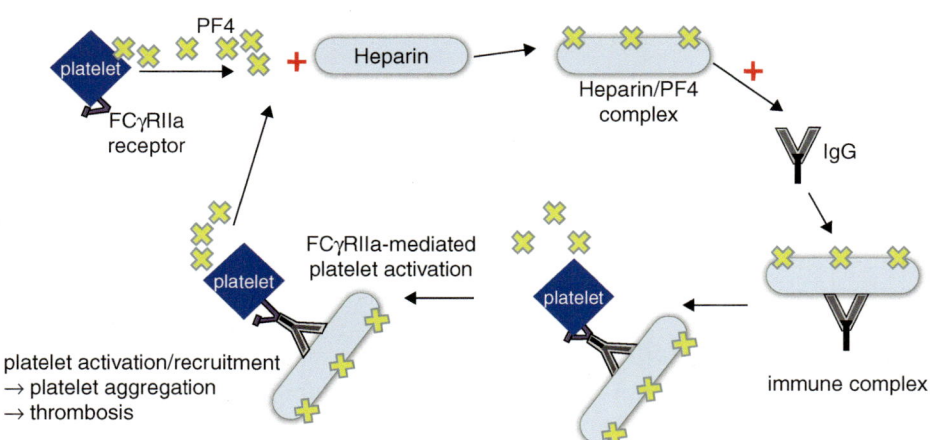

◘ **Figure 3.30**   Pathophysiology of heparin-induced thrombocytopenia (HIT-type-II). The platelets' α-granules release platelet factor 4 (PF4), that binds to heparin to form an antigenic complex (heparin-PF4). Immunoglobulin-G (IgG) antibodies are generated and form the heparin-PF4-IgG complex. The latter then leads to activation of free circulating platelets, inducing their aggregation, that results in both thrombocytopenia and endothelial injury, and with it, thromboembolic sequels. The cycle maintains itself (*adopted from* Donovan et al. 2010)

Impact of HIT on pregnancy

It is unlikely that the development of HIT-type-I affects pregnancy. Conversely, a HIT-type-II, that develops during pregnancy can be expected to have a negative impact on course and outcome of that pregnancy depending on the severity of the HIT-related complications. However, to the best of our knowledge, there are no reports that support such a supposition.

3.6.5 Thrombopathy

Thrombopathy or thrombasthenia refers to rare inherited platelet dysfunctions that lead to bleeding disorders of variable severity, mostly in mucous membranes and the skin. The most common thrombopathy is probably the autosomal recessive Glanzmann's thrombasthenia, a platelet adhesion disorder, typically diagnosed in early childhood with parents often being cousins. There is no reported prevalence, but the disorder is seen predominantly in certain ethnic groups (e.g. French gypsies, Jews, Jordanian tribes, Iraqi Arabs) (Chandrakala and Suthanthira 2014). Initial symptoms are easy bruising, petechiae, purpura, epistaxis/gum bleedings and in affected girls, menorrhagia. Carriers of Glanzmann disease are usually asymptomatic. The disorder often leads to iron deficiency anemia. Other types of thrombopathy are even rarer and detailed elsewhere (Nurden and Nurden 2008).

Impact of pregnancy on thrombopathy

The limited data available are case reports and suggest that pregnancy does not alter the severity of the symptoms of a preexistent thrombopathy (Samuelson-Bannow and Konkle 2018).

Impact of thrombopathy on pregnancy

Preexistent thrombopathy increases the overall bleeding risk, thus also during pregnancy. Over 50 % of affected women require intra- or postpartum blood transfusion. Pregnancy in some reported cases was complicated by fetal growth restriction. Details about management of these pregnancies have been reported recently (Samuelson-Bannow and Konkle 2018).

3.6.6 Abnormal circulating levels of clotting factors

Blood coagulation is a life-saving system, that – if not properly controlled can become life-threatening as observed in disseminated intravascular coagulation (DIC). Consequently, an efficient back-up safety system is in place that ensures restriction of clotting activation both with respect to location (vascular injury) and time (fibrin formation, that only plugs injured tissue), as detailed previously (Wolberg et al. 2012). Inherent to this safety system is that plasma levels of clotting factors do neither contribute to the extent, nor to the quality of hemostasis, as long as peripheral levels are above a critical threshold. In individuals with – often inherited – bleeding disorders, the level of a specific clotting factor is below that critical threshold. For instance, Von Willebrand disease (VWD) is a fairly common autosomal recessive bleeding disorder resulting from deficient Von Willebrand factor (VWF). It accounts for up to 90 % of bleeding disorders in women (James et al. 2016). The severity of bleeding events varies widely depending on the VWD-subtype. The highest reported VWD-prevalence in the general population is 1.3 %, equally distributed between men and women (Reynen and James 2016). Hemophilia A and B are X-linked recessive disorders caused by deficient levels of coagulation factors VIII and IX, respectively, and are much less common than VWD (Peyvandi et al. 2016). Besides hereditary bleeding disorders, deficiency in clotting factors may also be acquired. An example is the decline in all clotting factors together with platelets, due to their excessive consumption in a patient who suffers from DIC, which may complicate sepsis, trauma, a surgical procedure, or – in pregnancy – a specific pregnancy disorder (e.g. amniotic fluid embolism). Last but not least, VWD can also be acquired by autoimmune mechanisms as elaborated on elsewhere (James 2015; James et al. 2016).

Impact of pregnancy on subnormal circulating clotting factors

Pregnancy does not seem to alter the rate and severity of bleeding events in women with one of the bleeding disorders described above.

Impact of subnormal circulating clotting factors on pregnancy

Apart from possibly a slightly higher rate of early pregnancy losses, course and outcome of pregnancy in women with a hereditary bleeding disorder does not differ appreciably from that in unaffected controls, with respect to rate of preterm birth, hypertensive disorders and birthweight (Kadir et al. 1997; Skeith et al. 2017). On the other hand, childbirth in these women is associated with an increased risk of severe bleeding. The clinical management has been detailed elsewhere (Samuelson-Bannow and Konkle 2018).

3.6.7 Thrombophilia (TPh)

Thrombophilia (TPh) is an inherited or acquired *clinical* phenotype characterized by an increased risk of developing thrombosis at a younger age than the general population. The most common TPh-s to be found in pregnant women are the antiphospholipid syndrome (APS), APC-resistance, factor V Leiden mutation (FVL), hyperhomocysteinemia and deficiencies of the natural anticoagulants antithrombin, protein C and protein S. The pathophysiology of TPh consists of disruptions in the safety mechanism that limits the generation of thrombin from prothrombin at the site of activated hemostasis and thus results in a prothrombotic phenotype (O'Donnell et al. 2019). The pathophysiology of some of these disorders (e.g. APS) is not only limited to the proteins of the clotting cascade, but also involves the endothelium and complement system. This opposes the idea that their optimal management during pregnancy can be entirely achieved by only administering anticoagulants (Arachchillage and Laffan 2017). The pathophysiology of APS and its interactions with pregnancy have been detailed in ▶ sect. 3.5 (auto-immune disorders) of this chapter. In spite of a 4 to 5 times higher risk of developing thrombosis, the chance that a TPh-affected individual never develops thrombosis during his/her lifetime is probably much higher. The clinical criteria needed to diagnose TPh are not robust, which undermines reliable estimation of their prevalence.

Impact of pregnancy on TPh

Pregnancy is a hypercoagulable state generally thought to protect the woman from severe bleeding in case of miscarriage and during childbirth. However, the downside of this potential benefit is a 4 to 5-fold higher risk of thrombosis relative to nonpregnant women (James 2015). In TPh-affected women, this thrombosis risk is further raised to about 2–4 %, which is well above the 0.2 % absolute risk in the general obstetric population (James 2009).

Impact of TPh on pregnancy

Pregnant women with TPh due to an inherited disorder (FVL, factor-II mutation and deficiencies of prothrombin, protein S or C) are at increased risk of fetal loss, which can be effectively eliminated by anticoagulant prophylaxis (Folkeringa et al. 2007). Results of studies addressing previous claims that these TPh-s also predispose to placental abruption, placental syndromes and fetal growth restriction, have not been confirmed yet, partly because of poor study design and partly because of insufficient statistical power (De Santis et al. 2006; Battinelli et al. 2013). On the other hand, anticoagulant prophylaxis effectively prevents the development of a VTE during pregnancy in those TPh-affected women that do have an increased risk of developing a VTE. This applies to TPh-s caused by deficiency of prothrombin, protein C or protein S, homozygous for FVL (Croles et al. 2017) and APS (Arachchillage and Laffan 2017).

References

Acharya A. Management of acute kidney injury in pregnancy for the obstetrician. Obstet Gynecol Clin N Am. 2016;43:747–65.

Aggarwal N, Negi N, Aggarwal A, Bodh V, Dhiman RK. Pregnancy with portal hypertension. J Clin Exp Hepatol. 2014;4:163–71.

Alicic RZ, Rooney MT, Tuttle KR. Diabetic kidney disease, challenges, progress and possibilities. Clin J Am Soc Nephrol. 2017;12:2032–45.

Alkhunaizi A, Melamed N, Hladunewich MA. Pregnancy in advanced chronic kidney disease and end-stage renal disease. Curr Opin Nephrol Hypertens. 2015;24:252–9.

Anders H, Rovin B. A pathophysiology-based approach to the diagnosis and treatment of lupus nephritis. Kidney Int. 2016;90:493–501.

Antonelli A, Ferrari SM, Corrado A, et al. Autoimmune thyroid disorders. Autoimmune Rev. 2015;14:174–80.

Antovic A, Sennström M, Bremme K, Svenungsson E. Obstetric antiphospholipid syndrome. Lupus Sci Med. 2018;5. ▶ https://doi.org/10.1136/lupus-2016-000197. eCollection 2018. Review.

Arachchillage DRJ, Laffan M. Pathogenesis and management of antiphospholipid syndrome. Br J Haematol. 2017;178:181–6.

Arany Z, Elkayam U. Peripartum cardiomyopathy. Circulation. 2016;133:1397–409.

Arya R. Pregnancy outcome in women with mechanical prosthetic heart valves. Thromb Res. 2019;181(Suppl. 1):S37–40.

Atalla RK, Thompson JR, Oppenheimer CA, et al. Reactive thrombocytosis after caesarean section and vaginal delivery: implications for maternal thromboembolism and its prevention. Brit J Obstet Gynaecol. 2000;107:411–4.

Aubard Y, Darodes N, Cantaloube M. Hyperhomocysteinemia and pregnancy – review of our present understanding and therapeutic implications. Eur J Obstet Gynecol Reprod Med. 2000;93:157–65.

Audia S, Godeau B, Bonnotte B. Is there still a place for "old therapies" in the management of immune thrombocytopenia? Rev Med Interne. 2016;37:43–9.

Audia S, Mahévas M, Samson M, Godeau B, Bonnotte B. Pathogenesis of immune thrombocytopenia. Autoimmun Rev. 2017;16:620–32.

3

Balsells M, Garcia-Patterson A, Gich I, Corcay R. Maternal and fetal outcome in women with type 2 versus type 1 diabetes mellitus: a systematic review and meta-analysis. J Clin Endocrinol Metab. 2009;94:4284–91.

Banerjee D, Ventetuolo CE. Pulmonary hypertension in Pregnancy. Semin Respir Crit Care Med. 2017;38:148–59.

Banerji A, Riedl M. Managing the female patient with hereditary angioedema. Women's Health. 2016;12:351–61.

Battinelli EM, Marshall A Connors JM. The role of thrombophilia in pregnancy. Review. Thrombosis. 2013;9. ▶ https://doi.org/10.1155/2013/516420.

Belomo R, Kellum JA, Ronco C. Acute kidney injury. Lancet. 2012;380:756–66.

Bhagra C, D'Souza R, Silversides CK. Valvular heart disease and pregnancy part II: management of prosthetic valves. Heart. 2017;103:244–52.

Bissonnette J, Durand F, De Raucourt E, Ceccaldo PF, Plessier A, Valla D, Rautou PE. Pregnancy and vascular liver disease. J Clin Exp Hepatol. 2015;5:41–50.

Bove R, Alwan S, Friedman JM, Hellwig K, et al. Management of multiple sclerosis during pregnancy and the reproductive years. A systematic review. Obstet Gynecol. 2014;124:1157–68.

Braga AC, Vasconcelos C, Braga J. Pregnancy with autoimmune hepatitis. Gastroenterol Hepatol Bed Bench. 2016;9:220–4.

Bramham K. Diabetic nephropathy and pregnancy. Semin Nephrol. 2017;37:362–9.

Brucato A, Frassi M, Franceschini F, Cimaz R, et al. Risk of congenital complete heart block in newborns of mothers with anti-Rho/SSA antibodies detected by counter-immuno-electrophoresis. A prospective study of 100 women. Arthitis Rheum. 2001;44:1832–5.

Buyon JP, Hiebert R, Copel J, Craft J, et al. Autoimmune-associated congenital heart block: demographics, mortality, morbidity and recurrent rates obtained from a national neonatal lupus registry. J Am Coll Cardiol. 1998;31:1658–66.

Campos O, Andrade JL, Bocanegra J. Physiologic multivalvular regurgitation during pregnancy: a longitudinal Doppler echocardiographic study. Int J Cardiol. 1993;40:265–72.

Canobbio MM, Warnes CA, Aboulhosn J, et al. Management of pregnancy in patients with complex congenital heart disease. Circulation. 2017;135:e50–87.

Carapetis JR, Beaton A, Cunningham MW, et al. Acute rheumatic fever and rheumatic heart disease. Nat Rev Dis Primers. 2016 jan 14; 2:15084. ▶ https://doi.org/10.1038/nrdp.2015.84.

Castellano JM, Narayan RL, Vaishnava P, et al. Anticoagulation during pregnancy in patients with a prosthetic heart valve. Nature Cardiol. 2012;9:415–24.

Causey MW, Steele SR, Farris Z, Lyle DS, Beitler AL. An assessment of different scoring systems in cirrhotic patients undergoing nontransplant surgery. Am J Surg. 2012;203:589–93.

Chagnac A, Zingerman B, Rozen-Zvi B, Herman-Edelstein M. Consequences of Glomerular hyperfiltration: the role of physical forces in the pathogenesis of chronic kidney disease in diabetes and obesity. Nephron 2019;4:1–5.

Chandrakala M, Suthanthira K. Glanzmann's thrombasthenia complicating pregnancy. J Obstet Gynecol India. 2014;64:S3–5.

Chapman R, Fevery J, Kalloo A, Nagorney DM, Boberg KM, Shneider B, Gores GJ. Diagnosis and management of primary sclerosing cholangitis. Hepatology. 2010;51:660–78.

Chatterjee S, Khunti K, Davies MJ. Type 2 diabetes. Lancet. 2017;389:2239–51.

Chen B, Sun L, Zhang X. Integration of microbiome and epigenome to decipher the pathogenesis of autoimmune diseases. J Autoimmun. 2017;83:31–42.

Christensen JJ, Retterstol K, Godang K, et al. LDL cholesterol in early pregnancy and offspring cardiovascular disease risk factors. J Clin Lipidol. 2016;10:1369–78.

Cines DB, Cuker A, Semple JW. Pathogenesis of immune thrombocytopenia. Presse Med. 2014;43:e49–59.

Cooper N, Ghanima W. Immune thrombocytopenia. New Engl J Med. 2019;381:945–55.

Croles FN, Nasserinejad K, Duvekot JJ, et al. Pregnancy, thrombophilia and the risk of first venous thrombosis: a systematic review and Bayesian meta-analysis. BMJ. 2017;359:j4452. ▶ https://doi.org/10.1136/bmj4452.

Crousillat DR, Wood MJ. Valvular heart disease and heart failure in women. Heart Failure clin. 2019;15:77–85.

Cunningham FG, Byrne JJ, Nelson DB. Peripartum cardiomyopathy. Obstet Gynecol. 2019;133:167–79.

D'Cruz DP, Khamashta MA, Hughes GRV. Systematic lupus erythematosus. Lancet. 2007;369:587–96.

Dal-Bianco JP, Beaudoin J, Levine RA. Basic mechanisms of mitral valve regurgitation. Can J Cardiol. 2014;30:971–81.

De Leo S, Pearce EN. Autoimmune thyroid disease during pregnancy. Lancet Diabetes Endocrinol. 2018;6:575–86.

De Man YA, Dolhain RJEM, Van de Geijn FE, Willemsen SP, Hazes JMW. Disease activity of rheumatoid arthritis during pregnancy: results from a nationwide prospective study. Arthritis Rheum. 2008;59:1241–8.

De Santis M, Cavaliere AF, Straface G, et al. Inherited and acquired thrombophilia: pregnancy outcome and treatment. Reprod Toxicol. 2006;22:227–33.

Dekker RR, Schutte JM, Stekelenburg J, Zwart JJ, Van Roosmalen J. Maternal mortality and severe maternal morbidity from acute fatty liver of pregnancy in the Netherlands. Eur J Obstet Gynecol Reprod Biol. 2011;157:27–31.

Dendrou CA, Fugger L, Friese MA. Immunopathology of multiple sclerosis. Nat Rev Immunol. 2015;15:545–58.

De Vloo C, Nevens F. Cholestatic pruritus: an update (review). Acta Gastroenterol Belg 2019; 82: 75-82.

Dennis AT. Heart failure in pregnant women: is it peripartum cardiomyopathy? (focused review). Anesth Analg. 2015;120:638–43.

Dixon PH, Williamson C. The pathophysiology of intrahepatic cholestasis of pregnancy. Clin Res Hepatol Gastroenterol. 2016;40:141–53.

Donovan JL, Tran MT, Kanaan AO. An overview of heparin-induced thrombocytopenia. J Pharm Pract. 2010;23:226–34.

Dyson JK, Beuers U, Jones DEJ, Lohse AW, Hudson M. Primary sclerosing cholangitis. Lancet. 2018;391:2547–59.

Eapen DJ, Valiani K, Reddy S, Sperling L. Management of familial hypercholesterolemia during pregnancy: case series and discussion. J Clin Lipidol. 2012;6:88–91.

Effraimidis G, Wiersinga WM. Autoimmune thyroid disease: old and new players. Eur J Endocrinol. 2014;170:R241–52.

Eichholzer M, Tönz O, Zimmermann R. Folic acid: a public health challenge. Lancet. 2006;367:1352–61.

Elliott MA. Thrombocythaemia and pregnancy. Best Pract Res Clin Hematol. 2003;16:227–42.

Emmanuel Y, Thorne SA. Heart disease in pregnancy. Best Pract Res Clin Obstet Gynecol. 2015;29:579–97.

Fakhouri F, Roumenina L, Provot F, Sallée M, et al. Pregnancy-associated hemolytic-uremic syndrome revisited in the era of complement gene mutations. J Am Soc Nephrol. 2010;21:859–67.

Fakhouri F. Pregnancy-related thrombotic microangiopathies: clues from complement biology. Transfus Apher Sci. 2016;54:199–202.

Fischer MJ. Chronic kidney disease and pregnancy: maternal and fetal outcomes. Adv Chronic Kidney Dis. 2007;14:132–45.

Floreani A, Restrepo-Jimémenez P, Secchi MF, et al. Etiopathogenesis of autoimmune hepatitis. J Autoimmun. 2018;95:133–43.

Fogerty AE. Thrombocytopenia in pregnancy: mechanisms and management. Transfus Med Rev. 2018;32:225–9.

Fogo AB. The targeted podocyte. J Clin Invest. 2011;121:2142–5.

Fogo AB. Causes and pathogenesis of focal segmental glomerulosclerosis. Nat Rev Nephrol. 2015;11:76–87.

Folkeringa N, Brouwer JLP, Korteweg FJ, et al. Reduction of high fetal loss rate by anticoagulant treatment during pregnancy in antithrombin, protein C or protein S deficient women. Br J Haematol. 2007;136:656–61.

Franchini M, Veneri D, Lippi G. Thrombocytopenia and infections. Review. Expert Rev Hematol. 2017;10:99–106.

Franco V, Ryan JJ, McLaughlin VV. Pulmonary hypertension in women. Heart Failure Clin. 2019;15:137–45.

Fraser A, Lawlor DA. Long-term health outcomes in offspring born to women with diabetes in pregnancy. Curr Diab Rep. 2014;14:489, 8 pages.

Fremeaux-Bacchi V, Fakhouri F, Garnier A, et al. Genetics and outcome of a typical hemolytic uremic syndrome: a nationwide french series comparing children and adults. Clin J Am Soc Nephrol. 2013;8:554–62.

Fujioka K. Pathophysiology of type 2 diabetes and the role of incretin hormones and beta-cell dysfunction. JAAPA. 2007; Suppl 3–8.

Galiè N, Humbert M, Vachiery JL, et al. ESC/ERS guidelines for the diagnosis and treatment of pulmonary hypertension. Eur Heart J. 2016;37:67–119.

3

Geenes V, Williamson C. Intrahepatic cholestasis of pregnancy. World J Gastroenterol. 2009;15:2049–66.

George JN. Platelets. Lancet. 2000;355:1531–9.

Gerich JE. Contributions of insulin-resistance and insulin-secretory defects to the pathogenesis of type 2 diabetes mellitus. Mayo Clin Proc. 2003;78:447–56.

Giard JM, Terrault NA. Women with cirrhosis. Prevalence, natural history, management. Gastroenterol Clin N Am. 2016;45:345–58.

Gidding SS, Champagne MA, De Ferranti SD, et al. The agenda for familial hypercholesterolemia. A scientific statement from the American heart association. Circulation. 2015;132:2167–92.

Gilhus NE. Myasthenia gravis. New Engl J Med. 2016;375:2570–81.

Goldstein SA, Ward CC. Congenital and acquired valvular heart disease in pregnancy. Curr Cardiol Rep. 2017;19:96, 7 pages.

Gonzalez-Suarez ML, Kattah A, Grande JP, Garovic G. Renal disorders in pregnancy: core curriculum 2019. Am J Kidney Dis. 2018;73:119–30.

Goulielmos GN, Zervou MI, Vazgiourakis VM, Ghodke-Puranik Y, Garyfallos A, Niewold TB. The genetics and molecular pathogenesis of systemic lupus erythematosus (SLE) in populations of different ancestry. Genes. 2018;668:59–72.

GrØnbæk L, Vilstrup H, Jepsen P. Pregnancy and birth outcomes in a Danish nationwide cohort of women with autoimmune hepatitis and matched population controls. Alim Pharmacol Ther. 2018;48:655–63.

Grozovsky R, Giannini S, Falet H, Hoffmeister KM. Novel mechanisms of platelet clearance and thrombopoietin regulation. Curr Opin Hematol. 2015;22:445–51.

Gundlapalli AV, Scalchunes C, Boyle M, et al. Fertility, pregnancies and outcomes reported by females with common variable immune deficiency and hypogammaglobulinemia: results from an internet-based survey. J Clin Immunol. 2015;35:125–34.

Hague WM. Homocysteine and pregnancy. Best Pract Res Clin Obstet Gynaecol. 2003;17:459–69.

Hamel J, Ciafaloni E. An update: myasthenia gravis and pregnancy. Neurol Clin. 2018;36:355–65.

HAPO study cooperative research group; Metzger BE, et al. Hyperglycemia and adverse pregnancy outcomes. New Engl J Med. 2008;358:1991–2002.

Harrison CN, Bareford D, Butt N, et al. Guideline for investigation and management of adults and children presenting with thrombocytosis. Brit J Haematol. 2010;149:352–75.

Hassan A, Yasawi ZM. Myasthenia gravis: clinical management issues, before, during and after pregnancy. Sultan Qaboos Univ Med J. 2017;17:e259–67.

Hazes JMW, Coulie PG, Geenen V, Vermeire S, et al. Rheumatoid arthritis and pregnancy: evolution of disease activity and pathophysiologic considerations for drug use. Rheumatology. 2011;50:1955–68.

Head CEG, Thorne SA. Congenital heart disease in pregnancy. Postgrad Med J. 2005;81:292–8.

Helal I, Fick-Brosnahan GM, Reed-Gitomer B, Schrier RW. Glomerular hyperfiltration: definitions, mechanisms and clinical implications. Nat Rev Nephrol. 2012;8:293–300.

Heneghan MA, Yeoman AD, Verma S, Smith AD, Longhi MS. Autoimmune hepatitis. Lancet. 2013;382:1433–44.

Henry D, Gonzalez JM, Harris IS, et al. Maternal arrhythmia and perinatal outcome. J Perinatol. 2016;36:823–7.

Hernández-Gea V, Baiges A, Turon F, et al. Idiopathic portal hypertension. Hepatology. 2018;68:2413–23.

Hernández-Gea V, De Gottardi A, Leebeek FWG, Rautou PE, Salem R, Garcia-Pagan JC. Current knowledge in pathophysiology and management of Budd-Chiari syndrome and noncirrhotic non-tumoral splanchnic vein thrombosis. J Hepatol. 2019;71:175–99.

Hilfiker-Kleiner D, Sliwa K. Pathophysiology and epidemiology of peripartum cardiomyopathy. Nat Rev Cardiol. 2014;11:364–70.

Hilfiker-Kleiner D, Haghikia A, Berliner D, et al. Bromocriptine for the treatment of peripartum cardiomyopathy: a multicentre randomized study. Eur Heart J. 2017;38:2671–9.

Hogeveen M, Blom HJ, Den Heijer M. Maternal homocysteine and small-for-gestational age offspring. Am J Clin Nutr. 2012;95:130–6.

Holers VM, Girardi G, Mo L, Guthridge JM, et al. Complement C3 activation is required for antiphospholipid antibody-induced fetal loss. J Exp Med. 2002;195:211–20.

Horsley-Silva JL, Carey EJ, Lindor KD. Advances in primary sclerosing cholangitis. Lancet Gastroenterol Hepatol. 2016;1:68–77.

Huser M, Wagnerova K, Janku P, et al. Clinical mangement of pregnancy in women with Goodpasture syndrome. Gynecol Obstet Invest. 2015;79:73–7.

Imam MH, Gossard HH, Sinakos E, Lindor KD. Pathogenesis and management of pruritus in cholestatic liver disease. J Gastroenterol Hepatol. 2012;27:1150–8.

Ince-Ascan H, Dolhain RJEM. Pregnancy and rheumatoid arthritis. Best Pract & Res Clin Rheumatol. 2015;29:580–96.

Islam A, Khandker SS, Alam F, Kamal MA, Gan SH. Genetic risk factors in thrombotic primary antiphospholipid syndrome: a systematic review with bioinformatic analyses. Autoimmun Rev. 2018;17:226–43.

James AH. Venous thromboembolism in pregnancy. Arterioscler Thromb Vasc Biol. 2009;29:326–31.

James AH. Review: thrombosis in pregnancy and maternal outcome. Birth Defect Res C Embryo Today. 2015;105:159–66.

James AH, Eikenboom J, Federici AB. State of the art: von Willebrand disease. Haemophilia. 2016;22(suppl 5):54–9.

Jefferson JA, Shankland SJ. The pathogenesis of focal segmental glomerulosclerosis. Adv Chronic Kidney Dis. 2014;21:408–16.

Jim B, Garovic VD. Acute kidney injury in pregnancy. Semin Nephrol. 2017;37:378–85.

Jonsson R, Vogelsang P, Volchenkov R, et al. The complexity of Sjögren's syndrome: novel aspects on pathogenesis. Immunol lett. 2011;141:1–9.

Kadir RA, Economides DL, Braithwaite J, et al. The obstetric experience of carriers of haemophilia. Br. J Obstet Gynaecol. 1997;104:803–10.

Kahn SE, Hull RL, Utzschneider KM. Mechanisms linking obesity to insulin res stance and type 2 diabetes. Nature. 2006;444:840–6.

Karlsen TH, Folseraas T, Thorburn T, Vesterhus M. Primary sclerosing cho angitis – a comprehensive review. J Hepatol. 2017;67:1298–323.

Kassi E, Pervanidou P, Kaltsas G, Chrousos G. Metabolic syndrome: definitions and controversies. BioMed Central Medicine. 2011;9:48. ► http://www.biomedcentral.com/1741-7015/9/48.

Knotts RJ, Garan H. Cardiac arrhythmias in pregnancy. Semin Perinatol. 2014;38:285–8.

Korevaar TIM et al. The consortium on Thyroid and Pregnancy, Study Group on Preterm Birth. JAMA 2019;322:632–641.

Kuhn A, Wenzel J, Bijl M. Lupus erythematosus revisited. Semin Immunopathol. 2016;38:97–112 (Review).

Kusters DM, Lahsinoui HH, Van der Post JAM, et al. Statin use during pregnancy: a sytematic review and meta-analysis. Expert Rev Cardiovasc Ther. 2012; PMID 22390808.

Lane CR, Trow TK. Pregnancy and pulmonary hypertension. Clin Chest Med. 2011;32:165–74.

Lassi ZS, Salam RA, Haider BA, et al. Folic acid supplementation duirng pregnancy for maternal health and pregnancy outcomes (rev). Cochrane Database Syst Rev. 2013;3:CD006896.

Lateef A, Petri M. Systemic lupus erythematosus and pregnancy. Rheum Dis Clin N Am. 2017;43:215–26.

Lau E, Defaria Yeh D. Management of high-risk cardiac conditions in pregnancy: anticoagulation, severe stenotic valvular disease and cardiomyopathy. Trends Cardiovasc Med. 2019;29:155–61.

Lee GR. The balance of Th17 versus Treg cells in autoimmunity. Int J Mol Sci. 2018;19:730. ► https://doi.org/10.3390/ijms19030730 (14 pages).

Lee HJ, Li CW, Hammerstad SS, Stefan M. Immunogenetics of autoimmune thyroid diseases. A comprehensive review. J Autoimmun. 2015;64:82–90.

Lemus HN, Warrington AE, Rodriguez M. Multiple sclerosis: mechanisms of disease and strategies for myelin and axonal repair. Neurol Clin. 2019;36:11.

Li JM, Nguyen C, Joglar JA, et al. Frequency and outcome of arrhythmias complicating admission during pregnancy: experience from a high-volume and ethnically-diverse obstetrical service. Clin Cardiol. 2008;31(11):538–41.

Li J, Sullivan JA, Ni H. Pathophysiology of immune thrombocytopenia. Curr Opin Hematol. 2018;25:373–81.

Linnemann B. Antiphospholipid syndrome – an update. Vasa. 2018;47:451–64.

Liu L, Sun D. Pregnancy outcomes in patients with primary antiphospholipid syndrome: a systematic review and meta-analysis. Medicine (Baltimore). 2019 May;98(20). ► https://doi.org/10.1097/md.0000000000015733.

Liu Y, Ma X, Zheng J, Liu X, Yan T. A systematic review and meta-analysis of kidney and pregnancy outcome in IgA nephropathy. Am J Nephrol. 2016;44:187–93.

3

Liu J, Ghaziani TT, Wolf JL. Acute fatty liver of pregnancy: updates in pathogenesis. Diagnosis and Management. Am J Gastroenterol. 2017;112:838–46.

Llovet LP, Horta D, García Eliz M, Belenguer M, Fábrega E, et al. Pregnancy and autoimmune hepatitis: presentation and outcomes. Clin Gasteroenterol Hepatol. 2019, Jan 4 [Epub ahead of print].

Lohse AW, Mieli-Vergani G. Autoimmune hepatitis. J Hepatol. 2011;55:171–82.

Longhurst H, Cicardi M. Hereditary angio-oedema. Lancet. 2012;379:474–81.

Lopes van Balen VA, Spaan J, Ghossein C, et al. Early pregnancy circulatory adaptation and recurrent hypertensive disease. An explorative study. Reprod Sci. 2013;20:1069–74.

Ludvigsson JF, Bergquist A, Ajne G, Kane S, et al. A Population-based cohort study of pregnancy outcomes among women with primary sclerosing cholangitis. Clin Gastroenterol Hepatol. 2014;12:95–100.

Ma RCW, Tutino GE, Lillycrop KA, et al. Maternal diabetes, gestational diabetes and the role of epigenetics in their long-term effects on offspring. Progr Biophys Mol Biol. 2015;118:55–68.

Magee C, Grieve DJ, Watson CJ, Brazil DP. Diabetic nephropathy: a tangled web to unweave. Cardiovasc Drugs Ther. 2017;31:579–92.

Majak GB, Sandven I, Lorentzen B, Vangen S, Reisaeter AV, Henriksen T, Michelsen TM. Pregnancy outcomes following maternal kidney transplantation: a national cohort study. Acta Obstet Gynecol Scand. 2016;95:1153–61.

Malik GH, Al-Harbi HS, Al-Mohaya, Al-Wakeel S, et al. Repeated pregnancies in patients with primary membranous glomerulonephritis. Nephron. 2002;91:21–4.

Manns MP, Lohse AW, Vergani D. Autoimmune hepatitis–Update 2015. J Hepatol. 2015;62(1 Suppl): S100–11.

Marti-Carvajal AJ, Sola I, Lathyris D, et al. Homocysteine-lowering interventions for preventing cardiovascular events. The Cochrane Library. 2013; issue 1.

Mathiassen ON, Buus NH, Sihm I, et al. Small artery structure is an independent predictor of cardiovascular events in essential hypertension. J Hypertens. 2007;25:1021–6.

McCance DR. Diabetes in pregnancy. Best Pract Res Clin Obstet Gynaecol. 2015;29:685–99.

McDonald-Wallis C, Lawlor DA, Fraser A, et al. Blood pressure change in normotensive, gestational hypertensive, preeclamptic and essential hypertensive pregnancies. Hypertension. 2012;59:1241–8.

McInnes IB, Schett G. The pathogenesis of rheumatoid arthritis. N Engl J Med. 2011;365:2205–19.

Meng ML, Landau R, Viktorsdottir O, Banayan J, Grant T, Bateman B, Smiley R, Reitman E. Pulmonary hypertension in pregnancy. A report of 49 cases at four Tertiary North American Sites. Obstet Gynecol. 2017;129:511–20.

Metz TD, Khanna A. Evaluation and management of maternal cardiac arrhythmias. Obstet Gynecol Clin N Am. 2016;43:729–45.

Mignini LE, Latthe P, Villar J, et al. Mapping the theories of preeclampsia: the role of homocysteine. Obstet Gynecol. 2005;105:411–25.

Mikolasevic I, Filipec-Kanizaj T, Jakopcic I, et al. Liver disease during pregnancy: a challenging clinical issue. Med Sci Monit. 2018;24:4080–90.

Molodecky NA, Kareemi A, Parab R, Barkema HW, et al. Incidence of primary sclerosing cholangitis: a systematic review and meta-analysis. Hepatology. 2011;53:1590–9.

Moore JS, Teefey P, Rao K, et al. Maternal arrhythmia; a case report and review of the literature. Obstet Gynecol Survey. 2012;292–312.

Moroni G, Ponticelli C. Important considerations in pregnant patients with lupus nephritis. Expert Rev Clin Immunol. 2018;14:489–98.

Morton A, Laurie J. Physiological changes of pregnancy and the Swansea criteria in diagnosing acute fatty liver of pregnancy. Obstet Med. 2018;11:126–31.

Muir AJ. Understanding the complexities of cirrhosis. Clin Ther. 2015;37:1822–36.

Mulvany MJ. Small artery remodelling in hypertension. Basic Clin Pharmacol Toxicol. 2012;110:49–55.

Nandakumar KS. Targeting IgG in arthritis: disease pathways and therapeutic avenues. J Mol Sci. 2018;19:677. ► https://doi.org/10.3390/ijms19030677.

Nanna M, Stergiopoulos K. Pregnancy complicated by valvular heart disease: an update. J Am Heart Assoc. 2014 Jun 5;3(3). ► https://doi.org/10.1161/jaha.113.000712.

Naoum EE, Leffert LR, Chitilian HV, Gray KJ, Bateman BT. Acute fatty liver of pregnancy: pathophysiology, anesthetic implications and obstetric management. Anesthesiology. 2019;130:446–61.

Napoli C, D'Armiento FP, Mancini FP, et al. Fatty streak formation occurs in human fetal aortas and is greatly enhanced by maternal hypercholesterolemia. J Clin Invest. 1997;100:2680–90.

Napoli C, Palinski W. Maternal hypercholesterolemia during pregnancy influences the later development of atherosclerosis: clinical and pathogenic implications. Hotline editorial. Eur Heart J. 2001;22:4–9.

Neave L, Scully M. Microangiopathic hemolytic anemia and pregnancy. Transfus Med Rev. 2018;32:230–6.

Negro R, Mestman JH. Thyroid disease in pregnancy. Best Pract Res Clin Endocrinol Metab. 2011;25:927–43.

Nishimura RA, et al. 2014 AHA/ACC guideline for the management of patients with valvular heart disease. J Thorac Cardiovasc Surg. 2014;148:e1–132.

Nishimura RA, et al. 2017 focused update of the 2014 AHA/ACC guideline for the management of patients with valvular heart disease. J Am Coll Cardiol. 2017;70:259–89.

Nolan CJ, Damm P, Prentki M. Type 2 diabetes across generations: from pathophysiology to prevention and management. Lancet. 2011;378:169–81.

Novak J, Barratt J, Julian BA, Renfrow MB. Aberrant glycosylation of the IgA molecule in IgA nephropathy. Semin Nephrol. 2018;38:461–76.

Nurden P, Nurden AT. Congenital disorders associated with platelet disfunctions. Thromb Haemost. 2008;99:253–63.

O'Donnell JS, O'Sullivan JM, Preston RJS. Advances in understanding the molecular mechanisms that maintain normal haemostasis. Br J Haematol. 2019;186:214–36.

O'Shaughnessy MM, Jobson MA, Sims K, Liberty AL, Nachman PH, Pendergraft WF. Pregnancy outcomes in patients with glomerular disease attending a single academic center in North Carolina. Am J Nephrol. 2017;45:442–51.

Obican SG, Cleary KL. Pulmonary arterial hypertension in pregnancy. Seminar Perinatol. 2014;38:289–94.

Olsson KM, Channick R. Pregnancy in pulmonary hypertension. Eur J Respir Rev. 2016;25:431–7.

Op de Beeck A, Elzirik DL. Viral infections in type 1 diabetes mellitus – why the β-cells? Nat Rev Endocrinol. 2016;12:263–73.

Ope-Adenuga S, Moretti M, Lakhi N. Management of membranous glomerulonephritis in pregnancy: a multidisciplinary challenge. Case Rep Obstet Gynecol. 2015;2015:839376.

Orwat S, Diller GP, Van Hagen JM, et al. Risk of pregnancy in moderate and severe aortic stenosis. J Am Coll Cardiol. 2016;68:1727–37.

Ovadia C, Williamson C. Intrahepatic cholestasis of pregnancy: recent advances. Clin Dermatol. 2016;34:327–34.

Packham D. Thin basement membrane nephropathy in pregnancy. Semin Nephrol. 2005;25:180–3.

Paneni F, Costantino S, Cosentino F. Insulin resistance, diabetes and cardiovascular risk. Curr Atheroscler Rep. 2014;16:419, 8 pages.

Parikh P, Blauwet L. Peripartum cardiomyopathy and preeclampsia: overlapping diseases of pregnancy. Curr Hypertens Rep. 2018;20:69 (8 pages).

Pearce EN. Thyroid disorders during pregnancy and postpartum. Best Pract Res Clin Obstet Gynaecol. 2015;29:700–6.

Pellicoro A, Ramachandran P, Iredale JP, Fallowfield JA. Liver fibrosis and repair: immune regulation of wound healing in a solid organ. Nature Rev Immunol. 2014;14:181–94.

Petri M, Orbai AM, Alarcón GS, et al. Derivation and validation of systemic lupus international collaborating clinics classification criteria for systemic lupus erythematosus. Arthitis Rheum. 2012;64:2677–86.

Peyvandi F, Garagiola I, Young G. The past and future of haemophilia: diagnosis, treatments and its complications. Lancet. 2016;388:187–97.

Provan D, Stasi R, Newland AC, et al. International consensus report on the investigation and management of primary immune thrombocytopenia. Blood. 2010;115:168–86.

Puljic A, Salati J, Doss A, Caughey AB. Outcome of pregnancies complicated by liver cirrhosis, portal hypertension or esophageal varices. J Mat, Fetal, Neon Med. 2016;29:506–9.

Rahman T, Hamzan NS, Mokhsin A et al. Enhanced status of inflammation and endothelial activation in subjects with familial hypercholesterolaemia and their related unaffected family members: a case control study. Lipids Health Disease. 2017;16:81:PMID 28438163.

Rautou PE, Angermayr B, Garcia-Pagan JC, et al. Pregnancy in women with known and treated Budd-Chiari syndrome: maternal and fetal outcomes. J Hepatol. 2009;51:47–54.

Reese JA, Peck JD, Deschamps DR, et al. Platelet count during pregnancy. New Engl J Med. 2018;379:32–43.

Reynen E, James P. Von Willebrand disease and pregnancy: a review of evidence and expert opinion. Semin Thromb Hemost. 2016;47:717–23.

Rezk M, Masood A, Dawood R, et al. Improved pregnancy outcome following earlier splenectomy in women with immune thrombocytopenia: a 5 years observational study. J Matern Fetal Neonatal Med. 2018;31:2436–40.

3

Riess FC, Gross A, Budde U. Pulmonary embolism after cesarian section due to heparin-induced thrombocytopenia despite normal platelet count. Thorac Cardiovasc Surg. 2005;53:255–7.

Roeder HA, Kuller JA, Barker PCA, et al. Maternal valvular heart disease in pregnancy. Obstet Gynecol Survey. 2011;66:561–71.

Ronco P, Debiec H. Membranous nephropathy: a fairy tale for immunopathologists, nephrologists and patients. Mol Immunol. 2015;68:57–62.

Rosenn B, Miodovnik M, Combs CA, Khoury J, et al. Glycemic thresholds for spontaneous abortion and congenital malformations in insulin-dependent diabetes mellitus. Obstet Gynecol. 1994;84:515–20.

Rossier BC, Bochud M, Devuyst O. The hypertensive pandemic: an evolutionary perspective. Physiology. 2017;32:112–25.

Ruiz-Irastorza G, Crowther M, Branch W, Khamashta MA. Antiphospholipid Syndrome (Seminar). Lancet. 2010;376:1498–509.

Russell MA, Craigo SD. Cirrhosis and portal hypertension in pregnancy. Seminars Perinatol. 1998;22:156–65.

Samuelson-Bannow BS, Konkle BA. Inherited bleeding disorders in the obstetric patient. Transfus Med Rev. 2018;32:237–43.

Sanders DB, Wolfe GI, Narayanaswami P, et al. Developing treatment guidelines for myasthenia gravis. Ann NY Acad Sci. 2018;1412:95–101.

Sanhal CY, Kara O, Yucel A. Can fetal left-ventricular modified myocardial performance index predict adverse perinatal outcomes in intrahepatic cholestasis of pregnancy? J Matern fetal Neonatal Med. 2017;30:911–6.

Sankaran S, Robinson SE. Immune thrombocytopenia and pregnancy. Obstet Med. 2011;4:140–6.

Scaldaferri F, Pizzoferrato M, Ponziani FR, et al. Use and indications of cholestyramine and bile acid sequestrants. Intern Emerg Med. 2013;8:205–10.

Schafer AI. Thrombocytosis and thrombocytopenia. Blood Rev. 2001;15:159–66.

Schafer AI. Thrombocytosis: current concepts. New Engl J Med. 2004;350:1211–9.

Schuppan D, Afdhal NH. Liver cirrhosis. Seminar. Lancet. 2008;371:838–51.

Shah S, Prasoon V. Overview of pregnancy in renal transplant patients. Int J Nephrol. 2016;2016:4539342.

Shi-Min Yuan, Song-Li Yan. Mitral valve prolapse in pregnancy. Braz J Cardiovasc Surg. 2016;31:158–62.

Silver RM. Catastrophic antiphospholipid syndrome and pregnancy. Semin Perinatol. 2018;42:26–32.

Singh AG, Chowdhary VR. Pregnancy-related issues in women with systemic lupus erythematosus. Int J Rheum Dis. 2015;18:172–81.

Skeith L, Rydz N, O'Beirne M, et al. Pregnancy loss in women with von Willebrand disease: a single-center pilot study. Blood Coagul Fibrinolysis. 2017;28:393–7.

Sliwa K, Johnson MR, Zilla P, et al. Management of valvular heart disease in pregnancy: a global perspective. Eur Heart J. 2015;36:1078–89.

Smeele HTW, Dolhain RJEM. Current perspectives on fertility, pregnancy and childbirth in patients with rheumatoid arthritis. Semin Arthritis Rheum. 2019;49:S32–5.

Smok DA. Aortopathy in pregnancy. Semin Perinatol. 2014;38:295–303.

Smolen JS, Aletaha D, McInnes IB, Rheumatoid arthritis. (Seminar) Lancet. 2016;388:2023–38.

Smulders YM. The (non-)sense of the methionine loading test for detecting hyperhomocysteinaemia. Neth J Med. 2000;57:172–3.

Smyth A, Radovic M, Garovic VD. Women, renal disease and pregnancy. Adv Chronic Kidney Dis. 2013;20:402–10.

Soares MF, Roberts ISD. IgA Nephropathy: an update. Curr Opin Nephrol Hypertens. 2017;26:165–71.

Spaanderman M, Ekhart T, Van Eyk J et al. Preeclampsia and maladaptation to pregnancy. A role for atrial natriuretic peptide? Kidney Int. 2001;60:1397–406.

Spotti D. Pregnancy in women with diabetic nephropathy. J Nephrol. 2019;32:379–88.

Steegers-Theunissen RPM, Boers GHJ, Trijbels FJM, et al. Maternal hyperhomocysteinemia: a risk factor for neural-tube defects? Metabolism. 1994;43:1475–80.

Stojan G, Baer AN. Flares of systemic lupus erythematosus during pregnancy and the puerperium: prevention, diagnosis and management. Expert Rev Clin Immunol. 2012;8:439–53.

Tangren J, Nadel M, Hladunewich MA. Pregnancy and end-stage renal disease. Blood Purf. 2018;45:194–200.

Tao Z, Shi A, Zhao J. Epidemiological perspectives of diabetes. Cell Biochem Biophys. 2015;73:181–5.

Theocharidou E, Heneghan MA. Current and future perspectives in autoimmune hepatitis. Brit J Hosp Med. 2018;79:151–9.

Thomas E, Yang J, Jianjin X, Lima FV, Stergiopoulos K. Pulmonary hypertension and pregnancy outcomes: insights of the national inpatient sample. J Am Heart Assoc. 2017;6:1–12.

Thöne J, Thiel S, Gold R, Hellwig K. Treatment of multiple sclerosis during pregnancy – safety considerations. Expert Opin Drug Saf. 2017;16:523–34.

Tiniakos DG. Nonalcoholic fatty liver disease/nonalcoholic steatohepatitis: histological diagnostic criteria and scoring systems. Eur J Gastroenterol Hepatol. 2010;22:643–50.

Tong O, Delfiner L, Herskovitz S. Pain, headache and other non-motor symptoms in myasthenia gravis. Curr Pain Headache Rep. 2018;22:39 (review, 7 pages). ▶ https://doi.org/10.1007/s11916-018-0687-3.

Tran TT, Ahn J, Reau NS. ACG clinical guideline: liver disease and pregnancy. Am J Gastroenterol. 2016;111:176–94.

Tsiara S, Poppas A. Mitral valve disease in pregnancy: outcomes and management. Obstet Med. 2009;2:6–10.

Tsochatzis EA, Bosch J, Burroughs AK. Liver cirrhosis. Seminar. Lancet. 2014;383:1749–61.

Valera MC, Parant O, Vayssiere C, et al. Essential thrombocythemia and pregnancy. Eur J Obstet gynecol Reprod Biol. 2011;158:141–7.

Van de Boogaard E, Vissenberg R, Land JA, et al. Significance of (sub)clinical thyroid dysfunction and thyroid autoimmunity before conception and on early pregnancy: a systematic review. Human Reprod Update. 2011;17:605–19. (minor corrections on this report with no impact on outcome, were published in Human Reprod Update. 2016;22:532–3).

Van de Griend R, Biesma DH, Banga JD. Hyperhomocysteinaemia as a cardiovascular risk factor; an update. Neth J Med. 2000;56:119–30.

Van Hook JW. Acute kidney injury during pregnancy. Clin Obstet Gynecol. 2014;57:851–61.

Varner M. Myasthenia gravis and pregnancy. Clin Obstet Gynecol. 2013;56:372–81.

Vasavan T, Ferraro E, Ibrahim E, Dixon P, Gorelik G, Williamson C. Heart and bile acids – Clinical consequences of altered bile acid metabolism. Biochim Biophys Acta Mol Basis Dis. 2018;1864:1345–55.

Velásquez M, Rojas M, Abrahams VM, Escudero C, Cadavid AP. Mechanisms of endothelial dysfunction in antiphospholipid syndrome: associations with clinical manifestations. Front Physiol. 2018;9 (Dec 21, 2018). ▶ https://doi.org/10.3389/fphys.2018.01840. eCollection 2018.

Vellanki K. Pregnancy in chronic kidney disease. Adv Chronic Kidney Dis. 2013;20:223–8.

Vilas-Boas A, Bakshi J, Isenberg DA. What can we learn from systemic lupus erythematosus pathophysiology to improve current therapy? Expert Rev Clin Immuncl. 2015;11:1093–107.

Vivarelli M, Massella L, Ruggiero B, Emma F. Minimal change disease. Clin J Am Soc Nephrol. 2017;12:332–45.

Voskuhl R, Momtazee C. Pregnancy: effect on multiple sclerosis, treatment considerations, and breastfeeding. Neurotherapeutics. 2017;14:974–84.

Wellge BE, Sterneck E, Teufel A, Rust C, Franke A, Schreiber S, et al. Pregnancy in primary sclerosing cholangitis. Gut. 2011;60:1117–21.

Wender-Ozegowska E, Wroblewska K, Zawiejska A, et al. Threshold values of maternal blood glucose in early diabetic pregnancy – prediction of fetal malformations. Acta Obstet Gynecol Scand. 2005;84:17–25.

Westbrook RH, Dusheiko G, Williamson C. Pregnancy and liver disease. J Hepatol. 2016;64:933–45.

Wikström-Shemer EA, Stephansson O, Thuresson M, Thorsell M, Ludvigsson S, Marschall H-U. Intrahepatic cholestasis of pregnancy and cancer, immune-mediated and cardiovascular diseases: a population-based cohort study. J Hepatol. 2015;63:456–61.

Wolberg AS, Aleman MM, Leiderman K, et al. Procoagulant activity in hemostasis and thrombosis: Virchow's triad revisited. Anesth Analg. 2012;114:275–85.

Wu M-Y, Chen C-S, Yiang G-T, Cheng P-W, et al. The emerging role of pathogenesis of IgA nephropathy. J Clin Med. 2018 Aug 20;7:pii:E225 (16 pages).

Xiong H-F, Liu J-Y, Guo L-M, Li X-W. Acute fatty liver of pregnancy: over six months follow-up study of twenty-five patients. World J Gastroenterol. 2015;21:1927–31.

Yanagawa B, Whitlock RP, Verma S, et al. Anticoagulation for prosthetic heart valves: unresolved questions requiring answers. Curr Opin Cardiol. 2016;31:176–82.

Yancy CW, et al. ACCF/AHA guideline for the management of heart failure. Circulation. 2013;128:e240–327. (updated in 2017).

Yang LY, Thia EWH, Tan LK. Obstetric outcomes in women with end-stage renal disease on chronic dialysis: a review. Obstet Med. 2010;3:48–53.

Zakharia K, Tabibian A, Lindor KD, Tabibian JH. Complications, symptoms, quality of life and pregnancy in cholestatic liver disease. Liver international. 2018;38:399–411.

Zamanpoor M. The genetic pathogenesis, diagnosis and therapeutic insight of rheumatoid arthritis. Clin Genet. 2019;95:547–57.

3

Preexistent chronic disorders, often indirectly affecting pregnancy

Abstract

This chapter describes the impact of chronic disorders that do not directly interfere with placental development and function, but often have an *indirect* negative effect on the course and outcome of pregnancy. The most important primary organs targeted by these disorders are lungs (▶ sect. 4.1), GI-tract (▶ sect. 4.2), liver (partly) (▶ sect. 4.3), endocrine system (▶ sect. 4.4) and blood (▶ sect. 4.5). The final two sections describe the interaction of common psychiatric disorders with pregnancy (▶ sect. 4.6) and the effect of pregnancy on the pharmacokinetics of frequently used medication (▶ sect. 4.7). The adverse effects of these disorders on pregnancy are partly related to the impaired function of the chronically affected organs (such as reduced respiratory reserve capacity in women with severe asthma), and partly related to their negative effect on the cardiovascular and metabolic reserves normally available to accommodate pregnancy. These two features lower the threshold for activation of the stress response as detailed in ▶ Chaps. 1 and 2. Early activation of this stress response not only predisposes a pregnancy to preterm birth and/or placental dysfunction. It may also worsen the underlying chronic disorder and with it, indirectly amplify the stress response and its associated adverse effect on pregnancy. These inferences indicate that optimizing clinical management of the disorder prior to pregnancy can be expected to reduce the risk of these negative effects.

L. L. H. Peeters et al., *Pathophysiology of pregnancy complications*,
https://doi.org/10.1007/978-90-368-2571-9_4

4

> **Highlights**
>
> 1. Chronic disorders not directly affecting the reserve capacity of the circulation, volume regulation and immune function can still have an indirect adverse effect on pregnancy by disorder-related stress and associated stress response. These may increase the cardiovascular sympathetic tone and with it, the uterine vascular resistance. Occasionally, these disorders may also hamper the immune function and with it, adversely affect the microbiome in the genital tract. The latter is believed to increase the risk of facilitating hostile upstream colonization. Together, both effects predispose to placental syndromes and preterm labor;
> 2. Medical care of pregnant women with a chronic psychiatric disorder in the months after childbirth to support and secure the development of a healthy mother-infant relationship, is almost certainly beneficial;
> 3. Many women with a chronic disorder use medication for disease control. During pregnancy it requires critical evaluation, and in case of safety and/or efficacy issues during pregnancy, an alternative should be aimed for, ideally at least 3 months prior to conception.

4.1 Pulmonary disorders

4.1.1 Introduction

Pregnancy induces changes in both size of the various pulmonary compartments and pulmonary function. In the second half of pregnancy, functional residual capacity falls by about 20 %, due to a fall in expiratory reserve volume (ERV) and residual volume (RV) (▶ Chap. 1, ◻ fig. 1.20). This fall is a direct consequence of the higher upwards pressure exerted upon the diaphragm by the enlarged pregnant uterus. However, this mechanical effect does not alter diaphragmatic excursions, indicating that forced vital capacity (FVC) may be preserved. Maternal oxygen demand during pregnancy is raised, due to an approximate 15 % higher (maternal) basal metabolic rate and a 20 % higher oxygen uptake required to fuel fetal and placental metabolism and growth. The ±30 % rise in tidal volume during pregnancy relative to pre-pregnancy enables a pregnant woman to meet these higher oxygen demands.

4.1.2 Asthma and Chronic Obstructive Pulmonary Disease (COPD)

Asthma is an airway obstruction syndrome that partially overlaps with COPD, but differs from it by (1) type of inflammation (larger allergic component and no mast cell activation), (2) a more proximal location in the bronchial tree, and (3) being more reversible (Rogliani et al. 2016). It is a heterogeneous and complex disease resulting from gene-environment interactions, mostly occurring in early life. The pathogenesis of classic asthma is hyperresponsiveness of the airway to environmental triggers, followed by chronic airway inflammation. These events lead to repeated injury, repair and regeneration of the airway epithelium causing obstruction due to increased bronchial mucus production and bronchoconstriction (Papi et al. 2018). Common symptoms are cough, shortness of breath, wheezing and chest tightness. Asthma is often episodic with attacks often being triggered by viruses, allergens, irritants (smoke), exercise and temperature changes. It is a chronic disorder with the highest prevalence (> 15 %) among socially disadvantaged individuals. Recent studies indicate that classic asthma is easily confused with asthma-like disorders, such as non-obstructive dyspnea, dysfunctional breathing, airway sensory hyperreactivity, hyperventilation, postnasal drip, small airways disease, gastroesophageal reflux and vocal cord dysfunction. This confusion may explain the high proportion of misdiagnosis and treatment failures. The overall prevalence of asthma in pregnancy is around 9 % with a high level of interregional variation (Bonham et al. 2018; Papi et al. 2018).

Impact of pregnancy on asthma

The insights into the predictors and the mechanism that determines the severity of asthma exacerbations during pregnancy are limited. The asthma symptoms, experienced at conception, also determine their severity during pregnancy with symptoms improving, remaining unchanged, or worsening at about one-third each. However, some studies provide evidence for a higher deterioration rate in severe cases, irrespective of its heterogenous etiology (Vanders and Murphy 2015). Pregnancy induces five functional changes that may alter preexistent asthma symptoms.

1. With advancing pregnancy, the rising upward pressure exerted upon the diaphragm by the *growing uterus* progressively reduces respiratory functional residual capacity (▶ Chap. 1, ◻ fig. 1.20). However, it is unlikely that this factor alters the severity of asthma, as it neither affects FVC nor the cyclic diaphragmatic breathing excursions;

2. *The 30 % rise in tidal volume* during pregnancy results from a progesterone-induced rise in the PCO_2 sensitivity of the respiratory center in the medulla oblongata. Theoretically, this effect increases the friction during breathing exerted upon the bronchial mucosa and with it, the chance of mucosal irritation, mucus formation and coughing. Yet, the concomitant pregnancy-induced relaxation of the smooth muscle layer of the bronchial tree is likely to dampen this effect;

3. The *altered innate immune function* in pregnancy includes an upregulated Th-2 (favoring tissue repair) and a downregulated Th-1 response (favoring cytotoxicity). Presumably, this effect plays a role in the amelioration of various preexistent autoimmune disorders including asthma in some pregnant women (Lunjani et al. 2018);

4. *Pregnancy-induced nasal congestion*, presenting as rhinosinusitis and presumably triggered by the endocrine environment of pregnancy. This condition affects about 20 % of pregnancies (Ellegard 2006). It is likely that asthmatic- more than non-asthmatic women, suffer more from this complaint;

5. Pregnancy-induced *altered pharmacokinetics of asthma medication*. The higher metabolic rate in pregnancy may shorten the half-life of various drugs (see final section of this chapter) and with it, their efficacy to control symptoms (Murphy et al. 2017).

The exacerbation rate of asthma in pregnancy increases as a function of asthma severity at conception. An important risk factor for these events during pregnancy is discontinuation of medication, because of concerns about potential teratogenic effects. This factor

□ Table 4.1   Perinatal outcome in women with bronchial asthma

perinatal outcome	RR compared to women without asthma	95% CI	number studies	number of women studied
low birth weight	1.46	1.22–1.75	11	1,109,907
SGA	1.22	1.14–1.31	11	1,083,861
preterm birth	1.41	1.23–1.62	15	988,852
preeclampsia	1.54	1.32–1.81	14	1,178,958

Abbreviations: RR, relative risk; CI, confidence interval; SGA, fetal growth restriction (adopted from Giles et al. 2013).

comes on top of the impact of the physiologic changes in pharmacokinetics induced by pregnancy. Asthmatic women are also more likely to have intercurrent viral upper respiratory infections that can also trigger asthma exacerbations.

Impact of asthma on pregnancy

Poorly controlled asthma in pregnancy predisposes to fetal growth restriction (SGA), preterm birth and preeclampsia (□ tab. 4.1), disorders that predispose to a higher rate of cesarean birth and serious perinatal morbidity. It should also be kept in mind that the use of inhaled corticosteroids reduces fetal growth rate and with it, contributes to a higher incidence of SGA. Nevertheless, neonatal outcome is generally favorable with no higher perinatal mortality. Interestingly, epidemiological data indicate that pregnant women expecting a boy have a higher risk of adverse pregnancy outcome than their counterparts expecting a girl. On the other hand, for unknown reasons this latter group has a higher risk of worsening asthma during pregnancy than their counterparts expecting a boy (Murphy et al. 2005).

Management of asthma should be preceded by diagnostic exclusion of the asthma-like disorders. The main objective of management during pregnancy is to prevent exacerbations. Details about clinical management have been reported elsewhere (Murphy et al. 2017; Namazy and Schatz 2018).

4.1.3 Cystic fibrosis (CF)

Cystic fibrosis (CF) is an autosomal recessively inherited disorder of exocrine glands resulting in viscous secretions in lungs, pancreas and gut, often resulting in organ damage due to clogging secretions. Pulmonary infections are the primary cause of morbidity and mortality in patients with this disease. The prevalence of CF varies from 1 in 2,500 to 1 in 32,000 individuals in white and Asian populations, respectively (Shulman and Elias 2001). The carrier rate in whites is about 1 in 25 persons. The CF phenotype may be the outcome of over 1,400 defects in the CF gene located on chromosome 7 that encodes for the transport protein 'cystic fibrosis transmembrane conductance regulator' (CFTR). This protein regulates anion transport and mucociliary clearance from glands in the bronchial tree, pancreas and gut (Grasemann and Ratjen 2015). Functional failure of the CFTR protein results in mucus retention and epithelial cell dysfunction in the bronchial

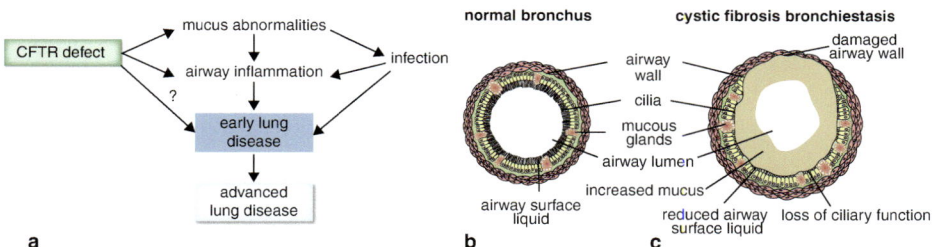

Figure 4.1 Pathogenesis of cystic fibrosis (CF) related lung disease. (**a**) Basic mechanism in CF eventually resulting in advanced lung disease; (**b**) normal bronchus; (**c**): bronchus in a patient with CF: Local factors acting in concert in damaging the airway wall. *Abbreviations: CFTR*, CF transmembrane conductance regulator (*adopted from* Grasemann and Ratjen 2015)

tree (leading to chronic bacterial lung infection), pancreas (malabsorption), liver (biliary cirrhosis), sweat glands (heat shock), and vas deferens (infertility).

Most of the morbidity and mortality in CF relates to pulmonary disease. In the lungs, regular spells of bronchial inflammation due to impaired mucus disposal is accompanied by the gradual development of bronchiectasis and obstruction of smaller airways, gradually evolving to advanced lung disease (fig. 4.1). In recent decades, effective treatment of intestinal obstruction in the newborn and pulmonary infections has markedly improved the CF prognosis and life expectancy. Treatment with drugs that improve bronchial mucus clearance and resolve secondary infection also corrects pancreatic insufficiency and undernutrition. This type of management has also improved the quality of life of CF patients.

Impact of pregnancy on CF

With a better clinical outcome and higher life expectancy of CF patients, their demand for reproductive care has risen. In male patients CF leads to infertility due to aspermia, because of atresia or bilateral absence of the vas deferens (Shulman and Elias 2001). However, the anatomy of the female reproductive tract is unaffected. Still, female fertility is somewhat reduced, because of sticky cervical mucus and impaired ovulatory function in a subset of CF women (Chen et al. 2012). This subfertility is reflected in a spontaneous pregnancy rate of only 50 % in CF women (Ahmad et al. 2013).

As discussed in the section on asthma, pregnancy increases tidal volume by about 30 %, relaxes the tracheobronchial smooth muscle layer, and – in advanced pregnancy – lowers the respiratory residual volume due to upwards pressure exerted upon the diaphragm by the growing uterus. The effect of these changes on maternal health is usually mild and transient (Ahluwalia et al. 2014), as long as the CF-affected woman has a predicted 'one-second forced expiratory volume' (FEV$_1$) of over 50 %, a body mass index over 18 kg/m^2 and no diabetes mellitus at the time of conception (Patel et al. 2015). Conversely, in the presence of at least one of these unfavorable features at conception, she will be at increased risk of developing a wide range of other complications as listed in tab. 4.2. Pregnancy-related alterations in cell-mediated immunity may increase both risk and severity of pulmonary infection and alter the typical persistent bacterial infection usually found in CF. Pregnancy in CF patients also poses an extra risk of developing gestational diabetes and associated complications.

4

□ **Table 4.2**   Medical conditions and events (n with [% incidence]) in nationwide in-patient sample in the US at childbirth among cystic fibrosis (CF) women compared to non-CF controls

medical condition or events	cystic fibrosis (n = 1119)	no cystic fibrosis (n = 12,627,627)	odd ratio (95 % CI)	p-value
asthma-like symptoms	165 [15 %]	411,451 [3%]	5.1 (4.3–6.1)	< 0.0001
anemia	154 [14 %]	1,363,611 [11%]	1.3 (1.1–1.6)	0.001
diabetes mellitus	147 [13 %]	134,209 [1%]	14.0 (11.8–16.7)	< 0.0001
pneumonia	75 [7 %]	13,150 [< 1%]	68.7 (54.3–86.9)	< 0.0001
card. conduction disorders	39 [4 %]	83,146 [< 1%]	5.5 (4.0–7.6)	< 0.0001
thrombophilia	36 [3 %]	71,418 [< 1%]	5.7 (2.7–12.1)	< 0.0001
mechanical ventilation	25 [2 %]	9003 [< 0.1%]	31.9 (21.4–47.5)	< 0.0001
acute respiratory failure	14 [1 %]	5450 [< 0.1%]	29.6 (16.7–48.0)	< 0.0001
acute renal failure	11 [1 %]	7075 [< 0.1%]	16.4 (8.9–30.4)	< 0.0001
death	11 [1 %]	921 [0.6%]	125 (67–2331)	< 0.0001

Abbreviations: CI, confidence interval; *OR*, odds ratio (*data derived from* Patel et al. 2015).

Impact of CF on pregnancy

The clinical presentation of CF varies widely between patients due to the many possible underlying CF gene mutations. This variability in types of CF mutations complicates identification of some less common mutations in different populations. With a CF carrier rate of 1 in 25 individuals, the risk of a CF-woman giving birth to a child with CF is 1:50 and even 1:2 if the partner was untested and later identified to be a CF carrier. This difference emphasizes the importance of preconceptional genetic counseling, that should also include the critical evaluation of medication used before pregnancy and nutritional advice. The type of CF-gene mutation determines phenotype. A mild and stable CF phenotype is associated with an acceptable prepregnant maternal lung function ($FEV_1 > 50$ %), nutritional state ($BMI > 18$ kg m^{-2}), absence of diabetes and a regular menstrual cycle. Most of these clinically stable CF women will probably have a normal pregnancy, albeit with an increased risk of preterm birth and fetal growth restriction (Schlüter et al. 2018). Pregnancy neither worsens the results of pulmonary function tests, nor the nutritional status and the rate of exacerbations. Malabsorption may be an issue requiring extra attention as detailed elsewhere (McArdle 2011). Pregnancy outcome in CF women with a less favorable phenotype is mostly determined by the degree and stability of lung dysfunction. Pregnancy outcome in these women will benefit from prepregnant optimization of lung function and – if indicated – the woman's nutritional state. Because of the increased risk of diabetes, it is recommended to evaluate glucose tolerance before or early in pregnancy to minimize the risk of diabetes-related birth defects. Obviously, optimal management of these women during pregnancy requires supervision by a team that includes a high-risk obstetrician, a pulmonary physician with expertise in CF and an intensive-care physician.

4.1.4 Respiratory infections

Lower respiratory tract infection refers to acute bronchitis, pneumonia and exacerbations of chronic lung disease. Community-acquired pneumonia (CAP) is a leading cause of morbidity and mortality worldwide, often presenting with symptoms of mild pneumonia (fever and productive cough), but sometimes also with symptoms of severe pneumonia, respiratory distress and sepsis. In most cases, CAP is caused by streptococcus pneumonia, hemophilus influenzae, mycoplasma pneumoniae or respiratory viruses (Goodnight and Soper 2005; Sheffield and Cunningham 2009). The rate of respiratory infections in women of reproductive age is low (about 0.1 %) irrespective of pregnancy (Brito and Niederman 2011), except for influenza virus pneumonia, which is more common in pregnancy (Kourtis et al. 2014). It follows that pregnancy-induced changes in lung structure and function, as detailed earlier in this chapter, do not necessarily raise the susceptibility to (bacterial) lung infections. However, the course of pneumonia during pregnancy is more severe, probably due to the altered immune function. Pregnancy is a period of immune paradox. The maternal immune system has to tolerate the presence of the semi-allogeneic fetus without compromising its function to prevent infections that may threaten her own health. Pregnancy shifts the balance of immune responses in favor of anti-inflammation (for details, see ▶ Chap. 1). Before the introduction of antibiotics in clinical medicine, pregnancy was a recognized risk factor for severe complications of pneumococcal pneumonia. Pregnant women are also at increased risk of severe illness from influenza pneumonia. Pneumonia is accompanied by the same symptoms in pregnant and non-pregnant women: cough, dyspnea, tachypnea, tachycardia (heart rate > 100 beats/min), fever (> 4 days), wheezing, chest pain and abnormal findings on physical examination. The diagnostic work-up for -, and clinical management of respiratory infections in pregnant women have been detailed elsewhere (Sheffield and Cunningham 2009; Torres et al. 2017a; Rac et al. 2018).

Impact of pregnancy on a respiratory infection

Pregnancy is associated with an increased risk of contracting pneumonia, most likely because of the adaptive changes in the innate immune function. The threshold for the development of pneumonia may also be lower during pregnancy due to the lower pregnancy-induced colloid-osmotic pressure in the circulating blood that facilitates fluid transfer from the vascular bed to the interstitial space. Women with preexistent disorders, such as anemia and asthma, are at increased risk of contracting pneumonia during pregnancy. Also, certain forms of clinical management during pregnancy, such as the intravenous administration of tocolytic agents and the (prolonged) use of corticosteroids, increases the risk of contracting pneumonia.

Impact of a respiratory infection on pregnancy

The maternal distress after contracting pneumonia, caused by the higher respiratory strain, along with a probably less efficient immune response to overcome the infection, is likely to lead to a more intense and protracted stress response, that may adversely impact the intrauterine conditions for fetal growth. This may explain why pneumonia predisposes to preterm birth and fetal growth restriction (Brito and Niederman 2011).

4.1.5 Acute pulmonary edema

Acute pulmonary edema refers to fluid accumulation in the pulmonary alveoli resulting from a fluid shift from the pulmonary microcirculation to the alveoli, triggered by either an imbalance in the Starling forces or increased capillary permeability in the pulmonary microcirculation (■ fig. 4.2). Since this complication interferes with the oxygen uptake, it is life-threatening, also because pulmonary edema frequently develops as a complication of a serious primary disorder, such as a hypertensive crisis or septic shock.

The normal hemodynamic and volume adaptation to pregnancy increases the vulnerability to develop pulmonary edema as a side-effect of specific conditions during pregnancy. Pregnancy is characterized by relative arterial underfilling as a consequence of the pregnancy-induced vascular relaxation. Compensatory mechanisms to prevent a fall in blood pressure include volume retention, hemodilution and activation of the arterial baroreceptors, the renin-angiotensin-aldosterone system and the sympathetic nervous system. These compensations result in a hypervolemic, hypo-osmotic and hypo-oncotic

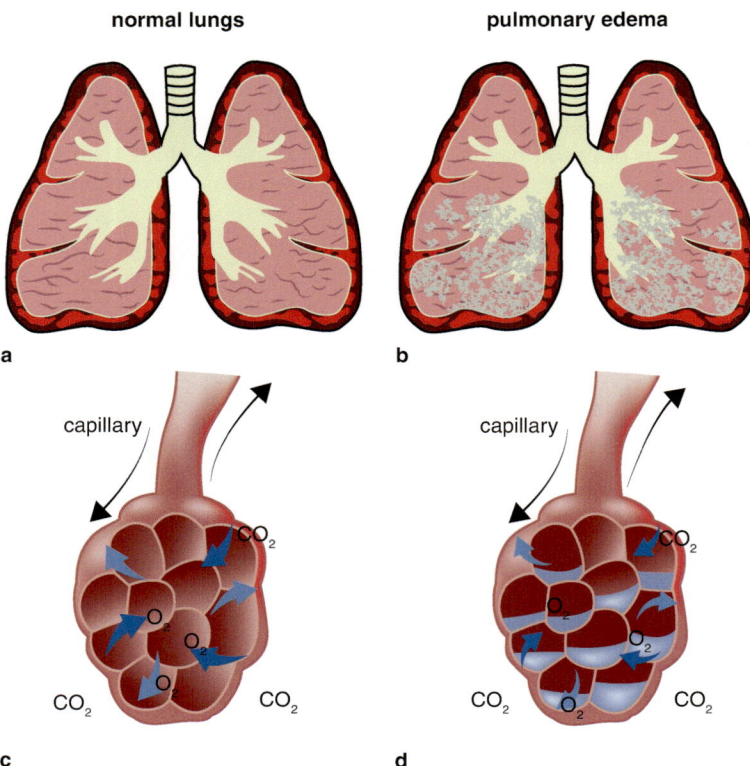

normal lungs   **pulmonary edema**

a   b

capillary   capillary

c   d

■ **Figure 4.2** Schematic representation of pulmonary edema. (**a**) Normal lungs and (**b**) pulmonary edema. (**c**) Aveoli of normal lungs. (**d**) Aveoli of lungs with pulmonary edema, characterized by impaired alveolar gasexchange

state of the cardiovascular bed with an extracellular compartment and plasma volume that are enlarged by about 50 % and 40 %, respectively. Near term, the plasma volume compartment is more than 50 % larger than before pregnancy. The latter is critical in preserving circulating volume, blood pressure and uteroplacental blood flow throughout pregnancy. The higher cardiovascular demands of pregnancy combined with the compensations in volume homeostasis, impose extra stress upon the pulmonary and cardiovascular systems, as also indicated by a higher risk of respiratory complications (Lumbers and Pringle 2014).

Impact of pregnancy on pulmonary edema

In pregnant women, acute pulmonary edema may complicate severe preeclampsia, particularly in women of advanced age, obesity, or a poorly-managed preexistent hypertensive disorder. In normotensive pregnant women, the development of acute pulmonary edema may be provoked e.g. by (1) the intravenous administration of large amounts of fluid or certain drugs (corticosteroids, β-mimetics), (2) in women with a chronic cardiac condition (cardiomyopathy, ischemic heart disease), who develop amniotic fluid- or thromboembolism complicated by left-ventricular failure, (3) during sepsis and (4) after aspiration (Adam 2017). Obviously, the development of acute pulmonary edema during pregnancy is a serious complication with a high risk of maternal and fetal mortality. Early recognition is key to ensure the timely initiation of treatment. Symptoms of acute pulmonary edema are breathlessness, ortho/tachypnea, agitation and cough, often accompanied by cardiac symptoms, such as tachycardia, crackles and wheeze on chest auscultation, cardiac S3 gallop-rhythm murmurs and reduced oxygen saturation. Transthoracic echocardiography is pivotal in diagnosing and managing lung edema as detailed elsewhere (Picano and Pelikka 2016). The diagnostic work-up and management of acute pulmonary edema in a pregnant patient, have been detailed elsewhere (Dennis and Solnordal 2012).

4.2　Gastrointestinal (GI) disorders

During pregnancy, concomitant adaptive changes in the maternal GI-tract (Drozdowski et al. 2009) and in the intestinal microbiome (Edwards et al. 2017) contribute to a higher intestinal uptake of nutrients. These adaptations seem to be triggered by higher demands for nutrients together with the growth-promoting endocrine environment of pregnancy (Drozdowski et al. 2009). This section provides an overview of the possible adverse effects of various common chronic GI-tract disorders on pregnancy and vice versa, whether the pregnancy-induced maternal adaptations alter the clinical symptoms and course of these preexistent chronic GI disorders.

4.2.1　Peptic ulcer disease (PUD)

The term "peptic ulcer" refers to open mucosal lesions in the upper GI-tract. Most peptic ulcers are located in the stomach or proximal duodenum, but occasionally they are also found in the esophagus. The most common symptom is epigastric pain, often accompanied by dyspepsia, abdominal fullness, nausea or early satiety. However, about two-thirds of patients with PUD are asymptomatic, and are only identified by complications, such as GI bleeding, gastric outlet obstruction or perforation (Kavitt et al. 2019). The lifetime prevalence of PUD in the general population ranges from 5 to 10 %, with a higher incidence observed in smokers, the elderly, and subjects with chronic medical conditions (Lanas and Chan 2017). Over the last three decades, the incidence of PUD has fallen markedly (Lanas and Chan 2017).

Ulcers may develop, because of an imbalance between gastric-acid production and pepsin, the enzyme that protects the gastric mucosa from the acid. In most cases, PUD is caused by an infection with Helicobacter (H) pylori, but it may also occur during treatment with non-steroidal anti-inflammatory drugs (NSDAIDs) or prednisone. The risk of H. pylori infection is raised, when a person, (1) lives in a crowded environment, (2) has restricted access to clean water, (3) lives with someone infected by H. pylori, and (4) uses NSAIDs chronically. Most H. pylori-infected subjects remain asymptomatic. This is not necessarily a good sign as H. pylori infection also predisposes to GI malignancy and mucosa-associated lymphoid tissue (MALT) lymphoma (Venerito et al. 2017).

Impact of pregnancy on peptic ulcer disease

Many pregnant women experience nausea and vomiting in early pregnancy and gastro-esophageal reflux disease (GERD) in more advanced pregnancy. These effects develop secondary to the pregnancy-induced functional changes in the GI tract. Nevertheless, most women with PUD improve during pregnancy, to deteriorate again postpartum (Frise and Nelson-Piercy 2012). Therefore, testing for H. pylori infection in pregnant women is recommended, if they have a history of (untreated) PUD, if they have nausea and/or vomiting that persists after the first trimester, or if they develop symptoms of GERD that are nonresponsive to treatment with a proton pump inhibitor (PPI) or histamin-2 (H2) receptor blocker (Clark et al. 2014). Pregnant women with GERD and severe unexplained anemia due to iron- or vitamin B12 deficiency may benefit from H. pylori testing as these deficiencies can be caused by chronic colonization with H. pylori, presumably as a consequence of asymptomatic PUD. This severe anemia and associated reduced circulatory reserve capacity may explain the increased risk of fetal growth restriction, placental syndromes and preterm birth in these pregnancies (Den Hollander et al. 2017).

Impact of pregnancy on peptic ulcer disease

Pregnancy does not alter the risk factors for PUD.

4.2.2 Inflammatory bowel disease (IBD)

Inflammatory bowel disease (IBD) consists of two major chronic inflammatory intestinal disorders, that are both characterized by flare-ups and clinical remission: ulcerative colitis and Crohn's disease. IBD arises from a complex interaction among genetic and environmental factors, dysregulated immune responses and alterations of the microbiome as illustrated in ◘ fig. 4.3.

Genome-wide association studies have identified more than 200 alleles to be associated with IBD with many affected genes involved in bacterial handling, suggesting that this feature may be key in the pathogenesis of IBD (Torres et al. 2017b; Rogler

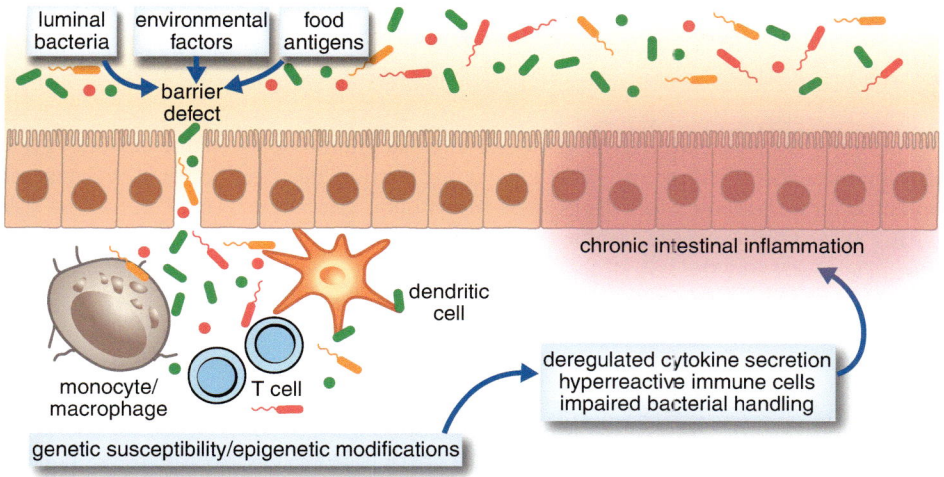

◨ Figure 4.3 Presumed pathogenesis of inflammatory bowel disease (IBD). Intestinal microbiota, environmental factors and food antigens either cause a leaky barrier or penetrate through a barrier leak into deeper, submucosal tissue layers. In a susceptible host, epigenetic modifications and dysregulation of the innate and adaptive immune response trigger intestinal inflammation (*adopted from* Rogler et al. 2018)

et al. 2018). In ulcerative colitis, the infection may be limited to the rectum, but can also extend to the more proximal segments of the colon. Symptoms of the disorder are normally bloody mucous diarrhea and occasionally also urgency, tenesmus and fecal incontinence. The disorder is diagnosed by colonoscopy combined with histological findings.

Patients with Crohn's disease usually have a transmural inflammatory process in the distal ileum, but this can be located anywhere in the GI tract. Disturbance of the gut microbiome or 'dysbiosis' refers to a shift in the balance of intestinal bacteria in favor of pathogenic (proinflammatory) bacteria, and at the cost of beneficial (anti-inflammatory) bacteria. Dysbiosis has emerged as an important contributor to its pathogenesis (Kostic et al. 2014; Ohkusa and Kiodo 2015). Stability, resilience and complexity of the microbiome differ in various phases of life. In a healthy gut, the microbiome is involved in the protection against pathogens, the digestion and the training of the immune system. The microbiome throughout its development is affected by genetics, diet and medication. Some of these factors can disrupt its complexity and stability, and with it, cause microbial dysbiosis.

Crohn's disease presents with abdominal pain, chronic diarrhea, weight loss, fatigue and (usually microscopic) blood loss in the stool (Torres et al. 2017b). Also, Crohn is diagnosed by a combination of endoscopy and histopathology. Nowadays improved CT imaging techniques facilitate the diagnostic work-up in Crohn patients (Taguchi et al. 2018). The onset of ulcerative colitis and Crohn's disease usually occurs between 15 and 40 years with a slight female predominance in Crohn's disease. Female predominance in this age bracket suggests involvement of hormones in the disease expression. Prevalence of both forms of IBD is highest in Europe and Canada (about 300 cases per 100,000). Family occurrence increases the risk 10-fold, mainly in first-degree relatives. Management of IBD in women that wish to conceive or are already pregnant, have been detailed elsewhere (Ungaro et al. 2017; Torres et al. 2017b; Van der Woude et al. 2015; Choden et al. 2018).

4

Impact of IBD on pregnancy

Crohn's disease, but not ulcerative colitis, may be associated with subfertility due to the fallopian tubes being obstructed by -, or being entangled in pelvic adhesions that develop as a sequel of infection. A woman with IBD that wishes to conceive is advised to counsel with her gastroenterologist prior to conception to evaluate the efficacy of her IBD maintenance therapy and whether her medication needs adjustment, because of potential teratogenicity. Most drugs used to maintain remission in IBD are of low risk during pregnancy, except for methotrexate, which is contraindicated. Active IBD during pregnancy increases the risk of fetal growth restriction, preterm birth, low birthweight and stillbirth. However, if pregnancy advances to term with preserved disease remission, there is no evidence of any extra risk for the infant. IBD is not associated with an increased risk of congenital anomalies in the offspring (Van der Woude et al. 2015).

Impact of pregnancy on IBD

Conception during active disease reduces the chance to achieve remission in the remainder of pregnancy (Van der Woude et al. 2015). This indicates that pregnancy does impact the course of IBD. On the other hand, conception during remission does not change the prepregnant risk of relapse. It is recommended that a near-term Crohn patient complicated by active perianal disease, should be delivered by cesarean section to minimize the risk of perianal sequels (Hatch et al. 2014). Postpartum flares are uncommon in women with Crohn's disease on maintenance therapy. In contrast, women with ulcerative colitis are at increased risk of a postpartum flare.

4.2.3 Gallstone disease

Stones commonly accumulate in the gallbladder, particularly in Western populations with risk factors such as older age, female gender, multiparity, dyslipidemia, type-2 diabetes, obesity and sedentary lifestyle. Postpartum studies have found gallstones in 12 % of men and 24 % of women of all ages (Chowdhury and Lobo 2011). However, incidental gallstones are commonly noted at routine imaging with as many as 80 % of cases remaining asymptomatic for the next 20 years. Therefore, gallstone or biliary 'disease' refers to the condition in about 20 % of subjects with gallstones that suffer of repeated, usually postprandial, right-upper quadrant abdominal pain, often lasting less than 30 minutes and sometimes accompanied by nausea and emesis (Portincasa et al. 2006; Chung and Duke 2018).

The rate of gallstones in women, who completed 2–3 pregnancies, is nearly 3 times higher than in their nulliparous age-matched counterparts. Moreover, around 5 % of women respond to pregnancy with neoformation of gallstones, often accompanied by biliary sludge, both effects usually redissolving again postpartum (Ko et al. 2005). Acute cholecystitis refers to inflammation of the gallbladder, in most cases resulting from a gallstone obstructing the cystic duct (◘ fig. 4.4). A patient with gallstone disease is at increased risk of complications, such as obstructive jaundice, acute cholecystitis, cholangitis, gangrene of the gallbladder, gallstone ileus and gallstone pancreatitis.

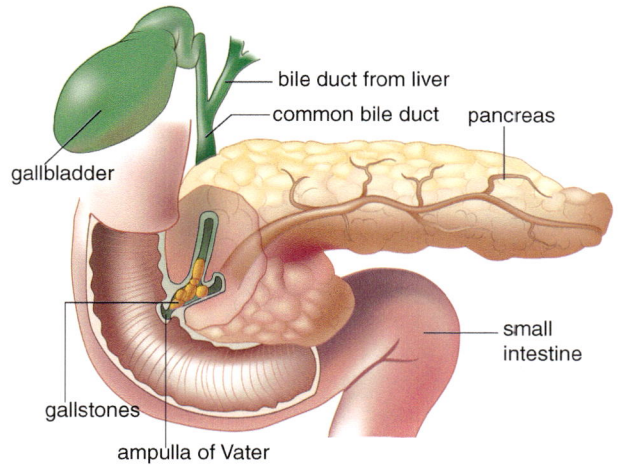

bile duct from liver

common bile duct

pancreas

gallbladder

small intestine

gallstones

ampulla of Vater

▫ **Figure 4.4**   Display of the biliary drainage system in its anatomic relaticn with the pancreas. Note how gallstones proximal to the sphincter of Oddi (ampulla of Vater) obstruct the common bile duct (choledocholithiasis). This condition predisposes to cholangitis and gallstone pancreatitis

Impact of gallstone disease on pregnancy

Episodic biliary (colic) pain, typical for gallstone disease, causes maternal stress, and with it, raises the sympathetic tone in the maternal cardiovascular system. It is conceivable that this effect contributes to the observed higher incidence of preterm birth in these women (Dhupar et al. 2010). It is unlikely that the usually asymptomatic pregnancy-induced increase in biliary sludge and bile lithogeny, and the lower fractional postprandial gallbladder ejection (Bolukbas et al. 2006) play a role in the higher risk of preterm birth. At any rate, when needed, invasive procedures, such as laparoscopic cholecystectomy are relatively well-tolerated if performed in the second trimester of pregnancy or postpartum (Dhupar et al. 2010).

Impact of pregnancy on gallstone disease

Gallstone formation is particularly facilitated in the third trimester of pregnancy, probably due to the pregnancy-induced relaxation of smooth muscles in all maternal tissues and organs with a smooth muscle wall, including the hepatobiliary system. In the latter system, smooth muscle relaxation lowers motility causing sludge and gallstone formation (Bolukbas et al. 2006). The also lower motility of the GI-tract magnifies this effect, as does the high hepatic cholesterol output during pregnancy, caused by the hepatic breakdown of the large amounts of placental steroids. Because of the high hepatic cholesterol production, the bile tends to become hyper-saturated with cholesterol. This effect facilitates gallstone formation, which is further enhanced by the concomitant relative overproduction of hydrophobic bile acids, that lower the bile's ability to dissolve cholesterol. Last but not least, the high circulating progesterone levels reduce gallbladder emptying, further promoting stone formation by causing bile stasis. Ultrasound is a reliable and safe method to identify gallstones and biliary sludge in pregnant women. The management of gallstone disease in pregnancy has been described in detail elsewhere (Date et al. 2008; De Bari et al. 2014).

4

4.2.4 **Acute appendicitis**

Appendicitis is an inflammation of the vestigial vermiform appendix located at the base of the cecum near the ileocecal valve. Once the appendix is obstructed by inflammation, the lumen fills with mucus and distends, increasing luminal and intramural pressure. This may lead to perforation of the appendix and with it, cause peritonitis. Classic symptoms of acute appendicitis are right-lower-quadrant abdominal pain (McBurney's point), anorexia, nausea and vomiting. However, many patients present with atypical or nonspecific symptoms, such as malaise, diarrhea and indigestion. Adolescents and young adults (< 40 years) are most vulnerable to develop appendicitis. The rate of (histologically confirmed) appendicitis is between 1 and 2 in 1,500 pregnancies and is the same as in the nonpregnant state (Pastore et al. 2006). Yet, acute appendicitis is the most common intestinal surgical emergency during pregnancy and also associated with a higher complication rate than in the nonpregnant state as e.g. reflected in the more than twice as high perforation rate relative to nonpregnancy (Tase et al. 2017). This is probably related to a higher incidence of atypical clinical and laboratory findings in the diagnostic work-up during pregnancy and may also explain the more than 25 % higher rate of histologically healthy appendices being removed surgically from pregnant – relative to age-matched nonpregnant patients (De Franca Neto et al. 2015). Besides, differential diagnosis of right-lower-quadrant abdominal pain in pregnancy is more complex as it also includes obstetrical complications. Acute appendicitis during pregnancy occurs most often in the second trimester and least often in the third trimester, with only half of affected pregnant women presenting with the typical right-lower-quadrant pain (Tase et al. 2017). After the first trimester, the location of the appendix migrates by about 5 cm upwards following the growing uterus toward the costal margin (◘ fig. 4.5). Since pain at this particular location can also be the most common complaint in other disorders, good clinical skills are needed to make a timely decision on appendectomy.

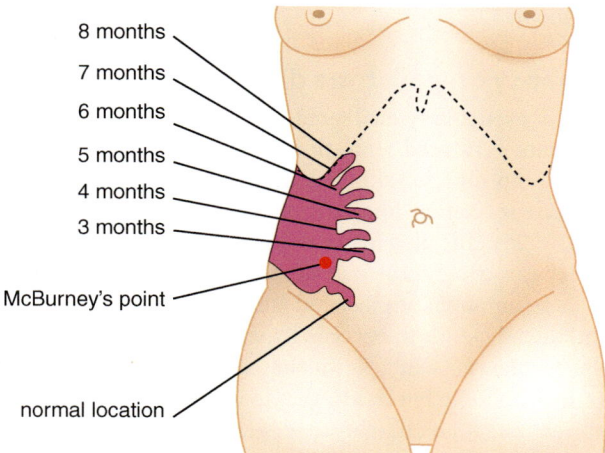

◘ **Figure 4.5**   With advancing gestational age, the appendix – along with the appendicitis-induced pain – migrates upwards towards the upper-right abdominal quadrant

Impact of appendicitis on pregnancy

In most patients, acute appendicitis induces uterine contractions, sometimes accompanied by cervical changes. Because of the high rate of complications associated with laparotomy in pregnancy, particularly in case of suspected appendicitis, prophylactic antibiotics are occasionally recommended, but their use in pregnancy is not without risk, particularly for the fetus (Pastore et al. 2006). About one-third of pregnant women that experience acute appendicitis in the first trimester will miscarriage after the appendectomy. Meanwhile, about 10 % of women having acute appendicitis followed by appendectomy in the second trimester of pregnancy, have their pregnancy complicated by preterm birth. This rate is almost twice as high as that observed in matched healthy controls (Ibiebele et al. 2019). Acute appendicitis that has developed in the third trimester is associated with a preterm birth rate as high as 20 % (Miloudi et al. 2012). A perforated infected appendix found during surgery does not predispose to more postsurgical pregnancy complications.

Impact of pregnancy on appendicitis

The most relevant impact of pregnancy on appendicitis is the often atypical clinical presentation and the lower specificity of laboratory tests in the diagnostic work-up. Recently, the value of MRI has increased markedly in the diagnostic work-up in pregnant women suspected of acute appendicitis, because of its high specificity and sensitivity at minimal risk for both mother and infant (Kave et al. 2019).

4.3 Liver disorders

4.3.1 Introduction

Pregnancy leads to a higher metabolic rate of the maternal liver, as a consequence of the extra metabolic demands associated with the breakdown of large amounts of placental products (lactate, alkaline phosphatase and α-fetoprotein and steroid hormones) and the removal of the metabolic waste products from the fetus, the placenta, along with the higher maternal basal metabolic rate. Also, the enhanced hepatic gluconeogenesis is pivotal in preventing maternal hypoglycemia developing in between meals and during the overnight fast. Therefore, liver diseases that are either associated with a lower hepatic metabolic reserve capacity (e.g. intra-hepatic cholestasis, certain genetic disorders, primary sclerosing cholangitis and hepatic cirrhosis), or result from autoimmunity (auto-immune hepatitis) have a negative impact on pregnancy. These disorders represent about 3 % of all severe pregnancy complications (Mikolasevic et al. 2018) and have been discussed in ▶ Chap. 3. Pregnancy-induced smooth-muscle relaxation lowers the motility and peristalsis of the GI tract, and with it, that of the gall bladder and biliary system. The resulting clinical effects have been discussed earlier in this chapter (▶ sect. 4.2).

Pregnancy neither alters hepatic blood flow nor liver function tests, except for those involved in the breakdown of placental products (alkaline phosphatase, α-fetoprotein). It is plausible that pregnancy-induced changes in the endocrine environment and/or those in the intestinal microbiome also alter gut-liver signaling, but if this is the case, the exact mechanism remains unclear (Dixon and Williamson 2016; Li Ren et al. 2019).

4.3.2 Acute viral liver infections during pregnancy

Viral hepatitis is associated with a substantial rate of morbidity and mortality worldwide. Even though acute infections may be self-limiting, unrecognized chronic infections and underutilization of guideline-based management contribute to rising rates of cirrhosis, liver cancer and death. Acute viral hepatitis is the most common cause of jaundice in pregnancy worldwide. Regarding acute viral hepatitis, it is important to identify the causal virus (hepatitis A, B, C, D, E, herpes simplex, varicella zoster, CMV and Epstein-Barr) to determine, whether the infection is primary or an exacerbation of a chronic viral hepatitis, and to determine, whether the infection is a sequel of another liver disorder, such as autoimmune hepatitis or acute fatty liver disease of pregnancy. Pregnancy increases the risk of hepatitis-related morbidity and mortality. The person-to-person transmission of hepatitis A and E is horizontal, by the fecal-oral route and from contaminated food and water. Hepatitis B and C are transmitted by exposure to infectious blood or body fluids. The worldwide rate of (vertical) mother-to-infant transmission of chronic hepatitis B and E is about 50 % and 5 %, respectively. Management of viral hepatitis in pregnancy requires assessing the risk of vertical transmission and the gestational age at the time of infection, along with the maternal risk of hepatic decompensation and the possible side effects of antiviral drugs (Shao et al. 2017).

Hepatitis A virus (HAV) infection

Hepatitis A virus (HAV) infection is a self-limiting, usually benign, viral infection with 1.4 million reported cases worldwide each year (Shao et al. 2017). After an incubation period of 30 ± 15 days, symptoms develop. These include malaise, anorexia, nausea, vomiting, jaundice, dark urine, abdominal pain and mild fever. Presence of the anti-HAV-immunoglobulin antibody (IgM) in the serum confirms the diagnosis. The jaundice and other symptoms usually recover gradually after about 6 weeks (Mohsen and Levy 2017). Hepatitis A in pregnancy is rare with a similar clinical course as in the nonpregnant state and no reported adverse impact on pregnancy outcome. Yet, fetal meconium peritonitis, neonatal cholestasis and preterm labor have been documented (Cho et al. 2013; Rac and Sheffield 2014). This has led to the recommendation to vaccinate high-risk women, for instance, those who consider to travel to HAV-endemic areas. HAV vaccines and immunoglobulin are safe in pregnancy. Immunoglobulin is available for post-exposure prophylaxis. There are no contra-indications against natural childbirth and breastfeeding in women with hepatitis A. Serologic testing by detection of anti-HAV immunoglobulin M (IgM) antibodies is performed in high-risk patients suspected of acute HAV infection. Prevention focuses on adherence to sanitary practices.

Hepatitis B virus (HBV) infection

Hepatitis B virus (HBV) infection is a major global health problem. Transmission occurs via parental or mucosal exposure to infected body fluids. Prevalence of HBV infection ranges from 0.4 % (USA) to 12 % in sub-Saharan Africa (Dunkelberg et al. 2014). About 240 million people worldwide have chronic HBV infection and mother to child (vertical) transmission is responsible for about half of the chronic HBV infections worldwide. Acute HBV infection during pregnancy is usually benign with no increased mortality or teratogenicity risk. Maternal symptoms are the same as in HAV. The infant is at increased risk of fetal growth restriction and preterm birth. The rate of vertical transmission of

HBV in early pregnancy is about 10 % and increases to around 60 % near term. Because of the high rate of vertical transmission and highly variable prevalence of symptom-free carriers, guidelines recommend testing of all pregnant women for hepatitis B surface antigen in the first trimester, or any time thereafter in the absence of early testing, even if they were vaccinated before pregnancy. Hepatitis B vaccination protects more then 90 % of the vaccinated, but over 5 % of individuals fail to respond to currently available vaccines. The impact of chronic HBV infection on pregnancy is probably small, although secondary liver damage (e.g. cirrhosis, portal hypertension) may adversely affect pregnancy (see ▶ Chap. 3). Acute HBV flares may occur during pregnancy and postpartum. Their management has been detailed elsewhere (Terrault et al. 2016).

A key objective in HBV is the prevention of vertical transmission, particularly during labor, when the risk is highest, particularly in women with a high viral load. To minimize vertical transmission, amniocentesis, use of scalp electrodes and prolonged rupture of membranes should be avoided. Cesarean birth does not prevent vertical transmission. Breastfeeding is not contraindicated, as the level of antiviral drugs excreted in breast milk is minimal and thus unlikely to cause toxicity. Therefore, breastfeeding is encouraged provided that the infant has received appropriate immunoprophylaxis. For women treated for cirrhosis or otherwise advanced liver pathology, antiviral therapy should be continued during pregnancy to prevent disease progression and hepatic decompensation. Pregnant HBV carriers do not require therapy. All infants should be vaccinated for HBV at birth, and all infants born to mothers who test positive for hepatitis B antigen should receive the HBV vaccine and the immune globulin within 24 hours postpartum. The vaccination program is to be completed within 6 months. Obviously, vaccination and passive immunoprophylaxis reduces the transmission risk substantially.

Chronic hepatitis C virus (HCV) infection

Chronic hepatitis C virus (HCV) infection is a blood-borne infection affecting about 150 million people worldwide. The global prevalence of HCV is 2–3 % (Shao et al. 2017; Rac and Sheffield 2014). The rate of vertical transmission in pregnant women with chronic HCV is 3–5 %, a rate that is twice as high in women co-infected with HIV. The most important risk factor for HCV infection is past or current intravenous drug use. The incubation time is 5–10 weeks. Other risk factors are the same as those in nonpregnant women, namely, contact with contaminated blood. Initial screening is by HCV antibody testing, and if inconclusive, by an HCV RNA test to confirm the diagnosis. HCV infection is usually asymptomatic and, therefore, identified either by screening high-risk patients or in patients with persistently elevated aminotransferase levels. Acute HCV infection during pregnancy is rare. During pregnancy, supportive treatment of HCV is sufficient as the impact on pregnancy is small. The risk of vertical transmission is minimal, if amniocentesis, the use of scalp electrodes and prolonged rupture of membranes are avoided. There is no vaccine or immune globulin for prevention. HCV infection should not influence mode of delivery and is not a contra-indication for breastfeeding.

Hepatitis delta or hepatitis D

Hepatitis delta or hepatitis D is a hepatitis caused by the hepatitis D (delta) virus (HDV), a small defective RNA virus that requires HBsAg for transmission and packaging (Mohsen and Levy 2017). Therefore, HDV is considered to be a sub-viral satellite, as it can only propagate in the presence of HBV. HDV has co- or superinfected about

4 % of the 350 million HBV carriers worldwide (Alvarado-Mora et al. 2013). Superinfection with HDV in an HBV carrier leads to the most severe form of viral hepatitis, as also indicated by a relatively high mortality rate (Yurdaydin 2017). The WHO recommends testing for HDV in HBV-positive pregnant women. Prevention of HDV infection requires prevention of HBV. Treatment of HDV in pregnancy is supportive (Shao et al. 2017).

Acute hepatitis E (HEV)

Acute hepatitis E (HEV) is caused by the hepatitis E virus (genotype 1 and 2) and affects about 20 million subjects worldwide yearly, predominantly in developing countries. The mortality rate in symptomatic patients is relatively high (2 %), often in conjunction with fulminant liver failure (Shao et al. 2017). Horizontal transmission is mainly by fecal-oral contamination. In an animal model, HEV infection was transmitted vertically to the fetus with HEV replication in the placenta. Pregnancy in HEV-infected women is at increased risk of stillbirth, preterm birth and antepartum bleeding, causing a high rate of adverse pregnancy outcomes. Management of acute HEV is supportive (Shao et al. 2017).

Herpes simplex (HSV) hepatitis

Herpes simplex (HSV) hepatitis is caused by HSV-1 (main target: oral mucosa, but nowadays increasingly also the genital tract mucosa) and HSV-2 (main target: genital tract mucosa) (Magawa et al. 2020). Both HSVs are common, contagious viruses spread by infected individuals. More than 60 % and 10 % of the world population under the age of 50 years, has experienced an infection with HSV-1 and -2, respectively. HSV-2 infection is one of the most common sexually transmitted infections. Because of their neurotrophy, the HSVs are able to persist in the body after the primary infection by hiding from the immune system within the neurons, to be re-activated any time after the primary infection. The disease onset is often abrupt with the typical appearance of multiple vesicular lesions. The primary infection may be accompanied by fever and malaise. Type-specific antibodies against HSV develop in the first weeks after the primary infection and persist indefinitely. In general, the course of re-activated herpes is much milder than the primary disease.

Immune-compromised patients are most susceptible to develop HSV hepatitis, but also pregnant women are at increased risk. HSV hepatitis in pregnancy has a very serious course and is associated with a high maternal and perinatal mortality (McCormack et al. 2019). This complication is to be suspected, whenever serum transaminases increase acutely, and are paralleled by the development of coagulopathy, high fever and malaise, without jaundice. About half of the patients also develops typical mucocutaneous lesions. The diagnosis HSV hepatitis is confirmed by a liver biopsy based on the presence of typical intranuclear inclusions and HSV antigens by immunofluorescence (◘ fig. 4.6). Vertical transmission from mother to fetus is exceptional in the presence of antibodies before pregnancy (Silasi et al. 2015). As a consequence, the highest rate of vertical transmissions occurs in pregnant women that lack these antibodies, but develop a primary HSV infection, the most vulnerable period being the third trimester of pregnancy (Lee and Nair 2017). Treatment with acyclovir should not be delayed if HSV hepatitis is suspected. The clinical management has been detailed elsewhere (McCormack et al. 2019).

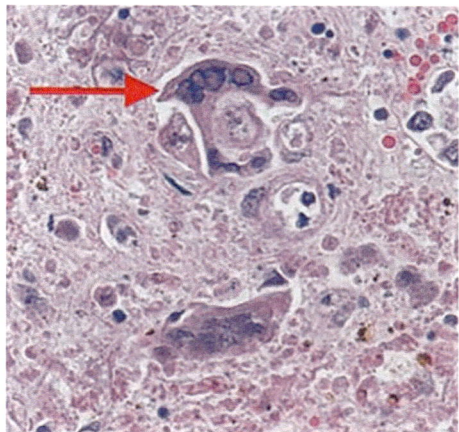

◘ Figure 4.6   HSV hepatitis liver biopsy, the hepatocytes (arrow) show multinucleation with intranuclear viral inclusions at the periphery of necrotic tissue

4.3.3 Wilson's disease

Progressive hepatolenticular degeneration or Wilson's disease (WD) is an autosomal recessive disorder giving rise to a molecular defect of the p-type ATPase ATP7B, which is an essential enzyme involved in copper transport across cellular membranes. Impaired biliary copper excretion leads to accumulation of copper (incorporated in ceruloplasmin) in the blood causing pathological hepatic and cerebral copper deposition and eventually, primarily hepatic and cerebral disease. The prevalence of WD ranges from 1 to 3 cases per 100,000 subjects (Ala et al. 2007) and the disease affects hepatic copper transport from birth onwards. The mean age at diagnosis is 13 years (ranging from 5 to 35 years). Typical Kayser-Fleischer rings, resulting from copper deposits in the corneal margins, are often present (◘ fig. 4.7). They reflect the high degree of copper storage in the body.

WD is usually diagnosed by a combination of blood tests (low serum copper and ceruloplasmin levels together with raised urinary copper excretion) and clinical findings (Kayser-Fleischer corneal ring), or by the detection of bi-allelic *ATP7B* pathogenic variants on molecular genetic testing. WD mostly leads to a combination of hepatic, neurologic and psychiatric symptoms. Acute liver failure in WD-affected subjects is often accompanied by hemolysis, a symptom that may also occur episodically, independent of liver failure. Liver disease may present itself by recurrent jaundice, simple acute self-limited hepatitis-like illness, autoimmune-type hepatitis, fulminant liver failure, or chronic liver disease. Neurologic presentations include movement disorders (e.g. poor coordination, tremors, loss of fine-motor control) or rigid dystonia (e.g. mask-like facies, rigidity, gait disturbance). Psychiatric disorders include e.g. neurotic behavior, depression and disorganized personality. Untreated WD is fatal, with most patients dying from liver disease, and a minority from complications of progressive neurologic disease. With chelation therapy and liver transplantation, prolonged survival has become the norm (EASL clinical practice guidelines 2012).

4

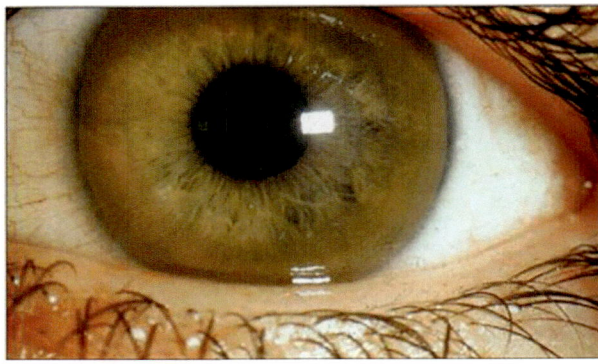

□ Figure 4.7   Kayser-Fleischer rings are brownish discolorations at the outer margins of the cornea due to copper deposition. They are pathognomic for Wilson's disease. These rings can only be identified reliably by a skilled observer using a slit-light (*adopted from* Ala et al. 2007)

At conception, the chance that a sibling of a WD-affected person is affected or a non-carrier, is 1 in 4. This sibling has also a 50 % chance of being an asymptomatic carrier. Once the pathogenic variant has been identified, carrier testing is possible for at-risk relatives, as is prenatal testing and preimplantation genetic diagnosis for pregnancies at increased risk of WD. The copper status in women with WD should be optimized prior to pregnancy. Identifying new WD patients in pregnancy is rare, but cases of reduced fertility and recurrent spontaneous miscarriages in untreated WD women have been reported.

Impact of pregnancy on WD

In asymptomatic WD patients that continue their chelation therapy in pregnancy, liver function only deteriorates transiently in about 6 % of cases, followed by complete recovery postpartum. In one study, the rate of *de novo* neurological complications during pregnancy in WP patients was just around 1 %. However, the typical symptoms (1x ataxia, 1x spasticity and 1x worsening tremor) did not recover postpartum. Importantly, 93 % of WD patients did not experience a change in health state during pregnancy (Pfeiffenberger et al. 2018).

Impact of WD on pregnancy course and outcome

The rate of first-trimester spontaneous abortion in WD patients – undiagnosed at the time of conception – is higher (41 % vs. 19 %, p < 0.001), and life birth rate lower (59 % vs. 82 %, p < 0.01) than in their (diagnosed) pregnant counterparts, who had chelation therapy throughout pregnancy (Pfeiffenberger et al. 2018). The rate of birth defects in both subgroups does not differ from that in the general population. Undiagnosed, untreated pregnant WP patients also have an increased risk of developing a hypertensive disorder in pregnancy, but without signs of fetal growth restriction (Malik et al. 2013). These data support the concept that pregnancy in WD-affected women benefits from continuing chelation therapy (Sternlieb 2000). Nevertheless, copper deficiency is a potential risk factor for birth defects. Therefore, over-chelating – or more precisely over-decoppering – should be prevented by calculating dose reduction of anti-copper drugs during pregnancy (Pfeiffenberger et al. 2018). Infants born from WP mothers are obligate carriers of the autosomal recessive genetic defect that causes WD (Dufernez et al. 2013) and their mothers should be informed about the need for screening their children for WD. The clinical management of WD has been detailed elsewhere (Ala et al. 2007; EASL clinical guidelines: Wilson's disease 2012).

4.3.4 Hepatocellular adenoma (HCA)

Hepatocellular adenoma (HCA) refers to a rare disorder, characterized by encapsulated benign liver nodules with a diameter ranging from 0.5 to 15 cm and with arterial vascularization, but no portal tract or cholangial proliferation. It develops from a rare proliferation of hepatocytes in an otherwise normal liver and is usually located in the right lobe. Proliferating hepatocytes often resemble normal cells that may be steatotic or show glycogen storage with only few mitoses (Bioulac-Sage et al. 2017). Over two-thirds of HCA nodules are solitary (◘ fig. 4.8). Insight into the pathogenesis of HCAs is still incomplete (Rebouissou et al. 2008). The available evidence suggests that environmental factors, such as exposure to steroids, high alcohol intake and obesity, may trigger mutations that initiate the development of a HCA (Vijay et al. 2015). The reported incidence of only 3 in a million individuals (Vijay et al. 2015) is most likely an underestimation of the true incidence, as many HCAs remain asymptomatic and therefore, are only diagnosed accidentally. The same applies to other benign liver masses, such as focal nodular hyperplasia (Cobey and Salem 2004).

Various studies have provided evidence for a causal role of estrogen in the development of HCA. HCAs usually regress after discontinuation of estrogen intake. The chance that HCA causes vague abdominal pain is size-dependent. Bleeding and malignant transformation are the most notorious complications. In general, it is recommended to perform preventive ablation or surgical removal, if the HCA diameter exceeds 5 cm, if only to minimize bleeding risk.

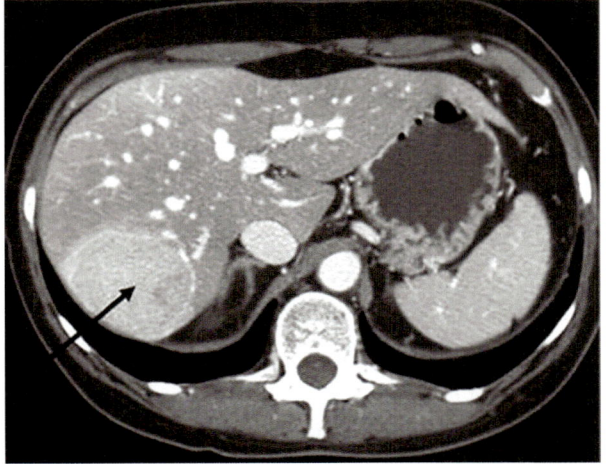

◘ **Figure 4.8**   CT scan of a large hepatocellular adenoma. (Source: Dept. Radiology, Div. Body Imaging, University of Washington Seattle [WA], USA)

Impact of pregnancy on HCA

In 1 in 4 women with a preexistent HCA, the adenoma grows during pregnancy, though, with minimal risk for mother and fetus, particularly, when the HCA is smaller than 5 cm (Gaspersz et al. 2020). Yet, preexistent HCAs should be monitored closely throughout pregnancy (with ultrasound or MRI) particularly if their initial size exceeds 5 cm and especially in the third trimester, when estrogen levels are highest and with it, the risk of HCA rupture. Rupture with hemorrhage, is potentially lethal for both mother and infant (Cobey and Salem 2004). Whether certain subtypes are more prone to complications during pregnancy is unknown, as most diagnosed HCAs are dormant at the time of discovery.

Impact of HCA on pregnancy

An HCA that does not rupture during pregnancy, has no appreciable negative impact on pregnancy course and outcome (Cobey and Salem 2004). If removal of an HCA during pregnancy is indicated and the intervention is performed and completed uneventfully, the impact on pregnancy course and outcome is probably small (Agrawal et al. 2015). Recently, some experts assembled a sub-classification system to serve as a guide in determining the optimal clinical management in various cases of HCA (Thomeer et al. 2016; Nault et al. 2017). HCAs smaller than 5 cm in diameter should be monitored with serial ultrasound, at least until one year postpartum as detailed elsewhere (Klompenhouwer et al. 2017).

4.4 Endocrine disorders

4.4.1 Introduction

The endocrine system is a chemical messenger system that consists of a set of endocrine glands secreting hormones, that together with the heart (α-ANP) and kidneys (renin, erythropoietin), play key roles in the regulation of blood pressure, red cell mass and intravascular volume, respectively. The hypothalamus forms the coordination center of the endocrine system and sends signals to the pituitary gland (hypothalamic-pituitary axis) by means of releasing and inhibiting factors, while also acting as a bridge between central-nervous and endocrine systems. It consolidates signals derived from the autonomic nervous system, the upper cortical inputs and the environment, such as light and temperature. Major endocrine glands are the pituitary gland, thyroid, parathyroid, adrenals, pancreas, kidneys and gonads. ◘ Figure 4.9 illustrates the functions of these endocrine organs (except for heart and kidneys). The hypothalamus is located at the base of the brain, below the third ventricle and just above the optic chiasm and pituitary gland. The pituitary gland regulates the function of various target organs by releasing hormones. A normal endocrine function is closely interlinked with a normal pregnancy. Endocrine disorders can be managed appropriately, as long as they are detected early (preferable preconceptionally).

Before and during pregnancy, endocrine dysfunction can be detected by screening and pragmatic counseling. Taking a detailed history and conducting a targeted physical examination is essential, when endocrine dysfunction is suspected on the basis of menstrual disturbances, frequent headaches, visual symptoms, galactorrhea, bone pains,

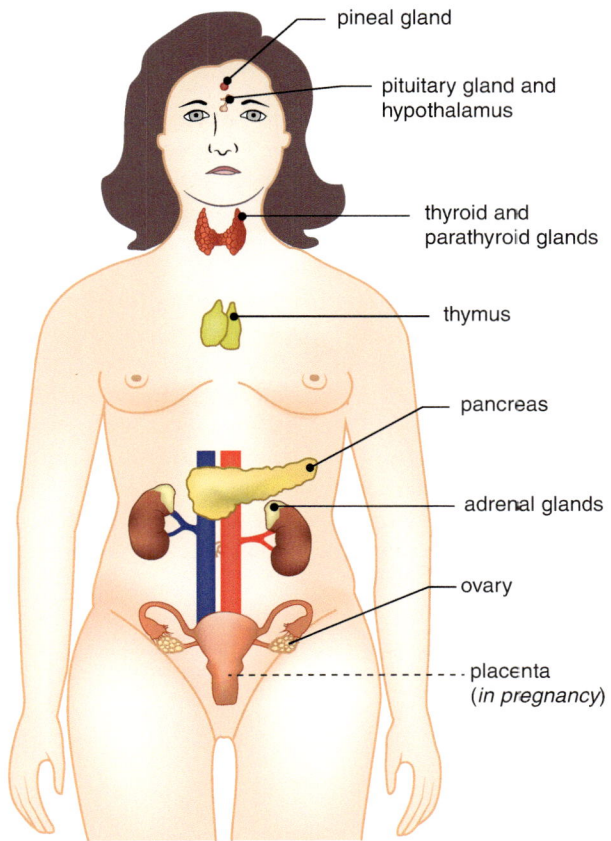

▣ Figure 4.9 The female endocrine system consists of various hormone-producing glands that regulate a wide range of body functions

muscle weakness, hirsutism, obesity/weight gain and signs of hypo- or hyperthyroidism. Women presenting with unintentional infertility, poor obstetric history or a previous history of endocrine dysfunction should be tested accordingly. Obviously, maternal and fetal outcomes benefit from optimizing a preexistent endocrine disorder prior to pregnancy. Endocrine disorders may interfere with pregnancy, not only by disrupting the placenta-induced cardiovascular and metabolic adaptive changes. Excessive circulating levels of certain hormones may also cross the placenta and adversely impact fetal development and/or fetal growth.

During pregnancy, the placenta produces large amounts of hormones, such as hCG, progesterone, estrogen, prolactin and placental lactogen (hPL), with maximum output of these hormones varying depending on the demands associated with each phase of pregnancy. For instance, in the 6–8 weeks post-implantation period, a rapidly rising output of hCG preserves luteal function by suppressing the hypothalamic axis and with it, the menstrual cycle. This luteal "rescue" has two crucial effects in early pregnancy. First, it maintains the progesterone output, which is key for successful implantation and second, it preserves and enhances the release by the corpus luteum of relaxin, a key factor in the institution of a high-flow and low-resistance circulation as detailed in ► Chap. 1. In mid-pregnancy, the placental endocrine function is mostly involved in securing the transplacental supply and demand of nutrients, oxygen and metabolic waste products. To this end, placental steroids, in concert with hPL and various growth factors initially induce maternal anabolism, building up sufficiently large glycogen and fat reserves, which are mobilized again in the second half of pregnancy to meet the then progressively increasing fetal demands. Meanwhile, in late pregnancy, the placental progesterone output declines in concert with a relative rise in placental estrogen output. This combination of steroid changes contributes to the eventual onset of labor.

These inferences support the concept that the placenta is a *dynamic* fetal organ, that 'intrudes' into the maternal endocrine system to serve primarily fetal interests and thus also includes avoiding maternal health risks. These fetal interests differ in the various phases of pregnancy. The quality of the placenta-induced adaptive changes depends on both maternal and fetal wellbeing. A normally functioning placenta integrates maternal and fetal signals in the various stages of pregnancy and uses its hormones mostly for two purposes: first, in early and late pregnancy, to create immune tolerance enabling embryo implantation and to prepare for labor, respectively, and second, throughout pregnancy, to build up and then later on, reallocate maternal nutrient resources in order to meet fetal nutrient requirements (◘ fig. 4.10).

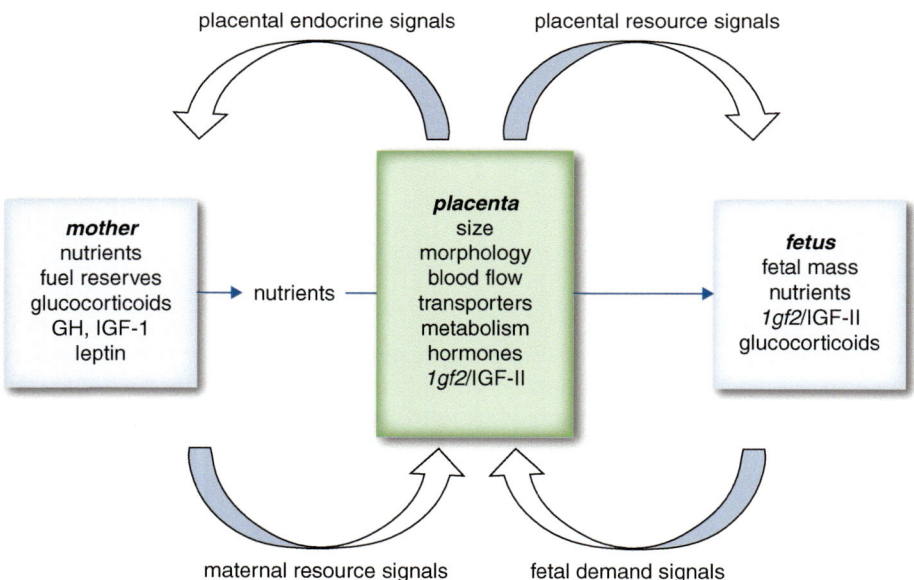

◘ Figure 4.10 Schematic diagram showing some of the maternal, placental and fetal factors that are involved in the transplacental resource allocation from mother to fetus. 1gf2 is a paternally-expressed imprinted gene encoding for the most potent fetoplacental growth factor, IGF-II (insulin-like growth factor II). In this context it is relevant to mention that the complex 1gf2/IGF-II plays a key role in resource allocation by identifying mismatches between fetal demand and placental supply of nutrients. *Abbreviations*: GH, growth hormone, IGF-I, insulin-like growth factor-I. (*for details: see article by* Fowden and Moore 2012)

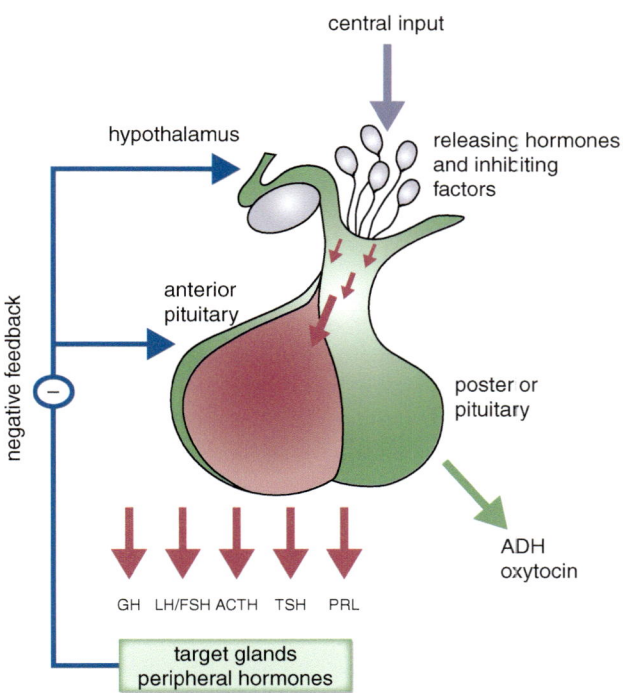

Figure 4.11 Interaction between hypothalamus and pituitary gland, and the various hormones released by the gland's two lobes. Feedback loops modulate hormone release in order to maintain homeostasis. (Schneider et al. 2007)

The *pituitary gland* is located in a bony cavity (sella turcica) at the base of the brain, and regulates the function of a number of target organs by releasing hormones, with feedback loops to modulate their release. The anterior pituitary lobe produces adreno-corticotropic hormone (ACTH), thyrotrophic hormone (TSH), luteinizing hormone (LH), follicle-stimulating hormone (FSH), prolactin (PRL) and growth hormone (GH). Their secretion is regulated by hypothalamic stimulating and inhibiting factors and by negative feedback inhibition of their peripheral hormones (■ fig. 4.11). The intermediate lobe secretes melanocyte stimulating hormone (MSH). The posterior pituitary lobe or neurohypophysis is functionally connected to the hypothalamus and acts as a storage site for hypothalamic hormones, antidiuretic hormone (ADH/vasopressin) and oxytocin.

During pregnancy, the placenta influences the pituitary gland with its endocrine arsenal, inducing both hyperplasia of the lactotroph cells and a rise in circulating prolactin levels. Placental estrogen accelerates the hepatic output of hormone-binding globulins, thus expanding the circulating pool of active placental steroids, cortisol, thyroxin and GH. This effect and that of other endocrine changes in pregnancy, may mask a suspected endocrine disorder, as symptoms of these disorders overlap with those of normal pregnancy and with it, complicate the diagnostic work-up. Pituitary disorders in pregnancy are rare (Chrisoulidou et al. 2015), but if present, may adversely affect pregnancy course and outcome. Therefore, clinical exploration of a suspected disorder, preferably before pregnancy, is crucial. Pregnancy may worsen some disorders, such as subclinical hypopituitarism or prolactinoma. Other hormone-producing pituitary adenomas are rare during childbearing age. Last but not least, the size of the pituitary gland more than doubles during pregnancy.

4.4.2 Hypopituitarism

Hypopituitarism refers to subnormal output of pituitary hormones due to diseases of the pituitary gland or the hypothalamus. The estimated prevalence and yearly number of new cases of hypopituitarism is about 1 in 25,000 (Higham et al. 2016). The true prevalence, though, is probably higher since clinical signs are usually nonspecific, which delays diagnosis. Pituitary diseases may result from a traumatic brain injury, ischemic stroke, infiltrative disorders (such as sarcoidosis), infections (such as meningitis), subarachnoid hemorrhage, pregnancy-related infarction (Sheehan syndrome), pituitary mass lesions (adenomas) or lymphocytic hypophysitis. If a pituitary disorder is caused by an adenoma, it is important to know, whether or not this mass produces hormones or only leads to mechanical pressure on the surrounding tissue. Below, only the two most common postpartum causes of hypopituitarism will be discussed.

Sheehan's syndrome

Sheehan's syndrome is caused by infarction and necrosis of the pituitary gland after postpartum hemorrhage complicated by hypotension (Diri et al. 2016). Due to improved obstetrical care in developed countries, the rate of severe postpartum hemorrhage has fallen markedly over the last decades. However, in developing countries Sheehan's syndrome remains a common cause of hypopituitarism. Women suspected of having developed this complication should be tested accordingly. Subnormal serum levels of prolactin, gonadotrophins, ACTH, GH and TSH confirm the diagnosis. Clinically, these women have both deferred postpartum onset of lactation and persistent amenorrhea postpartum. Subnormal levels of TSH, free T4 and free T3 indicate secondary hypothyroidism. About half of these women also have adrenal insufficiency reflected in early-morning subnormal serum cortisol levels (< 3 µg/dL or 80 nmol/L), often accompanied by hyponatremia and episodes of disturbed consciousness. At the time of diagnosis, half of the patients have complete hypopituitarism that coincide with the typical postpartum symptoms. The other half has partial hypopituitarism with only mild symptoms, sometimes only developing years later. Particularly, in case of adrenal insufficiency, replacement therapy should be started promptly. If the pituitary gland is partially infarcted and the diagnosis is still uncertain, additional tests may be needed. Routine testing for prolactin deficiency is not recommended, because of the limited specificity of subnormal serum prolactin levels.

Lymphocytic hypophysitis

Lymphocytic hypophysitis is a rare disorder of unknown autoimmune etiology often occurring in late pregnancy or postpartum (Joshi et al. 2018). The disorder is initially characterized by lymphocytic infiltration, an enlarged pituitary gland, followed by destruction of pituitary cells. Lymphocytic hypophysitis should be kept in mind in the differential diagnosis.

Effect of hypopituitarism on pregnancy

Pregnancy in an untreated patient with hypopituitarism is exceptional, because of infertility (Du et al. 2014). Suboptimal treatment of hypopituitarism predisposes to complications, such as miscarriage, preterm birth, hypertensive disorders, placental abruption and postpartum hemorrhage.

Effect of pregnancy on hypopituitarism

Patients with hypopituitarism using hormonal replacement therapy ought to be counselled preconceptionally to evaluate the quality of the hypothalamic-pituitary-adrenal axis and if needed, to optimize the dose of their medication. This may include GH replacement and adjustment of the levothyroxine dose to obtain high-normal free T4 levels. Properly-treated patients have no increased risk of maternal and fetal adverse effects. It is possible that the replacement medication needs to be adjusted during pregnancy, because of the effect of placental hormones.

4.4.3 Prolactinoma and hyperprolactinemia

Prolactin is a protein secreted by the lactotroph cells in the anterior lobe of the pituitary gland, regulated by endocrine neurons in the hypothalamus. Its role is to induce lactation in females. Lactotroph adenomas (prolactinomas) can produce excessive amounts of prolactin (Molitch 2011). In women of childbearing age, markedly raised serum prolactin levels (> 100 ng/mL or 100 µg/L) are typically associated with ovarian dysfunction. Amenorrhea, infertility, vaginal dryness, hot flushes, and occasionally galactorrhea are symptoms of ovarian dysfunction. Moderately elevated serum prolactin levels (levels of 50 to 100 µg/L) cause oligomenorrhea or amenorrhea, whereas mild prolactinemia (levels between 20 to 50 µg/L) causes luteal insufficiency. This implies that also mild hyperprolactinemia interferes with a woman's fertility. Hyperprolactinemia may also cause headaches, visual field defects, unexpected weight gain and reduced bone density. Ovarian dysfunction in hyperprolactinemia results from inhibition of LH, and perhaps FSH secretion, by inhibiting the release of gonadotropin-releasing hormone. Only symptomatic prolactin-secreting, pituitary adenomas require preconceptional treatment with dopamine agonists to lower prolactin levels, reduce tumor size, and restore ovary function.

Effect of hyperprolactinemia on pregnancy

Hyperprolactinemia does not directly affect pregnancy course and outcome. The use of dopamine agonists in pregnancy does not increase the risk of congenital malformations.

Effect of pregnancy on hyperprolactinemia

As mentioned above, the size of the pituitary gland almost doubles in the course of pregnancy (which may also apply to prolactin-secreting pituitary adenomas). This growth increases the risk of visual field defects due to pressure of the gland on the optic chiasm. It follows that these tumors should be evaluated preconceptionally and managed accordingly as detailed elsewhere (Varlamov et al. 2019).

4.4.4 **Thyroid**

The thyroid gland, located at the anterior side of the neck, secretes the hormones involved in the metabolism, thyroxine (T4), triiodothyronine (T3), and also calcitonin that opposes the effects of parathyroid hormone. The thyroidal T3/T4 output is regulated by TSH, secreted by the anterior lobe of the pituitary gland, that itself is regulated by thyrotropin-releasing hormone (TRH) from the hypothalamus (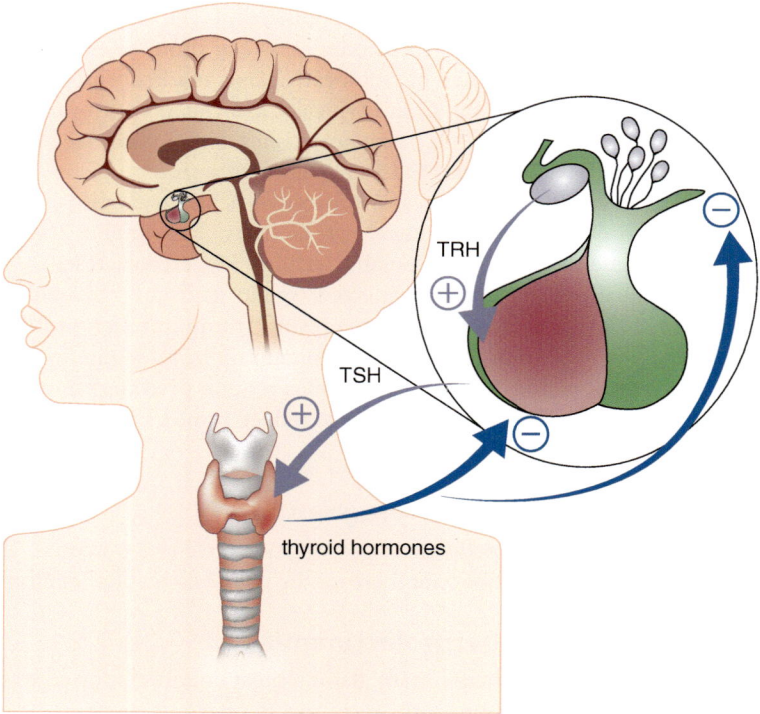 fig. 4.12). T3/T4 play key roles in the regulation of various metabolic processes important for growth and development in the infant, and remain important in regulating the metabolism in adulthood. The thyroid hormone status correlates with bodyweight and energy expenditure (Mullur et al. 2014).

T3 is the active thyroid hormone, and for about 80 % produced by the deiodination of T4. Over 99 % of T4 and T3 is protein-bound, mostly to thyroid-hormone-binding globulin (TBG). The unbound fractions of T3 and T4 are known as free T3 (FT3) and free T4 (FT4). A crucial mechanism of thyroid hormone regulation is its local activation from inactive T4 to active T3, which is essential in stimulating growth and development, besides its metabolic effects, which include inducing a higher basal metabolic rate, cardiac output, heart rate, respiratory rate and catabolism of carbohydrates and proteins. Iodine is an essential component required for the production of T3 and T4.

■ **Figure 4.12**   Feedback mechanisms between hypothalamus and pituitary gland, and between the pituitary – and thyroid gland regulating the release of thyroid hormones. *Abbreviations*: *TRH*, thyrotropin-releasing hormone; *TSH*, thyroid-stimulating hormone

Normal thyroid function during pregnancy

Normal thyroid function during pregnancy is pivotal for both mother and infant (Korevaar et al. 2017). The maternal iodide pool declines as a result of increased thyroid hormone production, transplacental iodine transfer to the fetus and increased renal iodine clearance due to renal hyperfiltration. It follows that iodine requirements during pregnancy are twice as high as before pregnancy. The recommended daily iodine intake in pregnancy is 250 μg. Iodine deficiency leads to thyroid insufficiency in both mother and fetus. In iodine-sufficient areas, women known with lactose intolerance, gluten intolerance, or use a low-carbohydrate or vegan diet are likely to require iodine supplementation during pregnancy. Pregnancy alters the thyroid function as follows (also illustrated in ◘ fig. 4.13):

– pregnancy leads to the doubling of the circulating TBG levels in response to an estradiol-induced higher hepatic TBG production combined with a slower peripheral metabolic TBG breakdown (Parkes et al. 2013). These two effects induce a compensatory rise in T3/T4 production throughout pregnancy.

– After embryo implantation, serum human chorionic gonadotropin (hCG) levels rise progressively to reach a peak by about 10 weeks pregnancy, followed by a decline afterwards. hCG binds to the TSH receptor on the thyroid-cell membrane and acts as a weak stimulant of T3/T4 production/output and with it, partly suppresses TSH. Presumably, because of the also higher serum TBG levels, most of the extra output of T3/T4 is bound to TBG with free T3/T4 serum levels remaining within the normal range and serum TSH levels somewhat suppressed. In late pregnancy, total circulating T4 has increased by about 50 % above the pre-pregnant level.

– Abundantly expressed deiodinase in the placenta, chorion, and amnion accelerates the T3/T4 degradation to inactive iodothyronine (reverse T3).

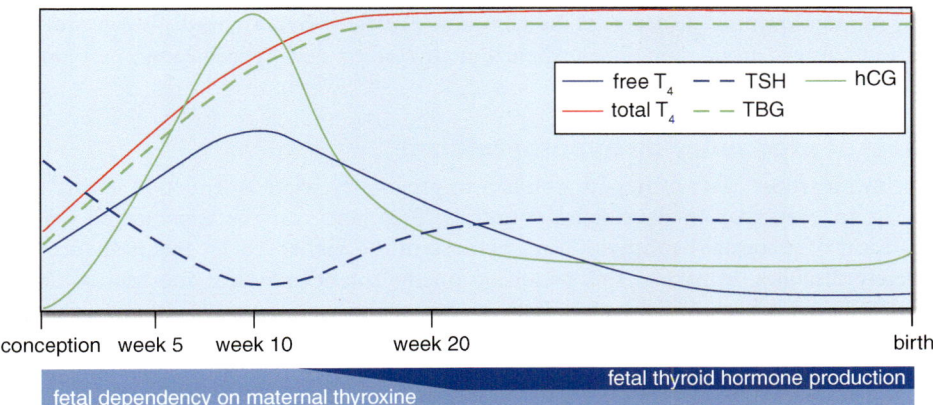

◘ **Figure 4.13**　Changes in thyroid function during pregnancy. In pregnancy, the functional efficacy of the available thyroid hormone (total T_4) is reduced by higher circulating levels of thyroxine-binding globulin (TBG), increased thyroxine uptake by the fetus and higher placental degradation. By increasing its output, the efficacy of functional thyroid hormone (free T_4) is maintained. Most of the upregulation in the first trimester results from thyroidal stimulation by human chorionic gonadotropin (hCG), which emphasizes the infant's dependence on maternal thyroxine in the first trimester (*adopted from* Korevaar et al. 2017)

During pregnancy, the normal range of peripheral TSH and T3/T4 levels are trimester-specific. The fetal thyroid only begins to concentrate iodine at around 10 weeks, with fetal pituitary TSH controlling T3/T4 synthesis and output only from 20 weeks onwards. It follows that the infant's growth and development until the 20th week depends almost entirely on maternal T4 supply reaching the fetus in small amounts to supplement embryonic thyroid function. Yet, at birth about 30 % of total T4 in cord blood is still from maternal origin.

4

4.4.5 Hypothyroidism

Hypothyroidism is diagnosed by abnormal lab tests, also because common symptoms lack specificity (fatigue, lethargy, weight gain, cold intolerance, bradycardia, irregular menstruation, constipation, change of voice, dry skin and muscle cramps). The prevalence of hypothyroidism in pregnant women in developed (iodine-sufficient) countries is about 2–3 % with overt hypothyroidism only observed in about 0.5 % of these cases (Pearce 2015; Chaker et al. 2017). Overt hypothyroidism refers to the combination of raised serum TSH and subnormal serum FT4 levels, whereas subclinical hypothyroidism refers to an isolated rise in serum TSH with serum FT4 still in the normal range. In women with central hypothyroidism due to hypothalamic or pituitary disease, both serum TSH and FT4 levels are low. Chronic autoimmune thyroiditis (Hashimoto's thyroiditis) is the most common cause of hypothyroidism in women living in iodine-sufficient areas. The prevalence of Hashimoto's thyroiditis is higher in females (7:1 versus males) and increases with age. It is clinically characterized by gradual thyroid failure with or without goiter formation due to autoimmune-mediated destruction of the thyroid gland. Nearly all patients with Hashimoto's thyroiditis have high circulating levels of antibodies against at least 1 thyroid antigen, particularly TPO-Ab or Tg-Ab. Details about autoimmune hypothyroidism (AITD) have been provided in ► Chap. 3, in the section on autoimmune disorders. Less common causes of hypothyroidism are previous thyroid surgery, neck radiation, postpartum thyroiditis and hypothalamic or pituitary disease.

Effect of pregnancy on hypothyroidism

Worldwide, most cases of hypothyroidism in pregnancy relate to endemic iodine deficiency, in particular in developing countries. Pregnancy can be expected to worsen this form of maternal hypothyroidism, because of the higher T3/T4 requirements. The severely disabling impact of this condition on the infant's physical and mental development is probably most relevant. Euthyroid pregnant women with either circulating antithyroid antibodies (TPO-Ab and Tg-Ab) or a history of post-hemithyroidectomy or treatment with radioactive iodine, are at increased risk that their often subclinical hypothyroidism evolves to overt hypothyroidism during pregnancy requiring thyroid hormone supplementation to prevent the adverse impact on the developing infant. The clinical management of hypothyroidism in pregnancy has been detailed elsewhere (Alexander et al. 2017).

Effect of hypothyroidism on pregnancy

Pregnancy in women with overt hypothyroidism, is rare as overt hypothyroidism reduces fertility. Rare pregnancies within this group usually end in a spontaneous miscarriage (Parkes et al. 2013). Meanwhile, pregnancy in women with subclinical hypothyroidism is more common (about 2 % in the US) and is at increased risk of a hypertensive disorder, and possibly also preterm birth, placental abruption and neonatal admission to an intensive care unit. Timely and adequate supplementation of levothyroxine normalizes these risks. In the first half of pregnancy, the infant depends on maternal FT4 that crosses the placenta and with it, preserves normal fetal thyroid development/function. Anti-TPO and anti-Tg antibodies do not cross the placenta.

Postpartum thyroiditis is an auto-immune disorder that affects about 8 % of pregnant women in the first year postpartum. Type-1 DM patients are particularly at risk, as are women with a history of postpartum thyroiditis or with circulating TPO antibodies. The disorder is accompanied by transient hyperthyroidism followed by transient or permanent hypothyroidism, often combined with the development of a small painless goiter. Most patients recover within a year, but the condition may relapse after a subsequent pregnancy. Between 20 % and 40 % of the cases will have developed permanent hypothyroidism within 3 to 12 years. Nearly all women with postpartum thyroiditis have TPO-antibodies.

4.4.6 Hyperthyroidism

Hyperthyroidism is a pathological disorder in which excess thyroid hormone is synthesized and secreted by the thyroid gland. If overt, it is characterized by excessive FT4 and/or FT3 levels along with subnormal circulating TSH levels. Subclinical hyperthyroidism is characterized by subnormal circulating TSH levels that coincide with normal serum FT4 and FT3 levels. In Europe and the US, the prevalence of hyperthyroidism is about 1 % and increases with age. It occurs 5 times more in females than in males (De Leo et al. 2016). In 80 % of the cases in iodine-sufficient areas, hyperthyroidism is caused by Graves' disease, an autoimmune disorder with circulating antibodies against the TSH receptor (Tr-Abs) confirming the diagnosis. The exact cause of Graves' disease is unclear, although it is generally believed that genetic and environmental factors are involved in causing loss of immunotolerance and the development of Tr-Abs. There is evidence for a genetic predisposition, though with a low penetrance as suggested by a concordance rate in monozygotic twins of less than one-third. Common clinical signs of hyperthyroidism include palpitations, tremor, dyspnea, weight loss, diarrhea, vomiting, polydipsia, dysphagia, heat intolerance with warm skin, increased sweating, anxiety and cognitive impairment. Only patients with Graves' disease have ophthalmopathy, but other eye symptoms such as stare and lid lag occur in all patients with hyperthyroidism. Clinical management has been detailed elsewhere (Alexander et al. 2017). Subclinical hyperthyroidism does not require treatment during pregnancy. hCG-mediated, overt hyperthyroidism (gestational transient thyrotoxicosis) does not require treatment with antithyroid drugs, because of its usually transient and mild nature, and only occasionally is supportive therapy required. Betablockers, such as metoprolol or propranolol (but not atenolol), can be used to treat symptoms, such as hyperthyroid-related tachycardia and tremor.

Effect of pregnancy on hyperthyroidism

Women managed for hyperthyroidism and intending to conceive are strongly advised to seek preconceptional counseling to critically evaluate the quality of disease control and the possible teratogenicity of their medication. The treatment objective is to maintain a state of mild maternal hyperthyroidism, to secure minimal risk of fetal hypothyroidism. In the first trimester of pregnancy, transient physiologic hCG-induced hyperthyroidism occurs in 1–3 % of all pregnancies. It is the most common cause of hyperthyroidism, but in some of the affected women, subclinical Grave's disease may become overt. Gestational hyperthyroidism is limited to the first half of pregnancy, is often associated with hyperemesis gravidarum and does not require treatment with antithyroid drugs. Women with subclinical Grave's disease can be identified by finding circulating Tr-Abs, with the presence of goiter or ophthalmopathy also raising suspicion of the diagnosis. Graves' disease, like many other autoimmune disorders, improves in pregnancy allowing a reduction in the dose of medication. Tr-Abs cross the placenta and may induce fetal or neonatal hyperthyroidism.

Effect of hyperthyroidism on pregnancy

Euthyroid women on levothyroxine after definitive therapy of Graves's disease with surgery or radioiodine, have a small risk of fetal hyperthyroidism from transplacental transfer of Tr-Abs. Poorly managed hyperthyroidism predisposes to miscarriage, preterm birth, hypertensive disorders, fetal growth restriction, low birthweight and stillbirth. It can lead to thyroid storm (overactive thyroid gland) in rare cases, which may be precipitated by preeclampsia, labor or infection. Thyroid storm may result in severe maternal left ventricular dysfunction and heart failure. When hyperthyroidism develops postpartum, the main diagnostic work-up consists of differentiating between Graves' disease, exacerbation of Hashimoto's thyroiditis and postpartum thyroiditis.

4.4.7 Parathyroid

The parathyroid consists of four small glands variably located posterior to the thyroid (fig. 4.14). Thyroid and parathyroid glands share blood supply and venous/lymphatic drainage. Parathyroid hormone (PTH) and its counterpart calcitonin from the thyroid, play key roles together with vitamin D, in keeping circulating levels of total- and ionized calcium within narrow limits by direct actions on bone and kidney, and an indirect effect on the intestine (Gafni and Collins 2019). PTH is also important in regulating phosphate metabolism by reducing renal phosphate reabsorption and increasing its uptake from the intestines and bones as shown in the figs. 4.14 and 4.15.

Pregnancy is associated with higher calcium demands (fig. 4.15), particularly in the third trimester, to enable the fetus to build up its skeleton. Table 4.3 lists the changes in calcium homeostasis during pregnancy. For adequate bone formation, the fetus requires about 30 g of calcium, along with 20 g phosphorus and 0.80 g magnesium daily (Kovacs 2016). To meet these higher demands, not only maternal calcium intake increases, but also the efficiency of intestinal calcium absorption. These effects are partly induced by a higher maternal circulating level of prolactin and placental lactogen, which also reduces urinary loss of calcium. The fetal demands for calcium and phosphorus have the potential to provoke maternal hypocalcemia and hypophosphatemia. Therefore, it is not surprising

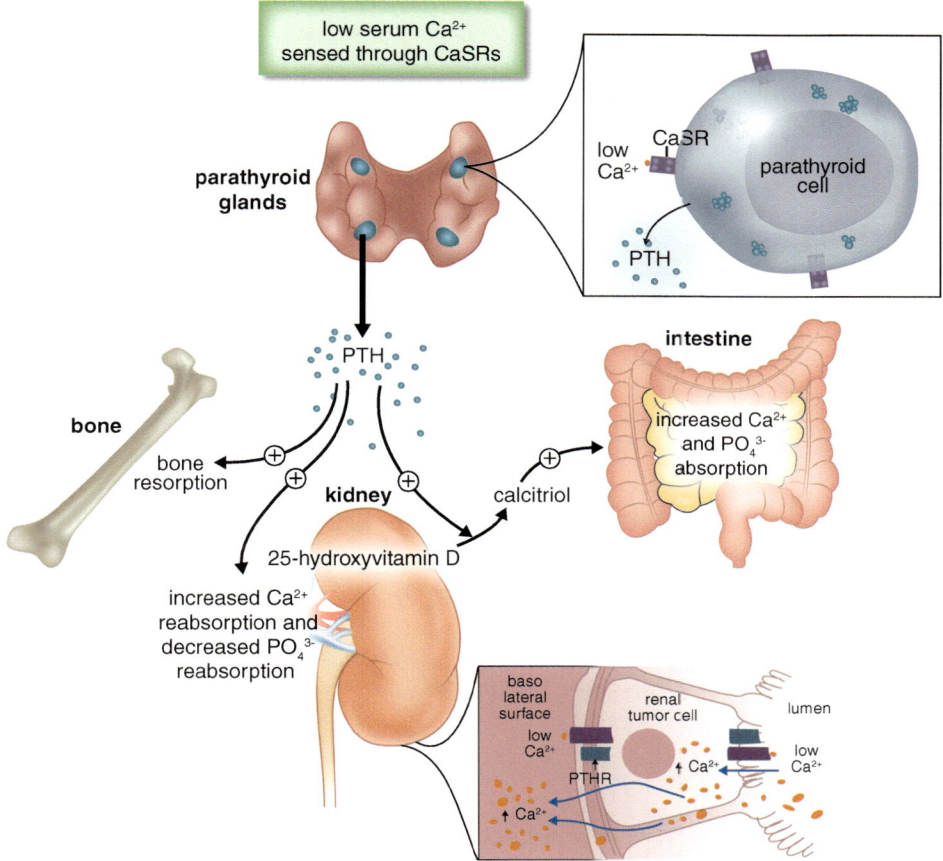

◘ Figure 4.14   Regulation of calcium homeostasis in the extra-cellular compartment by parathyroid hormone (PTH), calcium-sensing receptor (CaSR) and calcitriol (1,25(OH)$_2$D$_3$) (*adopted from* Gafni and Collins 2019)

that the placenta participates in securing the adequate availability of calcium and phosphorus by actively increasing the production of calcitriol, the activated form of vitamin D. Calcitriol both enhances intestinal calcium uptake and diminishes renal calcium loss.

Women with adequate nutritional calcium intake do not require extra calcium during pregnancy and lactation. The WHO recommends a daily intake of 1.5–2 g from the 20th week until childbirth. During pregnancy, total serum calcium declines in concert with serum albumin, but with no change in the level of ionized calcium. In the first trimester, the serum PTH level gradually falls to the lower end of the normal range, followed by stabilization or a small rise afterwards. During lactation, some calcium from the maternal skeleton is mobilized and added to the milk, an effect without any adverse long-term impact on the maternal skeleton. A newborn requires 200 mg calcium daily from milk in the first six months and 120 mg in the second 6 months. The average calcium content of human milk is ±200 mg/L.

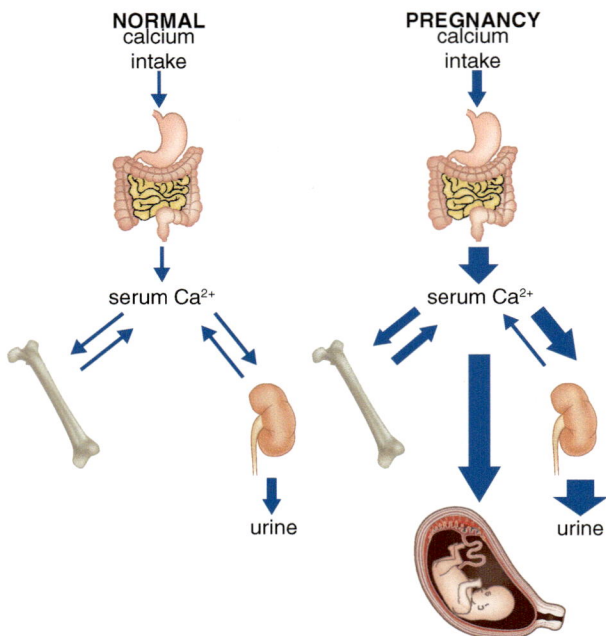

○ **Figure 4.15**   Pregnancy-induced change in calcium and bone homeostasis. The thickness of the blue arrows indicates the relative change to pre-pregnancy (*adopted from* Kovacs 2016)

○ **Table 4.3**   Pregnancy-induced change in calcium homeostasis

calcium & related substances	pregnancy-induced change
serum calcium	total $\downarrow$; ionized $\leftrightarrow$
urinary calcium	$\uparrow$
parathormone (PTH)	$\uparrow/\leftrightarrow$
PTH-related peptide	progressively $\uparrow$
25-vitamin D	$\leftrightarrow$
1,25-dihydroxyvitamin D	progressively $\uparrow$
calcitonin	$\uparrow$

4.4.8 Hypoparathyroidism

Hypoparathyroidism refers to PTH deficiency sufficient to cause hypocalcemia. The estimated prevalence is about 30 cases in 100,000 persons, developing in 80 % of cases as a complication of thyroid surgery, most often occurring in older women. Nonsurgical forms of hypoparathyroidism are often autoimmune-related (Gafni and Collins 2019). PTH is critical in maintaining circulating calcium within narrow limits through actions on bone, kidney and intestine. Its secretion is primarily regulated by the calcium-sensing receptor CaSR in the parathyroid chief cells (○ fig. 4.14). Symptoms can be absent or mild, consisting of paresthesia's of hands and feet, perioral numbness, muscle cramps and prolongation of the corrected QT interval on ECG. The quality of life is often reduced due to nonspecific symptoms, such as general fatigue, lack of focus, depression, anxiety and other neuropsychiatric disorders. Some HPT patients may develop severe, often acute symptoms, such as papilledema, tetany, arrhythmias, kidney stones, focal and generalized seizures and laryngospasm. Hypoparathyroidism in pregnant women is rare.

Effect of pregnancy on hypoparathyroidism

During pregnancy, the placenta reduces the effect of hypoparathyroidism on maternal calcium homeostasis by producing both calcitriol and PTH-related protein (PTHrP) (Leere and Vestergaard 2019). This protein has weak affinity to the PTH receptor, but because of abundant placental production and a concomitant synergistic effect of estradiol, PTHrP raises maternal circulating calcium levels, primarily by enhancing urinary calcium reabsorption. These actions raise calcium availability for transplacental transfer and dampen the negative effects of the hypoparathyroidism. Postpartum, the mammary glands take over placental PTHrP production to secure calcium availability for the infant.

Effect of hypoparathyroidism on pregnancy

Maternal hypocalcemia predisposes to miscarriage, stillbirth, preterm birth and neonatal morbidity, such as respiratory distress syndrome and secondary hyperparathyroidism in the neonate, leading to neonatal skeletal demineralization, subperiosteal bone resorption and osteitis fibrosa cystica. Signs of reactive parathyroid hyperplasia were found in fetuses that died in utero. Preterm birth in these patients may be related to hypocalcemia-induced myometrial irritability on top of a reduced myometrial resting potential throughout pregnancy. Other complications found in infants of mothers with hypoparathyroidism were intracranial bleeding, rickets, skeletal demineralization, subperiosteal bone resorption, osteitis fibrosa cystica, and subsequent intrauterine fractures. Clinical management of pregnant patients with hypoparathyroidism has been reviewed recently (Khan et al. 2019).

4.4.9 Hyperparathyroidism (HPT)

Hyperparathyroidism (HPT) is an endocrine disorder of the calcium metabolism defined by hypercalcemia combined with either an inappropriately normal (primary) or an increased serum PTH level (secondary). Most cases of *primary* HPT result from a benign parathyroid adenoma, giving rise to PTH being inappropriately secreted in a condition of already raised level serums of total or ionized calcium (Bilezikian et al. 2018). On the other hand, in *secondary* HPT, the parathyroid responds appropriately to a reduced level of serum calcium, which is subnormal, because of another serious condition, such as renal failure, impaired calcitriol production, inadequate calcium intake or absorption. Also, individuals with vitamin D deficiency or with gastrointestinal diseases causing malabsorption are at risk to develop secondary HPT. Primary HPT is typically a disorder of middle-aged and older women with the incidence in women of reproductive age (20 to 39 years) being only about 5 cases per 100,000. The so-called classical symptoms of primary HPT are known as "bones, stones, abdominal moans & psychic groans",

4

although its clinical course in nonpregnant women is usually relatively benign. By contrast, the clinical impact of primary HPT on pregnancy may be severe. In primary HPT, early recognition and timely surgical cure before pregnancy are crucial. On the other hand, in secondary HPT the emphasis is to be put on appropriate treatment of the primary disorder as detailed elsewhere (Bilezikian et al. 2018).

Effect of pregnancy on hyperparathyroidism

During pregnancy, placental hormones along with PTHrP may aggravate symptoms, and with it, lead to an increased risk of the pregnancy complications, as specified below.

Effect of hyperparathyroidism on pregnancy

Primary HPT in pregnancy is a rare condition and has an aspecific clinical presentation. Untreated primary HPT during pregnancy predisposes to maternal and fetal complications. The most common maternal complications are hyperemesis, nephrolithiasis, pancreatitis and hypercalcemic crisis. The most common complications affecting the infant are miscarriage, midtrimester fetal death, preterm labor, placental syndrome, fetal growth restriction, neonatal tetany and neonatal death (Norman et al. 2009; Rigg et al. 2019). The course of pregnancy in properly managed, mild primary HPT, does not differ appreciably from that in healthy controls (Abood and Vestergaard 2014).

4.4.10 **Adrenals**

The adrenal glands are located on top of the kidneys and consist of an outer cortex and an inner medulla. The adrenal cortex is subdivided into the zona glomerulosa, the zona fasciculata and the zona reticularis, as shown in ◘ fig. 4.16.

The adrenal cortex produces 3 main types of steroid hormones: mineralocorticoids, glucocorticoids, and androgens. Mineralocorticoids, particularly aldosterone, are produced in the outermost layer, the zona glomerulosa, and play a central role in the regulation of blood pressure and the electrolyte balance. The intermediate layer, the zona

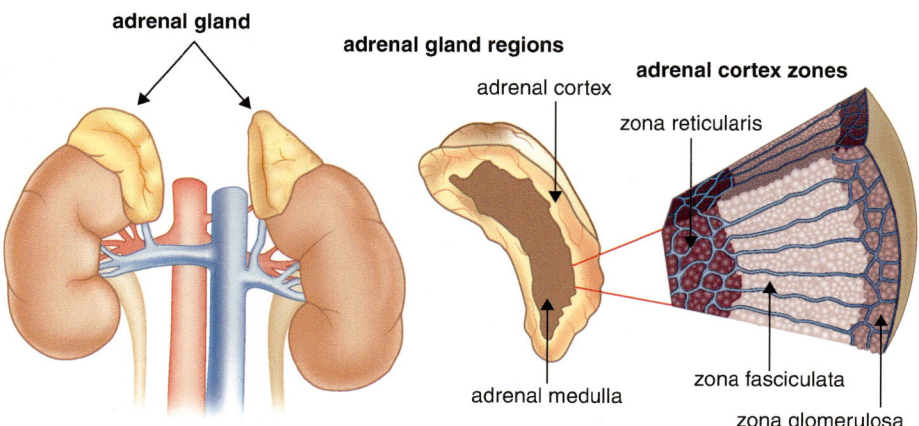

◘ **Figure 4.16**   The anatomical sites and global structure of the adrenal glands

fasciculata, produces the glucocorticoids cortisol and corticosterone, that are primarily involved in the regulation of the metabolism, but can also suppress the immune function in specific circumstances. Finally, the innermost layer of the cortex, the zona reticularis, produces androgens that are to be converted to functional sex hormones in the gonads and other target organs. The adrenal medulla produces the catecholamines, adrenaline (epinephrine), noradrenaline (norepinephrine) and dopamine. These hormones serve to generate a rapid response throughout the body during exposure to stress. Adrenal dysfunction leads to a number of endocrine diseases. Excessive cortisol production results in Cushing's syndrome, whereas deficient cortisol production results in Addison's disease. Congenital adrenal hyperplasia is a genetic disease produced by dysregulation of endocrine control mechanisms.

During pregnancy, the fetoplacental unit plays a key role in fetal adrenal growth and maturation by releasing large amounts of corticotropin-releasing hormone (CRH) into the fetal circulation (Rainey et al. 2004). In the meantime, it also stimulates the maternal hypothalamic-pituitary-adrenal (HPA) axis and with it, maternal steroid homeostasis, inducing a state of physiological hypercortisolism in the mother, reflected in three-fold higher circulating levels of ACTH, CRH and cortisol relative to their normal nonpregnant upper limit level. Besides, placental estrogen induces an approximately similar rise in cortisol-binding globulin (CBG) in the maternal plasma. The concomitant rises in cortisol and CBG both enlarge the plasma cortisol pool and extend the cortisol half-life. Maternal free serum cortisol level increases from the 11th pregnancy week onwards. Interestingly, these marked changes in plasma levels do not affect the circadian rhythm of plasma cortisol throughout pregnancy (Kamoun et al. 2014). Until the 33rd week, over 90 % of fetal cortisol is produced by the maternal adrenals, with the fetal adrenal contribution rapidly increasing afterwards, gradually replacing maternal cortisol. From the 8th week of pregnancy onward the activity of the maternal renin-angiotensin-aldosterone system (RAAS) increases, presumably to promote volume expansion and with it, increase cardiac preload, thus compensating for the circulatory effects of the early-pregnancy fall in systemic vascular resistance (as detailed in ▶ Chap. 1).

4.4.11 Adrenal insufficiency

Adrenal insufficiency may result from diseases of the adrenal glands (primary), impaired pituitary ACTH output (secondary), or impaired hypothalamic CRH secretion (tertiary). In primary adrenal insufficiency or 'Addison's disease', clinical signs only develop, when more than 90 % of adrenal cortical cells are destroyed. The most common cause of Addison's disease is an autoimmune disorder (Husebye et al. 2014), with less common causes being bilateral adrenal injury, hemorrhage, infarction or infection (CMV, tuberculosis). The prevalence of Addison's disease is only 120 per 100,000 persons (Ten et al. 2001). The severity of symptoms depends upon rate and extend of adrenal function loss, whether or not aldosterone production is preserved, and the amount of stress experienced. The onset of adrenal insufficiency is often gradual and may remain undetected until an illness or other acute stress factor, such as e.g. a circulatory shock, triggers an adrenal crisis. The symptoms of a slowly progressing development of adrenal insufficiency are often nonspecific, such as anorexia, fatigue, abdominal pain, weakness, nausea, vomiting, lethargy, fever, confusion, or coma. Hyperpigmentation of Addison's disease involves non-exposed parts of skin and creases of hands, extensor surfaces and mucous membranes, and may be paralleled by sites with vitiligo (▫ figs. 4.17 and 4.18).

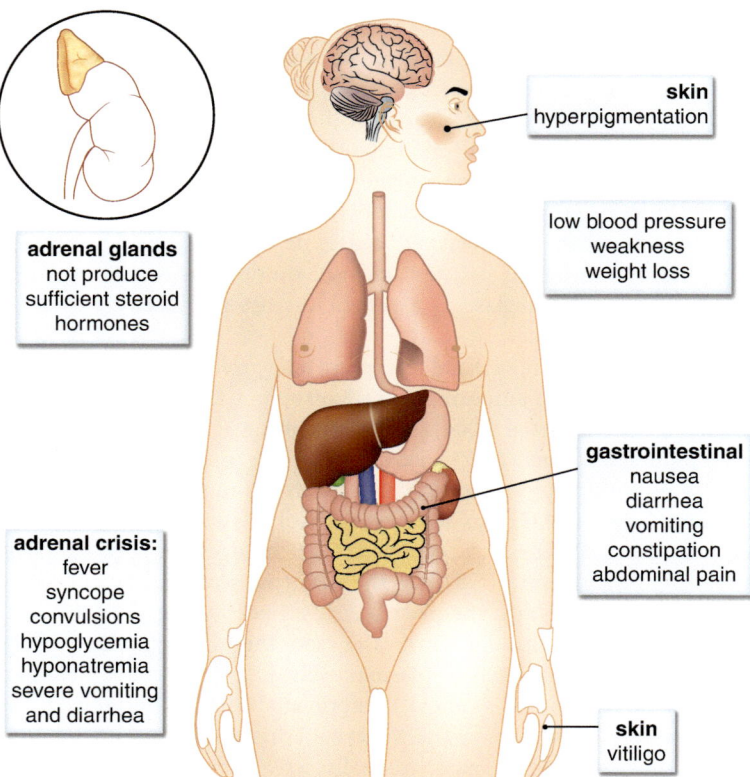

adrenal glands
not produce
sufficient steroid
hormones

skin
hyperpigmentation

low blood pressure
weakness
weight loss

gastrointestinal
nausea
diarrhea
vomiting
constipation
abdominal pain

adrenal crisis:
fever
syncope
convulsions
hypoglycemia
hyponatremia
severe vomiting
and diarrhea

skin
vitiligo

◘ Figure 4.17   Common signs and symptoms of Addison's disease

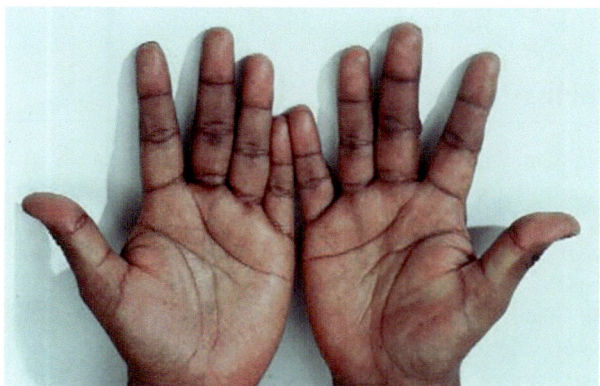

◘ Figure 4.18   Typical hyperpigmentation of the hands' creases in patients with Addison's disease

This effect is caused by the accompanying elevated circulating levels of melanocyte-stimulating hormone (MSH). Salt craving, hyponatremia with a > 5 mmol/L fall in plasma sodium along with metabolic acidosis are other typical signs of adrenal insufficiency. In chronic adrenal insufficiency regardless of clinical signs, a personal or family history of autoimmune disease should arouse clinical suspicion. Diagnostic work-up and clinical management have been detailed elsewhere (Anand and Beuschlein 2018; Manoharan et al. 2019). The prevalence of Addison's disease in pregnancy ranges from 5 to 10 cases per 100,000 pregnancies (Manoharan et al. 2019).

Effect of pregnancy on adrenal insufficiency

Replacement therapy used by pregnant patients with known adrenal insufficiency can be inadequate, because of too low daily doses of glucocorticoid and/or mineralocorticoid, or because of failure to increase the dose of glucocorticoid during superimposed stress due to an infection or other major illness, such as persistent vomiting or diarrhea. In rare cases, stressful events in pregnancy, such as hyperemesis gravidarum, infections, surgery or childbirth, may trigger an adrenal crisis, thus uncovering a yet unidentified patient. Pregnant women on cortisol replacement therapy should be administered hydrocortisone (100 mg) at the time of delivery or if labor is prolonged. Additional details about the management of pregnant and postpartum patients with adrenal insufficiency have been reported elsewhere (Kamoun et al. 2014; Anand and Beuschlein 2018; Manoharan et al. 2019).

Effect of adrenal insufficiency on pregnancy

New-onset adrenal insufficiency during pregnancy is extremely rare. Before glucocorticoid replacement therapy became available, pregnancy in women with adrenal insufficiency was associated with a high rate of maternal mortality and fetal growth restriction. At present, pregnancy course and outcome in almost all adequately managed patients with adrenal insufficiency does not differ from that in their healthy counterparts. However, pregnancy in women with unrecognized adrenal insufficiency is associated with a high rate of complications, such as fetal growth restriction, increased rate of cesarean section due to fetal malpresentation and postpartum hemorrhage. Lactation itself can be affected by comorbidities of adrenal insufficiency, like pituitary insufficiency. The physiological dose of glucocorticoid required to substitute for maternal adrenal insufficiency, is unlikely to cause harm in breast-fed children.

4.4.12 Cushing's disease (CD)

Cushing's disease (CD) refers to hypercortisolism and has a prevalence of about 40 cases per million persons, with 1.5 to 2 new cases per million persons yearly (Lonser et al. 2017). The median onset is at 41 years of age with a female to male ratio of 3 to 1 (Lacroix et al. 2015). Some CD cases are exogenous, indicating that they result from chronic exposure to therapeutic doses of glucocorticoids. However, most cases are endogenous, with about 20 % resulting from excessive glucocorticosteroids excretion by bilateral adrenal hyperplasia or adrenal tumors and the remaining 80 % resulting from exposure to excessive ACTH, produced by a pituitary adenoma (◘ fig. 4.19) or an ectopic (non-pituitary) source.

4

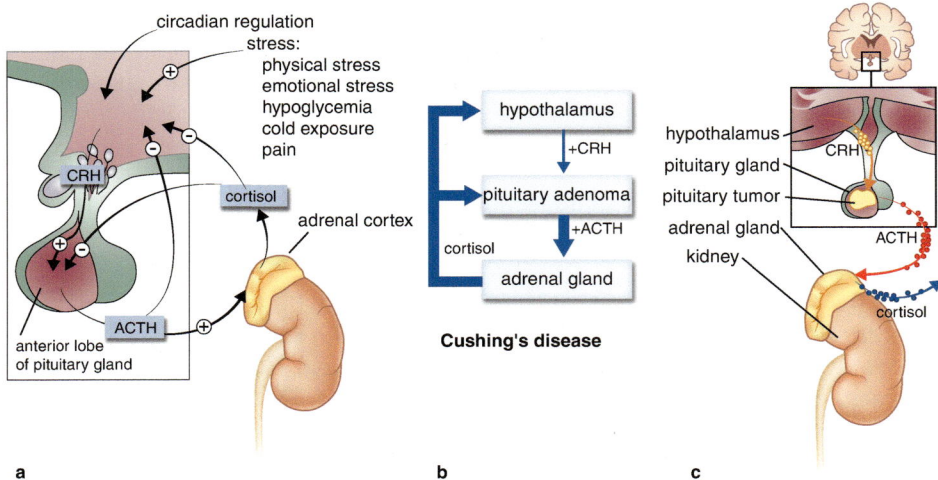

a   b   c

■ **Figure 4.19**   Pathophysiology of Cushing's disease. (a) Normal hypothalamic-pituitary-adrenal axis. (b) Pathophysiologic mechanism leading to Cushing's disease, and ACTH-producing pituitary adenoma releasing excessive amounts of ACTH unresponsive to cortisol-driven negative feedback. (c) Site of adenoma in the anterior lobe of the pituitary gland (*adopted from* Lonser et al. 2017)

Adult CD patients have both physical symptoms (e.g. diabetes, hypertension, obesity, moon face, facial plethora) and neuropsychiatric issues (such as depression, anxiety, learning impairment, memory deficits) (■ fig. 4.20). Most female patients with CD caused by excess ACTH secretion, are amenorrhoeic and infertile, because of excess androgen secretion. Conversely, women with CD resulting from a cortisol-producing adrenal adenoma have normal fertility, as their circulating androgen levels are normal. Therefore, it is extremely rare that a woman diagnosed in pregnancy with CD, has an ACTH-producing disorder. Diagnosing CD during pregnancy is challenging, not only because pregnancy itself stimulates the HPA-axis, leading to raised circulating levels of CRH, ACTH, CBG, total and free serum cortisol, and higher urinary cortisol excretion. Neither the early CD symptoms do arouse suspicion, as they resemble normal signs of a healthy pregnancy, such as weight gain, abdominal striae, edema and fatigue. Besides, some early CD symptoms may easily be confused with those of gestational diabetes and preeclampsia. At any rate, CD during pregnancy predisposes to severe maternal and perinatal morbidity. Therefore, a high level of clinical awareness is needed to avoid those complications. How to deal with the diagnostic hurdles in a pregnant woman suspected of CD, has been detailed elsewhere (Manoharan et al. 2019).

Effect of pregnancy on CS

CS in a pregnant patient often develops secondary to an adrenal adenoma producing pure cortisol. It is plausible that pregnancy by itself worsens (the effects of) a still unrecognized CS by activating the HPA-axis, as delineated in the previous paragraph. This could even lead to fetal/maternal mortality as suggested previously (Lindsay and Nieman 2005). However, to date there are no reports that confirm this severe outcome.

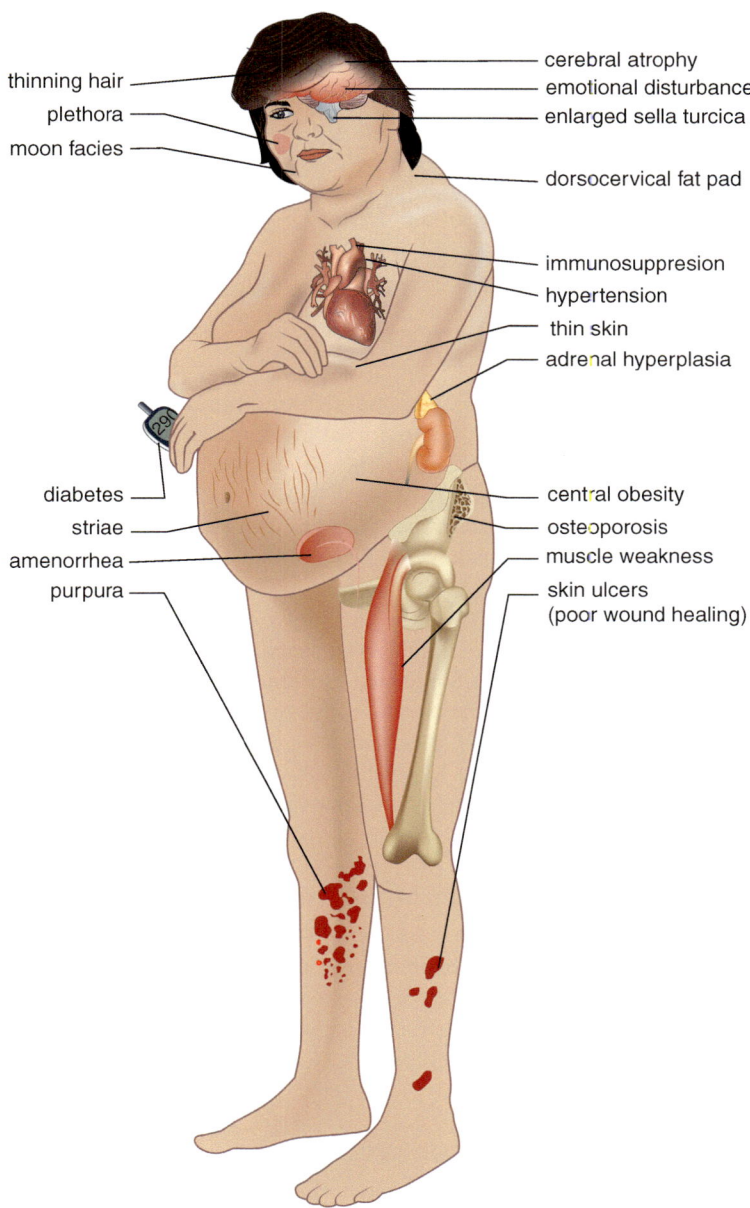

thinning hair
plethora
moon facies

cerebral atrophy
emotional disturbance
enlarged sella turcica

dorsocervical fat pad

immunosuppresion
hypertension
thin skin
adrenal hyperplasia

diabetes
striae
amenorrhea
purpura

central obesity
osteoporosis
muscle weakness
skin ulcers
(poor wound healing)

▣ Figure 4.20   Common signs and symptoms in women with Cushing's disease (*adopted from* Lonser et al. 2017)

Effect of CS on pregnancy

CS increases the risk of maternal morbidity as reflected in increased rates of hypertensive disorders and gestational diabetes (Manoharan et al. 2019). Also, perinatal morbidity and mortality are increased as indicated by the high rates of miscarriage, preterm birth, fetal growth restriction, stillbirths. The fetus is partially protected against the effects of hypercortisolism as the placenta converts most maternal cortisol to inactive cortisone. The clinical management of a pregnant CS-affected patient has been detailed elsewhere (Manoharan et al. 2019).

4.4.13 Pheochromocytoma (PCC)

Pheochromocytoma (PCC) is a catecholamine-secreting tumor arising from chromaffin cells in usually, the adrenal medulla. The reported incidence in the general population is 0.05 % (Iijima 2019). Only half of PCC patients have symptoms, such as transient episodes of severe hypertension or sustained hypertension, tachycardia, headache, sweating and palpitations with hypertensive crises being most typical. Less frequent symptoms are arrhythmia, hypostatic hypotension, weight loss, visual blurring, polyuria and polydipsia. If not detected and treated, PCC may become life-threatening because of complications, such as myocardial infarction, cardiomyopathy, cerebral hemorrhage, or pulmonary edema. A critical factor in PCC is to suspect it in the first place. Once suspected, the diagnosis of PCC can be confirmed by demonstrating a 4-fold rise in plasma fractionated metanephrines above the normal range or a raised 24h urinary fractionated metanephrines (Farrugia et al. 2017). Biochemical confirmation of PCC should be followed by radiological exploration to locate the tumor. Pregnancy in a PCC-patient is extremely rare as indicated by a reported incidence that ranges from 0.0002 % to 0.007 % (Iijima 2019).

Effect of pregnancy on pheochromocytoma

Although PCC symptoms in pregnant and nonpregnant women are similar, they may worsen in advanced pregnancy due to increasing pressure exerted upon the tumor by the growing pregnant uterus (Iijima 2019). Besides, PCC-related hypertension is episodic and not accompanied by proteinuria, as opposed to e.g. preeclampsia. However, if proteinuria does coincide with hypertension, PCC may be difficult to differentiate from preeclampsia.

Effect of pheochromocytoma on pregnancy

Pregnancy in a woman with a yet unrecognized PCC is at high risk of both fetal/maternal morbidity and mortality (Van der Weerd et al. 2017). Fetal risks are primarily related to the negative impact of the elevated maternal catecholamines on the uteroplacental perfusion, leading to complications such as spontaneous abortion, fetal growth restriction, preterm birth, fetal asphyxia and fetal demise. If a PCC-patient is properly treated from early pregnancy onward, her pregnancy is likely to evolve uneventfully (Van der Weerd et al. 2017). The clinical management of PCC in pregnancy has been detailed previously (Van der Weerd et al. 2017; Iijima 2019; Calina et al. 2019).

4.4.14 Primary aldosteronism (PA, Conn syndrome)

Primary aldosteronism (PA, Conn syndrome)refers to the high-aldosterone/low-renin state resulting from "autonomous" aldosterone synthesis/release, indicating that the latter events are no longer under the control of ACTH and associated renin suppression (◘ fig. 4.21). PA leads to volume expansion and with it, induces reflex vasoconstriction and hypertension.

PA is the most common endocrine cause of high blood pressure. Only a minority are familial, often related to a genetic cause. However, sporadic cases are much more commonly caused by some obscure mechanism, characterized by persistingly excessive aldosterone production in spite of high blood pressure, sodium retention, RAAS suppression and low potassium levels. Only in the last decade, it has been discovered that functional mutations of potassium channels were responsible for preserved aldosterone synthesis by adrenal cortical cells in spite of the presence of the usual inhibitors mentioned above (Stowasser and Gordon 2013).

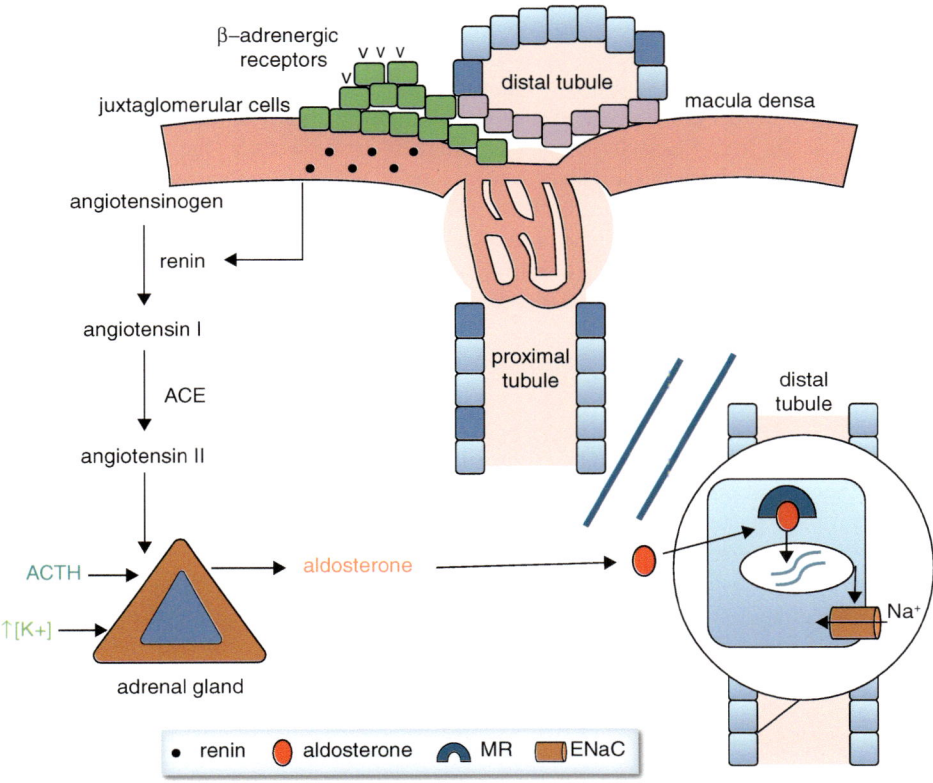

◘ **Figure 4.21** Physiology of aldosterone synthesis, secretion and actions. Juxtaglomerular (JG) cells detect hypovolemia and low Na$^+$ levels, which induces the release of renin. Renin then, catalyzes the conversion of angiotensinogen into angiotensin-I, followed by angiotensin-converting enzyme (ACE) that converts angiotensin-I into angiotensin-II. Angiotensin-II acts in concert with hyperkalemia and ACTH to stimulate the aldosterone synthesis/release from the zona glomerulosa. Then, aldosterone binds to its mineralocorticoid receptor (MR) in the distal tubule, translocates to the nucleus to raise the expression of Na$^+$ channels (ENaC) on the epithelium (*adopted from* Galati et al. 2013)

4

The prevalence of PA among patients with essential hypertension and identified by a too high plasma aldosterone/renin ratio, is as high as 20 % (Stowasser and Gordon 2013). More than half of PA cases result from bilateral adrenal hyperplasia, whereas about a third are caused by an aldosterone-producing adrenal adenoma. Less than half of PA-affected patients have hypokalemia. The female-to-male ratio is 2 to 1. PA results in more severe cardiovascular and renal morbidity than expected from direct mechanical damage from the high blood pressure. It also reduces the quality of life, because of symptoms such as lethargy, fatigue, difficulty to concentrate, anxiety disorders and depression (Stowasser and Gordon 2013). Cardiovascular and renal morbidity as well as the latter neuropsychiatric sequels improve markedly after the appropriate surgical or medical treatment. This emphasizes the importance of early diagnosis and appropriate management as detailed elsewhere (Funder et al. 2016).

Effect of pregnancy on a preexistent (untreated/unrecognized) PA

During pregnancy, the cardiovascular function becomes "hyperdynamic", a condition with cardiac output about one-third higher and peripheral vascular resistance correspondingly lower than before pregnancy (detailed in ▶ Chap. 1). This adaptive response is accompanied by a rise in cardiovascular sympathetic activity, but – more importantly – also by activation of the renin-angiotensin-aldosterone system (RAAS) to induce a compensatory rise in plasma volume. From a theoretical point of view, the pregnancy-induced rise in RAAS activity in a PA patient is irrelevant for the institution of a hyperdynamic circulation. Therefore, it seems unlikely that a preexistent, untreated PA deteriorates shortly after conception. Unfortunately, there are no scientific data supporting this concept. On the other hand, a woman with preexistent PA intending to conceive has often hypertension with associated reduced cardiovascular reserves, a condition by itself that increases her risk of various complications in pregnancy (see below).

Effect of primary hyperaldosteronism on pregnancy

The estimated rate of PA among pregnant women is 0.6–0.8 %, but most likely underdiagnosed in pregnant women with essential hypertension, as confirmation of the diagnosis PA in pregnancy is hampered by the pregnancy-induced activation of the RAAS-axis. From a theoretical point of view, the high circulating levels of progesterone during pregnancy can be expected to suppress the effect of aldosterone, as progesterone also binds to the aldosterone receptor. Yet, PA can be expected to cause end-organ damage reducing maternal cardiovascular reserve capacity prior to pregnancy and with it, its ability to adapt to pregnancy. Therefore, it is not surprising that pregnancy in PA-affected women is associated with a high rate of both maternal morbidity (pulmonary edema, superimposed preeclampsia, renal failure) and fetal morbidity (intrauterine fetal demise, preterm birth, fetal growth restriction, placental abruption and low birthweight) (Morton 2015; Landau and Amar 2016).

4.5 Red blood cell disorders

4.5.1 Introduction

Chronic hematological disorders refer to an abnormal quantity or function of the cellular components of the blood. For the red cells, this refers to anemia/polycythemia and disorders, such as thalassemia or sickle cell disease, etc. In this section, the most common disorders of red blood cells will be discussed, their possible impact on pregnancy and how pregnancy may affect them. Meanwhile, disorders of the platelets refer to thrombopenia, thrombocytosis, thrombopathy, together with conditions that cause a thrombophilic phenotype. These disorders and how they may interact with pregnancy, have been discussed in ▶ Chap. 3. Finally, diseases of white blood cells reflected in an abnormal number and/or composition of various types of white cells, are more complex to address as a separate hematological entity, as they frequently develop in response to some form of inflammatory trigger. Therefore, these disorders have been incorporated in the sections on immunological and infectious diseases in the preceding chapters.

4.5.2 Anemia

Anemia is the most common hematological disorder observed in pregnancy. Early recognition and effective management reduce the increased risk of adverse maternal and fetal outcomes (Jung et al. 2019). According to WHO data, anemia affects around 40 % of pregnant women worldwide, particularly in countries with poor resources (Di Renzo et al. 2015; Lopez et al. 2016). The three most common causes of anemia are poor nutrition (deficient intake of iron, folic acid, and vitamins A and B12), inherited hemoglobinopathies (sickle cell disease and thalassemia) and infections, such as malaria, schistosomiasis and HIV. Less frequent causes of anemia in pregnancy are autoimmune hemolysis and hypothyroidism. Women with subnormal iron stores at conception, are particularly prone to develop iron-deficiency anemia during pregnancy, because of a dramatic rise in the maternal iron requirements to satisfy her extra demands to expand her red cell volume, and to build up those of the conceptus (Breymann 2015). The diagnose of anemia differs between pregnant and nonpregnant women, and between different phases of pregnancy. The latter relates to the impact of pregnancy-induced hemodilution on the threshold value for a subnormal hematocrit (Hct) in midpregnancy relative to that in early and late pregnancy (◼ fig. 4.22).

The two most common forms of anemia (iron-deficiency and hemoglobinopathies) will be discussed in more detail below. Less common causes of anemia that often develop as a side-effect of some primary disease (infection and autoimmune – or endocrine disorders) have similar symptoms and effects on pregnancy, in addition to the symptoms and effects of the primary disorder. Therefore, relevant details of these anemias are discussed in the related sections (infections, auto-immune and endocrine disorders) in ▶ Chap. 3.

4

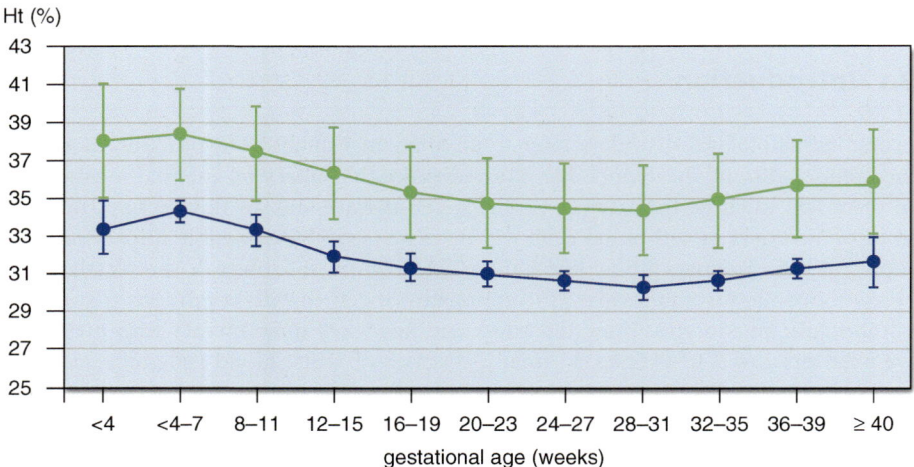

○ **Figure 4.22**   Hematocrit (Ht, %) as a function of gestational age. Mean (green line) and 5th centile (blue line) are presented with means ± SD. Note the 10 % fall in Ht between early and midpregnancy (*adopted from* Chiossi et al. 2019)

4.5.3 **Iron-deficiency anemia**

Iron-deficiency anemia (before and during pregnancy) may lead to symptoms, such as low physical and mental capacity, fatigue, dizziness, cold intolerance, spoon-shaped nails, mucosal paleness, leg cramps, headache and angular stomatitis (Lopez et al. 2016). The diagnosis of iron-deficiency anemia is confirmed by the presence of a subnormal circulating levels of hemoglobin (Hb), iron, transferrin and ferritin along with a raised total iron-binding capacity. Measurement of the Hb and serum ferritin levels suffice to identify anemic patients without underlying inflammation. To diagnose anemia that has developed during chronic inflammation requires additional testing (DeLoughery 2017). The C-reactive protein (CRP) level in many healthy pregnant women exceeds 3.0 mg/L and with it, the upper level of the nonpregnant adult reference range. As CRP is also an acute-phase reactant, these patients require additional diagnostic work-up for their anemia as detailed elsewhere (Lopez et al. 2016). Prevention and treatment of iron-deficiency anemia in pregnancy and anemia, caused by insufficient intake of other micronutrients (vitamin A, folic acid, vitamin B12) has been elaborated elsewhere (Muñoz et al. 2018).

Impact of pregnancy on iron deficiency anemia

The higher need for iron in pregnancy magnifies a preexistent iron-deficiency anemia and with it, contributes to the pregnancy complications listed below.

Impact of iron-deficiency anemia on pregnancy

Iron-deficiency anemia during pregnancy may lead to various maternal and perinatal complications. Epidemiologic data indicate a twice as high rate of preterm birth and a three-fold higher rate of placental insufficiency with low birthweight infants being the most common complication (Scholl and Reilly 2000; Savajols et al. 2014). Obviously, infants born from these anemic mothers can be expected to have insufficient iron stores, which increases their susceptibility to malaria and invasive bacterial infections. Besides, insufficient iron availability also predisposes them to impaired CNS myelination and with it, permanent defects in mental development and performance, thus reducing their learning abilities (Di Renzo et al. 2015).

The impact of iron-deficiency anemia on pregnant women includes subnormal physical functioning, higher susceptibility to infections and increased risk of cardiac failure and related death, particularly during labor – e.g. in conjunction with her reduced capacity to tolerate postpartum hemorrhage – but also hemorrhage afterwards (Azulay et al. 2015). The mother's limited physical functional capacity also persists postpartum, leading to less milk production, and with it, ongoing subnormal iron supply to the infant during breastfeeding. These effects may also explain her increased risk of developing postpartum depression and emotional instability (Di Renzo et al. 2015).

4.5.4 Hemoglobinopathies

Inherited hemoglobin disorders, such as sickle-cell disease, thalassemia and glucose-6-phosphate dehydrogenase deficiency (G6PDD), are the most common monogenic diseases worldwide and are not only an important cause of (hemolytic) anemia, but also of other health issues.

4.5.5 Sickle cell disease (SCD)

Sickle cell disease (SCD) is a multisystem disorder, caused by a single gene mutation that leads to the production of sickled hemoglobin (HbS). As soon as HbS becomes deoxygenated, the molecule polymerizes causing red blood cells to dehydrate and shrink. As a result, these cells become rigid and adopt a sickling shape (◘ fig. 4.23). These stiff, sickled red cells also express adhesion molecules and exhibit abnormal rheologic properties. Functionally, these erythrocytes are prone to hemolysis resulting in hemolytic anemia and because of their stiffness, also cause vascular occlusion of small blood vessels leading to ischemic tissue damage of any organ, an effect that may induce severe pain. Finally, SCD-affected persons are also at increased risk of venous thromboembolism (Piel et al. 2017). Splenic infarctions lead to functional hyposplenism early in life and with it, a higher susceptibility to infection. Each year, about 300,000 infants, homozygous for the HBS gene are born worldwide, mostly in Nigeria, Democratic Republic of Congo and India. Both survival and quality of life of affected persons has improved markedly since the introduction of various effective management strategies (Piel et al. 2017). Yet, life expectancy is still reduced, which partly relates to our incomplete insight into the contributions of genetic and nongenetic factors to the widely varying phenotype.

Impact of pregnancy on SCD

Pregnancy tends to increase the number of episodes of pain, infections, pulmonary complications and thromboembolic events, presumably also contributing to the about 6 times higher maternal mortality rate and about 4 times higher stillbirth rate than in a healthy reference population (Oteng-Ntim et al. 2015; Ware et al. 2017). Sickled red blood cells are more prone to lysis, which explains the worsening anemia during pregnancy. The accelerated hemolysis and worsening anemia lead to a higher sympathetic

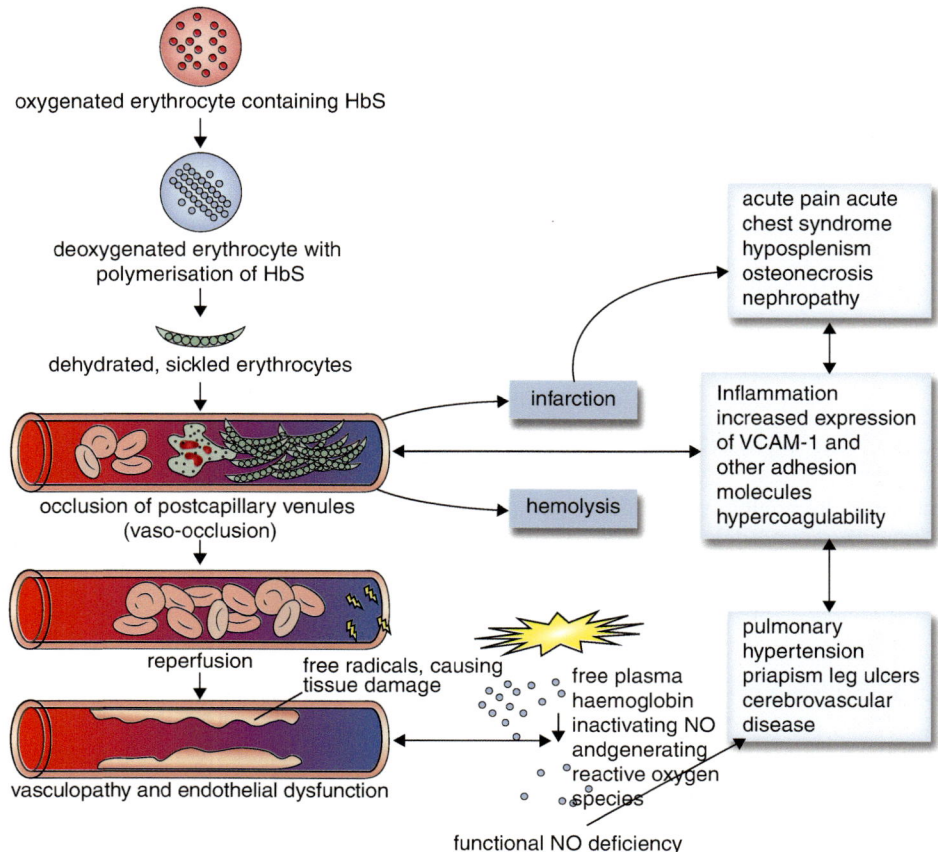

oxygenated erythrocyte containing HbS

deoxygenated erythrocyte with
polymerisation of HbS

dehydrated, sickled erythrocytes

infarction

acute pain acute
chest syndrome
hyposplenism
osteonecrosis
nephropathy

occlusion of postcapillary venules
(vaso-occlusion)

hemolysis

Inflammation
increased expression
of VCAM-1 and
other adhesion
molecules
hypercoagulability

reperfusion   free radicals, causing
tissue damage

free plasma
haemoglobin
inactivating NO
andgenerating
reactive oxygen
species

pulmonary
hypertension
priapism leg ulcers
cerebrovascular
disease

vasculopathy and endothelial dysfunction

functional NO deficiency

□ Figure 4.23   The pathophysiology of sickle cell disease (SCD) includes HbS-polymerization, hyperviscosity, hemolysis, vaso-occlusion and endothelial dysfunction and with it, a widely varying clinical
phenotype due to vasculopathy, tissue damage and thrombophilia (*adopted from* Rees et al. 2010)

tone in the cardiovascular system. Presumably, this may induce the cardiac output to be
redistributed at the expense of non-vital tissues, which also includes the uteroplacental
vascular bed. This concept is not only supported by the higher rate of chronic hypertension in SCD patients and the higher rate of placental syndromes and poor fetal growth in
pregnant SCD-patients. It is also supported by the beneficial effect of blood transfusions
on pregnancy course and outcome in SCD patients (Malinowski et al. 2015).

Impact of SCD on pregnancy

Relative to healthy controls, SCD-affected pregnant women show a higher rate of placental syndromes (Kuo and Caughey 2016), fetal growth restriction, low birthweight and
perinatal mortality (Boafor et al. 2016). Blood transfusions during pregnancy improve
pregnancy outcome (Malinowski et al. 2015), at least in part, because it alleviates the
adverse effects of severe anemia and vaso-occlusive disease in pregnancy. It is conceivable that the rigid and deformed sickled erythrocytes not only interfere with blood rheology in the vascular bed, but also hinders the institution of a high-flow/low-resistance
circulation. The increased risk of poor maternal and perinatal outcomes in SCD-affected

women emphasizes the importance of preconceptional counseling and professional medical care during pregnancy by a team of experts in both SCD and high-risk obstetrics (Howard and Oteng-Ntim 2012; Boga and Ozdogu 2016).

4.5.6 Thalassemia

Thalassemia is the other common monogenetic hemoglobinopathy and – similar to SCD – mostly observed in (sub)tropical regions with a high prevalence of malaria. This association relates to the fact that particularly heterozygosity of this disorder (but also of SCD) gives variable protection against malaria (Taylor et al. 2012). The WHO estimates that 1.5 % of the world's population may be β-thalassemia carriers and that each year, 60,000 severely affected infants are born. In higher-income countries, immigration has increased the prevalence of SCD and β-thalassemia over the last decades.

More than 200 thalassemic mutations have been reported, leading to defects in the α-like (α-thalassemia) or β-like (β-thalassemia) globin chains that form the tetramers of hemoglobin A (α2/β2). These defects create imbalances in the α/β-globin chain ratio, which – most importantly – reduces the red cell lifespan. The spectrum of thalassemia's is wide with one end comprising thalassemia minor, characterized by a mild hypochromic microcytic anemia and virtually no clinical symptoms, and the other end comprising thalassemia major, characterized by severe anemia requiring regular transfusions from early childhood onward. In these patients, rapid red cell turnover results in chronic hemolytic anemia. However, the compensatory accelerated erythropoiesis is ineffective, because of the underlying disease. ◘ Figure 4.24 summarizes the global pathophysiology and clinical manifestations of the various forms of thalassemia (Tahel et al. 2018).

A common complication of thalassemia is the development of splenomegaly that worsens the already existing anemia and with it, the need for more blood transfusions. The disorder may also lead to iron overload causing iron toxicity, affecting cardiac function and damaging primarily endocrine organs (Lao 2017). Infections and other causes of oxidative stress may trigger occasional superimposed hemolytic crises that further aggravate the anemia.

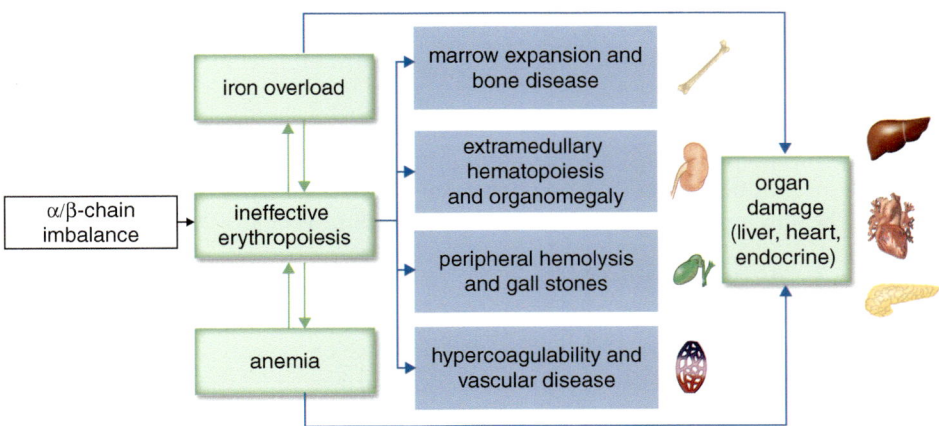

◘ **Figure 4.24** Pathophysiology and clinical manifestations of thalassemia (*adopted from* Tahel et al. 2018)

Impact of pregnancy on thalassemia

Pregnancy tends to worsen the preexistent hemolytic anemia of thalassemia, as the already subnormal erythropoiesis is further stretched to enable red cell volume expansion. Pregnancy may also worsen the chronic hemolysis, as the relatively fragile red blood cells are exposed to the higher shear forces that prevail in the circulation.

Impact of thalassemia on pregnancy

Anemia-related adverse pregnancy outcome due to prematurity, fetal growth restriction and low birthweight are more common in thalassemia-affected women. In addition, the chronically enhanced hemolysis leads to higher circulating levels of free hemoglobin that deplete a large fraction of the circulating nitric oxide (NO) and with it, increase peripheral vascular resistance, possibly contributing to the relatively high incidence of preeclampsia. With respect to the mother, particularly splenectomized patients are at increased risk of thromboembolic events, whereas transfusion-dependent patients are at extra risk of the maternal complications of thalassemia, such as iron toxicity that may affect the heart, immune system and liver functions (Carlberg et al. 2017). The obstetrical management of a thalassemia-affected woman has been detailed elsewhere (Petrakos et al. 2016; Carlberg et al. 2017; Lao 2017).

4.5.7 Glucose-6-phosphate-dehydrogenase-deficiency (G6PDD)

Glucose-6-phosphate-dehydrogenase-deficiency (G6PDD) is the most common human enzyme defect caused by a mutation in the G6PD gene. It is present in more than 400 million people worldwide with a higher prevalence among persons of certain ethnicities (Negroid, Mediterranean and Asian). G6PD generates NADPH that protects erythrocytes from oxidative injury. G6PDD is an X-linked, hereditary disorder leading to widely variable clinical manifestations ranging from asymptomatic to severe complications (e.g. neonatal jaundice and acute hemolytic anemia), usually triggered by an exogenous agent, like eating fava beans that can trigger a severe hemolytic attack in genetically susceptible persons as delineated elsewhere (Cappellini and Fiorelli 2008; Luzzatto and Aresi 2018). The most effective management of G6PDD is to prevent the hemolysis triggered by oxidative stress. Identification of G6PDD and patient education regarding safe and unsafe medications and foods is critical to prevent (future) hemolytic episodes.

Impact of pregnancy on G6PDD

Certain medications, such as nitrofurantoin (Van de Mheen et al. 2014), given during pregnancy, e.g. to treat a urinary infection, may trigger a severe hemolytic crisis in an otherwise healthy, pregnant woman with a high-risk ethnic profile.

Impact of G6PDD on pregnancy

About 20 % of the infants of mothers with an ethnic risk profile consistent with G6PDD and born uneventfully after a normal pregnancy develop severe, idiopathic neonatal jaundice that resulted from severe hemolytic anemia triggered by G6PDD (Christensen et al. 2013).

4.5.8 Erythrocytosis

Erythrocytosis refers to the quite rare condition with the hematocrit (Hct) being higher than 60 % and 56 % in men and women, resp. (McMullin 2016), due to accelerated development of multipotent stem cells into mature enucleated erythrocytes in the bone marrow (Zivot et al. 2017). In contrast to anemia, erythrocytosis raises blood viscosity by increasing total red cell mass. Erythrocytosis may develop because of a higher sensitivity of erythroid progenitors to erythropoietin (polycythemia vera, PV), primary familiar congenital polycythemia (PFCP), or induced by external stimuli (living at high altitude or triggered by a chronic hypoxic cardiac or pulmonary disease). Most of these individuals have no complaints, provided their condition is well-controlled and they adhere to preventive measures (optimal hydration, occasional venesection) that minimize their risk of developing the hyperviscosity syndrome (headache, dizziness, fatigue, apathy, slow mentation, paresthesia, myalgia, visual and auditive disturbances), thromboembolism, arterial hypertension and associated risk of stroke and cardiac disease.

Impact of pregnancy on erythrocytosis
Besides a fall of the elevated Hct in response to the pregnancy-induced hemodilution, there are no known other effects of pregnancy on the preexistent erythrocytosis.

Impact of erythrocytosis on pregnancy
PFCP-induced erythrocytosis is rare with only scarce information on its impact on pregnancy. Also, PV is rare, particularly in women of reproductive age, as reflected in a rate of only 0.3 cases in 100,000 individuals (Srour et al. 2016). Case reports indicate no adverse impact on pregnancy with newborns having normal birthweight, provided appropriate thromboprophylaxis had been instituted, with Hct closely monitored and kept below target (about 50 %) by occasional venesection, along with optimal fetal and maternal surveillance (McMullin et al. 2015; McMullin 2016).

4.6 Psychiatric disorders

Common mental disorders (CMDs) during pregnancy, such as depressive and anxiety disorders, may adversely impact the health of both mother and infant (Jha et al. 2018). However, in contrast to the disorders discussed in ▶ Chap. 3 and in the preceding sections of this chapter, mental disorders are more difficult to classify, because of the generally poor insight into their cause and pathophysiology (Phillips et al. 2012), and the fact that they are also often interrelated as shown in ◘ fig. 4.25 (Smoller 2013).

About 1 in 8 pregnant or postpartum women from high-income countries suffer from some form of nonpsychotic mental health issue (Fisher at al. 2012), a level at least twice as high as that in low and middle-low income countries. These problems usually coincide with the presence of risk factors, such as (in order of impact), a history of mental health issues, insufficient emotional and practical support, socioeconomic hardship, unintentional or unwanted pregnancy, unmarried and/or being of a young age (Fisher

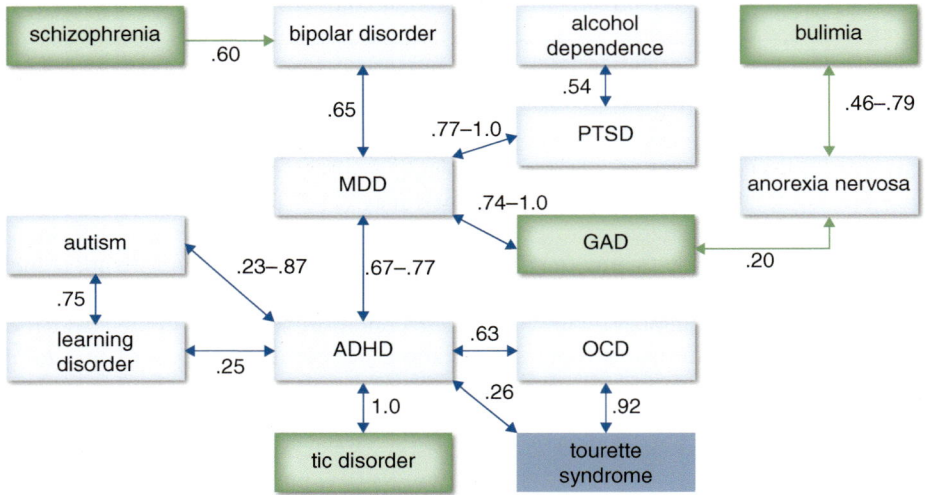

■ **Figure 4.25**   Genetic correlations among psychiatric disorders. The numbers next to the arrows are correlation coefficients that indicate the extend of genetic interrelationship between two disorders, estimated based on data from twin studies. *Abbreviations. GAD*, generalized anxiety disorder; *MDD*, major depressive disorder; *PTSD*, post-traumatic stress disorder; *OCD*, obsessive compulsive disorder; *ADHD*, attention deficit/hyperactivity disorder (*adopted from* Smoller 2013)

et al. 2012; Jha et al. 2018). We know that around 20 % of maternal mortality cases in developed countries occur in women challenged by at least one of these risk factors, which – tragically – correlate strongly with mental health issues (Kassenbaum et al. 2014; Lega et al. 2020).

Most cases of suicide in the perinatal period occur in women with a CMD, and is, together with CMD-related morbidity, often preventable if care providers during pregnancy are aware of the risk factors, enabling them to initiate timely preventive interventions (Mangla et al. 2019). In the section below, the most common chronic psychiatric disorders (bipolar disorder, depression, PTSD, schizophrenia, anxiety- and personality disorders) will be discussed, along with their possible impact on pregnancy and how pregnancy may affect the course of the preexistent CMD. A global mechanism which considers how a CMD may negatively impact the fetus, relates to the level of CMD-associated maternal stress experienced during pregnancy and mediated by hyperactivity of the HPA-axis, as shown in ■ fig. 4.26 and detailed elsewhere (Glover et al. 2018).

4.6.1 Bipolar disorder (BD)

Bipolar disorder (BD), formerly known as 'manic depressive illness' is a neuroprogressive recurrent chronic illness characterized by mood waves fluctuating between episodes of depression and inflated mood (mania), intermixed with periods of euthymia (■ fig. 4.27). The most recent estimate for the worldwide prevalence of BD is 2.4 %, irrespective of nationality, ethnic origin and socioeconomic status (Merikangas et al. 2011).

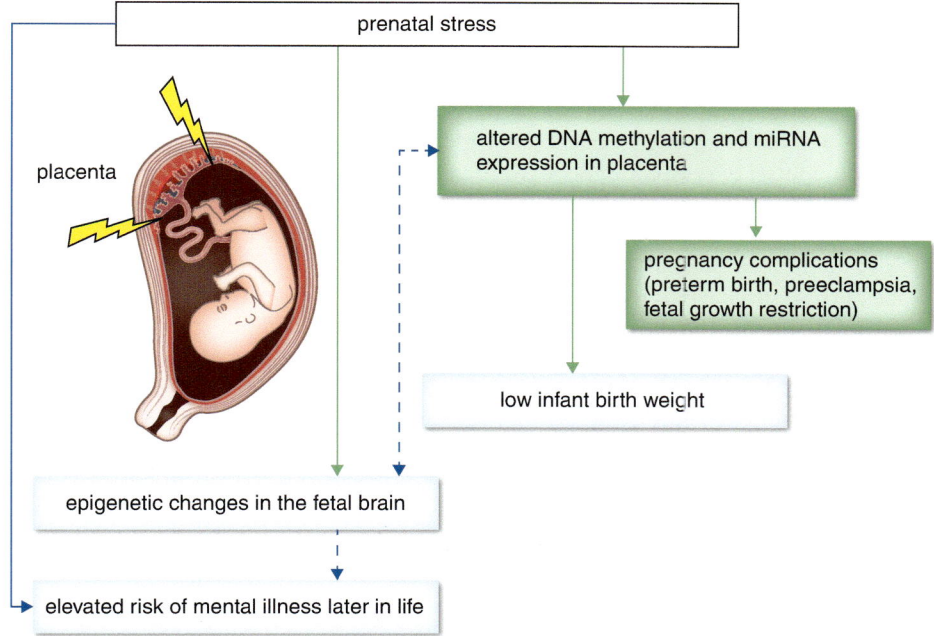

◘ Figure 4.26   Association between prenatal stress and mental health. Prenatal stress is thought to affect essential miRNA expression and DNA methylation in both placenta and brain development. Disruption of these epigenetic mechanisms in the placenta predisposes to fetal growth restriction and preterm birth. However, it is unknown, whether stress-induced epigenetic changes in placenta and fetal brain are causally related (Faa et al. 2016). Therefore, it is also unknown, whether these abnormal intrauterine effects predispose to a mental disorder later in life (Babenko et al. 2015)

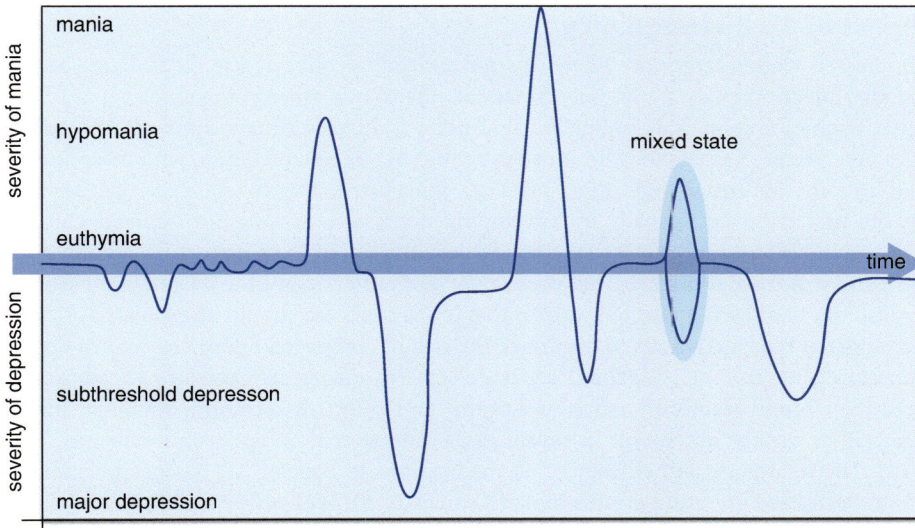

◘ Figure 4.27   Life chart showing the timeline of a bipolar disorder. According to severity, manic and hypomanic symptoms are registered above the state of euthymia (normal mood state), whereas depressive symptoms are depicted below (*adopted from* Grande et al. 2016)

BD usually begins in adolescence and worsens with age. It is an important cause of disability among the young and gradually leads to cognitive and functional impairment along with increased mortality, particularly from suicide (about 10 % of affected persons). The risk of suicide is heightened by the presence of risk factors such as depression, substance use disorder, psychiatric co-morbidity, history of self-harm, recent disease onset, abrupt onset of symptoms, no active treatment and young age (< 25 y). Combined with excess mortality due to natural causes, average life expectancy is about 15 years lower than in healthy controls. BD-affected persons typically have a high rate of psychiatric and medical co-morbidities (Harrison et al. 2018).

The current insight into the pathogenesis of BD is still frustratingly limited. Genetic susceptibility is a major risk factor, as reflected not only in a 10-fold higher risk of a child to develop BD if a parent is affected, but also based on the results of twin studies, that estimate a heritability of 0.7–0.8. The results generated by genomic studies suggest that abnormal calcium signaling plays a role in the pathogenesis of the disorder (Harrison et al. 2018). Also, environmental factors contribute to the development of BD, such as experiencing a misfortune in childhood. Because of the poor insight in the pathogenesis of BD, no valid biomarkers are available to early identify an affected person. Therefore, the disorder is to be diagnosed by clinical assessment based on widely accepted diagnostic criteria (Grande et al. 2016). Obviously, management of the disorder requires up-to-date knowledge of the evolving pharmacological and psychological options, as detailed elsewhere (Sharma et al. 2019), particularly in the complex condition of pregnancy and the highly vulnerable postpartum period.

Impact of pregnancy on BD

BP is a major risk factor for postpartum psychosis, a risk that may be magnified in the presence of additional risk factors, such as a family history of postpartum psychosis, primiparity and sleep deprivation (Khan et al. 2016).

Impact of BD on pregnancy

BD-affected women are more likely to smoke, drink alcohol or use illicit drugs, factors that also affect pregnancy adversely. Since the rate of unplanned pregnancies in a BD-affected woman is high, it is important that her psychiatrist timely discusses the advantages of a 'planned' pregnancy. In most euthymic BD-affected women, who discontinued their mood-stabilizing medication prior to conception, the BD quickly relapses during the first trimester, usually by developing depressive or dysphoric-mixed episodes (Khan et al. 2016). If a depressive episode develops in an early-pregnant woman without history of mental disease, that event may be the first sign of a yet undiagnosed BD. Medication, used by BD-affected women that try to conceive, should be evaluated critically and adjusted if needed, so as to minimize the risk of congenital anomalies and to uphold remission. The risk of congenital birth defects secondary to exposure to commonly prescribed mood stabilizers, such as lithium and selective serotonin reuptake inhibitors (SSRIs) may be acceptable in severe cases (Susser et al. 2016; Brummelte and Galea 2016). The teratology and efficacy of all medications to control BD has been elaborated in the specialized literature on this topic (Khan et al. 2016; Ornoy et al. 2017).

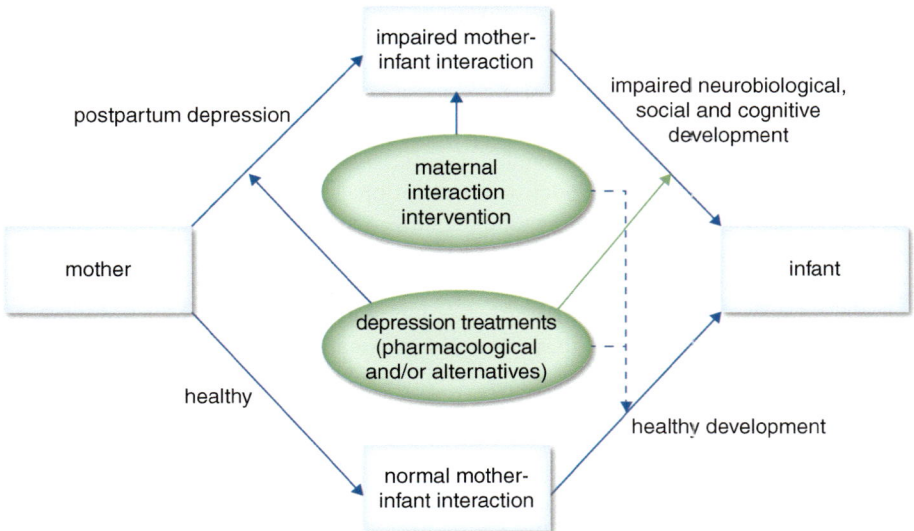

Figure 4.28 Potential relationship between postpartum depression (PPD), maternal-infant interaction and child outcome. PPD may contribute to a disturbed neurobiological development of the child. Improving both, maternal depressive symptoms and mother-infant interaction (blue arrows) may be important to enable a healthy development of the child (blue dotted arrow). However, *pharmacological* treatment of the maternal depression carries a small risk of adversely affecting the child's development and outcome (green arrow) (*adopted from* Brummelte and Galea 2016)

The rate of placental syndromes, including fetal growth restriction, is higher in BD-affected women than in non-affected healthy controls (Rusner et al. 2016), presumably by the mechanism shown in ⬛ fig. 4.26. The maternal depression that may develop postpartum requires special attention, as it is associated with a high risk of developing an unhealthy post-partum mother-infant relationship. Therefore, the postpartum focus of BP management is to prevent or at least to alleviate maternal postpartum depression, while also providing the measures and/or conditions that endorse the development of a long-term healthy relationship between the mother and her developing child (⬛ fig. 4.28) (Brummelte and Galea 2016; Gentile 2017).

4.6.2 Perinatal depression (PD)

Perinatal depression (PD) refers to a non-psychotic depressive episode of mild to moderate severity, during pregnancy or in the first 12 months postpartum (Gelaye et al. 2016). Pregnancy is a major life event accompanied by social, psychological and hormonal changes. These changes may trigger depressive episodes with serious impact for both mother and infant. The prevalence of PD in high-income countries has been reported to gradually rise from about 7 % in the first trimester to about 13 % in the third trimester of pregnancy, with an even higher rate postpartum (Howdeshell and Ornoy 2017).

Despite its rate being more than twice as high as that in low- and middle-income countries and its enormous economic and personal burden, PD remains under-recognized and undertreated in these countries (Gelaye et al. 2016). The risk of developing PD is influenced by external factors, such as the discontinuation of antidepressant medication, somatic symptoms, little social support, poor nutrition, poor antenatal care, increased substance use, exposure to partner violence, unintentional pregnancy and a history of a high relapse rate. The same applies to the emotional impact of an unfavorable pregnancy outcome, e.g. because of pregnancy complications, such as placental syndrome, fetal growth restriction or preterm birth. Untreated depression during pregnancy is of major concern, as it increases the risk of developing postpartum depression with its negative effects on the infant's neurocognitive development secondary to a disturbed mother-infant relationship. It follows that screening for depression in pregnant/postpartum women is of utmost importance, as is the recent development of new forms of psychotherapy and non-drug treatment modalities (Johansen et al. 2019).

Impact of pregnancy on PD

The effect of pregnancy on PD is similar to that described for BD.

Impact of PD on pregnancy

Depression during pregnancy has been associated with preterm birth, gestational diabetes and placental syndromes, including fetal growth restriction (Becker et al. 2016). Indirect evidence supports the view that untreated depression may lead to dysregulation of the hypothalamic-pituitary-adrenocortical axis, disrupting the normal release of catecholamines and cortisol. This endocrine disfunction has a negative impact on placental perfusion increasing the risk of developing a placental syndrome and preterm birth (Becker et al. 2016). Postpartum, the infant of a PD-affected mother is at increased risk of disruption of the normal mother-child bonding (Serati et al. 2016), which predisposes to impaired neurocognitive development (◻ fig. 4.28).

4.6.3 Post-traumatic Stress Disorder (PTSD)

About 1 to 2 % of pregnant women develop a PTSD postpartum, usually after a traumatic birth experience or an obstetric emergency associated with complications during childbirth. Other risk factors associated with postpartum PTSD are a history of PTSD or depression, psychological difficulties during pregnancy, fear of childbirth, poor health, lack of support during labor, neonatal complications and previous traumatic experiences (Andersen et al. 2012). Postpartum, PTSD is associated with an inability to cope with stress, and highly co-morbid with depression (Ayers et al. 2016) as illustrated in ◻ fig. 4.29.

Impact of PTSD on maternal health and mother-infant interactions

Postpartum PTSD resembles PD since it also predisposes to a disrupted development of mother-child bonding (Serati et al. 2016). If PTSD develops in a BD-affected woman in remission and the preceding pregnancy was complicated by fetal growth restriction, the latter may also have led to epigenetic imprinting affecting fetal brain development, similar to that described for BD. This risk emphasizes the value of timely and proactively

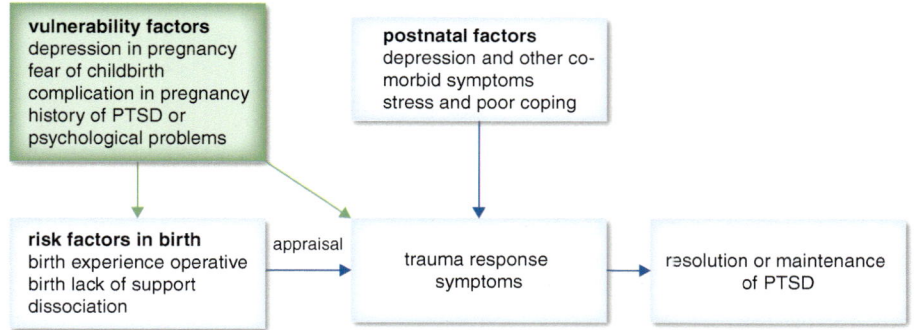

□ Figure 4.29 Vulnerability-stress model, which is the starting point for the potential development to birth-related PTSD (*adopted from* Ayers et al. 2016)

screening for PTSD, if possible before pregnancy. It enables the timely detection of a risk patient and the earliest initiation of preventive measures. For this strategy to be successful, collaboration of professionals across disciplines is essential (Cirino and Knapp 2019).

4.6.4 Schizophrenia (SZ)

Schizophrenia (SZ) is a chronic, disabling mental disorder with a lifetime prevalence of 0.7 % worldwide (Owen et al. 2016). SZ-symptoms usually develop between 16 and 30 years of age and consist of (1) positive symptoms, expressed in delusions, hallucinations and disorganized thinking; (2) negative symptoms, such as social withdrawal, less spontaneous speech, impaired motivation and melancholia, and (3) abnormal motor behavior and cognitive deficits resulting in limited attention span, working memory and executive function (Owen et al. 2016). Schizophrenia is diagnosed based on the DSM-5 criteria, as detailed elsewhere (Tandon et al. 2013).

SZ-affected individuals display a complex heterogenous behavior and cognition, which is the final outcome of a disrupted brain development resulting from a combination of genetic and environmental factors (□ fig. 4.30). The development of psychotic symptoms partly relates to dysfunctional glutamatergic neurotransmission with the widespread involvement of other brain areas and circuits (Owen et al. 2016; Howes et al. 2017; Stilo and Murray 2019). About half of SZ-affected persons have intermittent long-term psychiatric problems with 20 % of this subgroup having chronic symptoms or disability. Most SZ-affected individuals are unemployed. Life expectancy of a SZ-affected individual is reduced by as much as 10–20 years (Owen et al. 2016).

Impact of pregnancy on SZ

It is an ethical dilemma, whether SZ-affected women should continue their antipsychotic medication during pregnancy, as the evidence for the safety of this medication for the infant is still limited (Teodorescu et al. 2017). Pregnant SZ-affected women are quite often admitted for psychiatric reasons, particularly in the first trimester, at least in

4

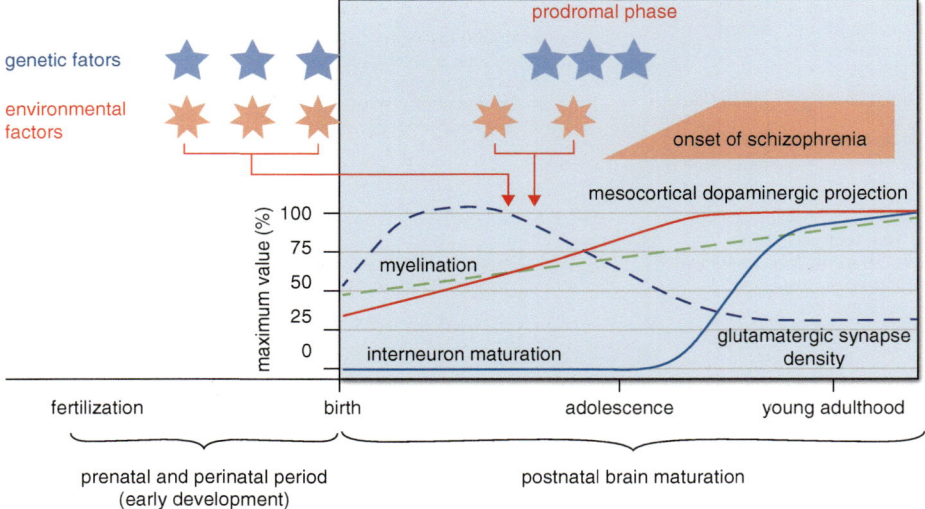

■ **Figure 4.30**   Interaction of genetic and environmental risk factors in the pathophysiology of schizophrenia (*adopted from* Owen et al. 2016)

part, because conception in many SZ-affected women was unintentional. The high rate of psychiatric admissions during pregnancy is accompanied by poorer prenatal care and a higher rate of adverse psychosocial outcomes for mother and child. The rate of obstetric complications does not differ from that in non-SZ-affected women, except for a slightly higher rate of fetal growth restriction (Harris et al. 2019). It is conceivable that the latter relates to the extra stress that these women experience during pregnancy, which adversely impacts placental perfusion (see ■ fig. 4.26). Yet, the rate difference relative to controls was small and could also be explained by the often-higher rate of smoking, substance abuse and unfavorable socio-economic conditions in SZ-affected women (Bennedsen 1998).

Impact of SZ on pregnancy

The modern antipsychotic medication currently used by SZ-patients to maintain remission, has a small risk of congenital anomalies, when continued during the 1st trimester of pregnancy. On the other hand, discontinuation of this medication increases the risk of relapse of psychotic episodes by 50 %. This dilemma requires close consultation between patient and the multidisciplinary team of care providers consisting of a psychiatrist, an obstetrician and a neonatologist. The only pregnancy complication observed at a higher rate in SZ-affected women is fetal growth restriction, as mentioned above.

4.6.5 Anxiety disorder (AD)

Pregnancy anxiety is observed in up to two-thirds of pregnancies (Williams and Koleva 2018) and refers to the interplay between a woman's emotions and the physiological experience of her pregnancy. It consists of a distinct feeling of worry related to pregnancy and upcoming motherhood, often including concerns about the baby's health, labor, caring for the baby after discharge and finances. However, a perinatal AD differs from pregnancy anxiety by virtue of intensity and persistence of excessive fear and worry, to such an extend, that it adversely impacts a woman's behavior and psychosocial functioning. ADs are often diagnosed based on the DSM-5 criteria as elaborated elsewhere (Williams and Koleva 2018). Their prevalence in the perinatal period ranges from 2 to 10 % (Williams and Koleva 2018).

Impact of pregnancy on an AD

The state of pregnancy may simply trigger the development of an AD. Timely recognition and treatment of a perinatal AD is crucial to both improve maternal well-being and reduce the rate of adverse pregnancy outcome. This requires the timely screening for an AD at least once during pregnancy (Williams and Koleva 2018; Sinesi et al. 2019), followed by the institution of the appropriate management to improve pregnancy outcome. In most cases, management consists of prescribing first-line psychotropic anxiety medication along with evidence-based psychotherapy as detailed elsewhere (Nillni et al. 2018; Thorsness et al. 2018).

Impact of an AD on pregnancy

During pregnancy, an AD predisposes to preterm labor, placental syndromes and after childbirth, to maternal postpartum depression. The child is at increased risk for adverse neurodevelopmental, cognitive and behavioral outcomes, such as language delay, attention deficit-hyperactivity disorder (ADHD) and an emotion regulation disorder (Thorsness et al. 2018).

4.6.6 Borderline Personality disorder (BPD)

A Borderline Personality disorder (BPD) is a psychiatric disorder characterized by a pattern of instability in interpersonal relationships, identity, impulsivity, along with emotion dysregulation. The diagnosis of the disorder is usually based on the DSM-5 diagnostic criteria (Evans and Simms 2018). Unstable relationships and a tendency to consider suicide or self-injury are the most useful indications for making a correct diagnosis. BPD-affected persons typically elicit both high rates of suicide and comorbid mental disorders (mostly mood/anxiety disorders and substance abuse), in addition to severe functional impairment and intensive use of treatment. These disorders are often associated with increased levels of economic and socio-cultural costs for society.

The estimated prevalence of BPD in the community is about 4.4 % (Kendall et al. 2009), but is as high as 10 % among psychiatric outpatients (Leichsenring et al. 2011). The most supported etiopathology of BPD is, that the disorder results from interactions between biological and psychosocial factors, in particular between biologically-based temperamental vulnerabilities, and adverse and traumatic experiences during childhood (fig. 4.31). An abnormality in the serotoninergic function has been suggested to form the underlying footing for the impulsive aggressive symptoms and that this defect may be associated with specific genetic risk factors (Leichsenring et al. 2011). The backbone treatment of BPD is psychotherapy with adjuvant pharmacotherapy to abate state-specific symptoms in periods of acute decompensation as detailed elsewhere (Kendall et al. 2009).

4

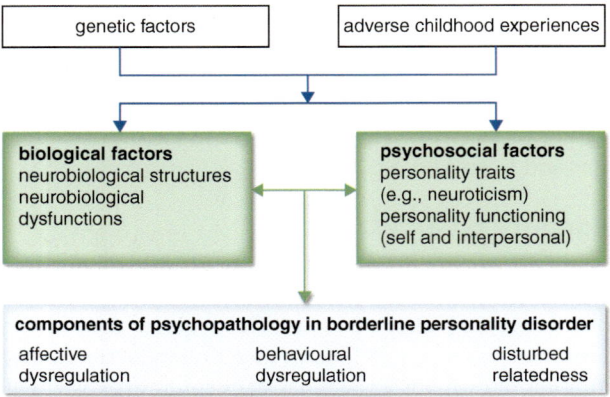

□ **Figure 4.31**   The biopsychosocial model of borderline personality disorder (*adopted from Leichsenring et al. 2011*)

Impact of pregnancy on BPD

Women affected by a BPD are at increased risk of both teenage – and unintended pregnancies (De Genna et al. 2012). Their risk behavior with respect to smoking and substance abuse increases the risk for the infant (fetal growth restriction) during pregnancy.

Impact of BPD on pregnancy

Pregnant women diagnosed with a BPD are at increased risk to develop gestational diabetes, preterm birth and venous thromboembolism, probably partly in conjunction with their higher rate of smoking and substance use (Pare-Miron et al. 2016). Postpartum, BPD-affected mothers are at increased risk of developing a maladaptive interaction with their infants, characterized by insensitive, overprotective and hostile parenting, when compared to mothers without BPD. This may eventually result in adverse offspring outcomes (Eyden et al. 2016). To prevent and enable timely management of these severe effects, those mothers should be closely monitored by a multidisciplinary team, preferable already from before pregnancy and until after childbirth.

In summary, the impact of chronic mental disorders (CMD) on pregnancy in an affected woman can be huge, (1) because of the extra stress the CMD-affected mother experiences during pregnancy, (2) because of the social and societal implications, and (3) because of the potential adverse effect of the CMD on the postnatal interrelation between mother and infant, and associated risk regarding the infant's neurodevelopmental, cognitive and social development.

4.7 Pharmacotherapy during pregnancy

▶ Chapters 3 and 4 focused on the course and outcome of pregnancy in women with a preexistent chronic disorder. Most of these disorders are managed by prescription drugs. Historically, concerns about fetal safety have limited pharmacotherapy during pregnancy, and with it, performing sufficient drug studies during pregnancy. Although these concerns are understandable, particularly the subgroups of pregnant women described in ▶ Chap. 3 (and in this chapter), often require medications to manage their various chronic medical conditions and, the state of pregnancy does not eliminate that requirement. Clinical management of these patients during pregnancy is not a topic addressed in this book, but the interested reader is provided with references to guidelines and review articles that specify this management, including the possible necessity to switch to alternative medication, e.g. because of proven or suspected teratogenic properties of (one of) the prescription drugs used in the non-pregnant state.

The *teratology* of various prescription drugs during pregnancy is beyond the scope of this book. Data on birth defects and changes in the rate of specific malformations are reported on the website of the International Clearinghouse for Birth Defects Surveillance and Research (ICBDSR or Clearinghouse in short), a voluntary non-profit International Organization affiliated with WHO (▶ www.icbdsr.org). The reported data are based on information collected worldwide, with data from several million newborns. Other sources are ENTIS (European Network of Teratology Information Services: ▶ www.entis-org.eu) and OTIS (Organization of Teratology Information Specialist: ▶ www.mothertobaby.org).

Besides teratologic properties of various medications, it is also possible that a prescription drug used before pregnancy becomes less effective post-conceptionally, due to pregnancy-related changes in the *pharmacokinetics* of that medication, as elaborated in the section below.

Recent studies on pharmacology during pregnancy highlight the complexity of drug distribution and response during pregnancy, as maternal adaptations, instituted to support fetal growth and development, also affect drug absorption, distribution, metabolism, elimination and transport (◼ fig. 4.32) and thus also their clearance, half-life and bioavailability (Ward and Varner 2019). Therefore, detailed pharmacologic information is important to adjust therapeutic treatment during pregnancy. Insight in both pregnancy physiology and the pharmacology of different agents is critical to achieve effective treatment at minimal risk for mother and infant. Treatment and dosing in pregnancy are often based on standard adult doses, usually derived from information obtained in healthy, mostly male, individuals. Information on the pharmacokinetic and -dynamics

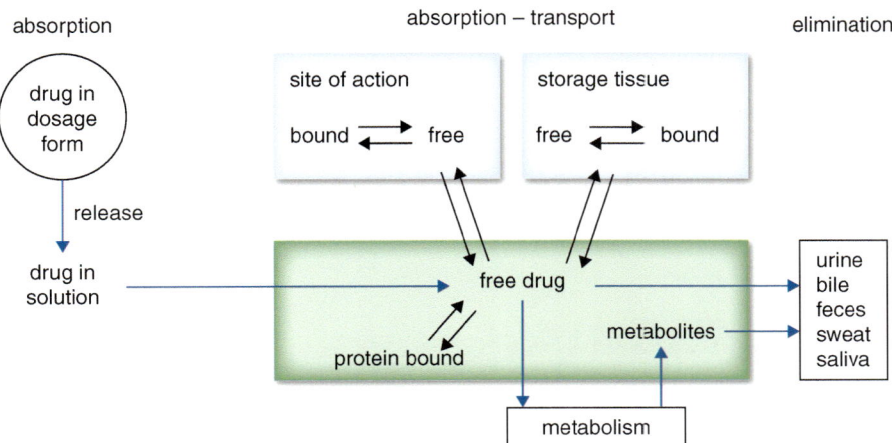

◼ **Figure 4.32**   The pharmacokinetic process (*adopted from* Feghali et al. 2015)

of many drugs during pregnancy and breastfeeding is lacking, even though it has been shown that these conditions modulate their pharmacokinetic and pharmacodynamic properties to such an extent, that dose adjustment would be needed (Larsson et al. 2008).

Information on the transplacental transfer of drugs, as can be derived from cord blood levels at birth and levels in mother milk, are important to limit health risks for the fetus in late pregnancy and the infant during breastfeeding. The following section provides an overview of the potential impact of pregnancy-induced maternal adaptations on efficacy and possible side effects of various common prescription drugs.

4

4.7.1 Drug absorption

Drug absorption is the movement of a drug from the site of administration to the systemic circulation and is a prerequisite for its pharmacologic action (■ fig. 4.33). Drug absorption is often confused with bioavailability, the fraction of intact, active drug that

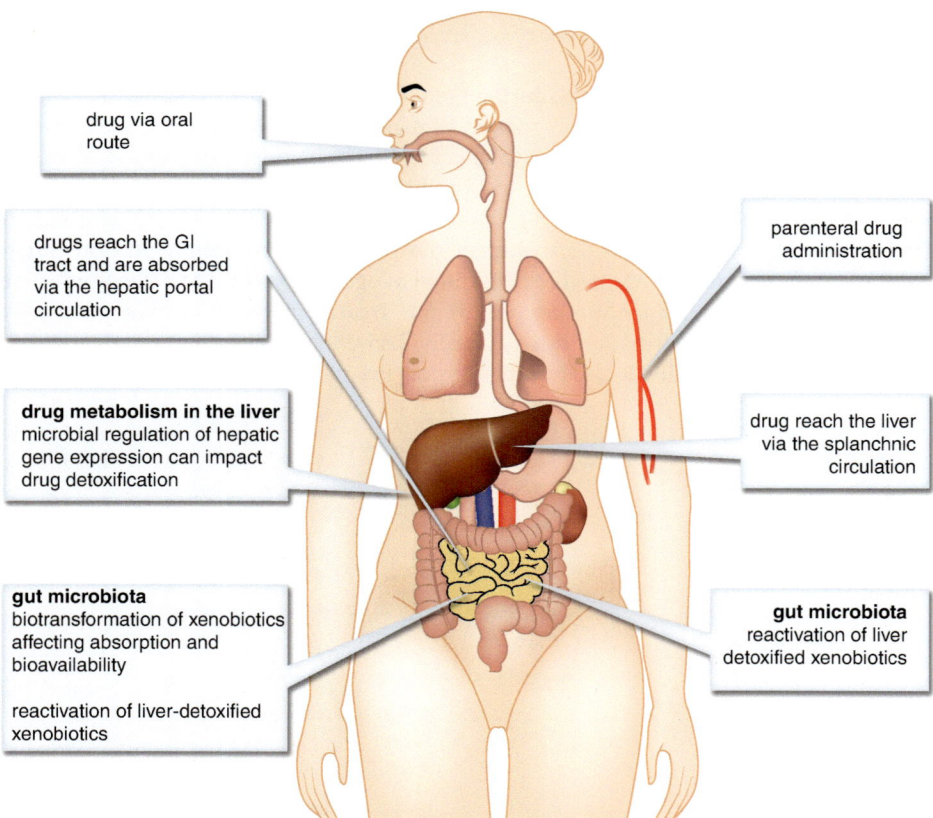

drug via oral route

parenteral drug administration

drugs reach the GI tract and are absorbed via the hepatic portal circulation

drug metabolism in the liver
microbial regulation of hepatic gene expression can impact drug detoxification

drug reach the liver via the splanchnic circulation

gut microbiota
biotransformation of xenobiotics affecting absorption and bioavailability

reactivation of liver-detoxified xenobiotics

gut microbiota
reactivation of liver detoxified xenobiotics

■ **Figure 4.33**   Oral (left-side boxes) versus parenteral (right-side boxes) drug administration route. The uptake of most highly-soluble drugs takes place in the upper small intestines, where the direct impact of drug-microbiome interactions is not yet fully uncovered (*adopted from* Clarke et al. 2019)

reaches the systemic circulation, irrespective of route of administration. Drugs that are administered intravascularly, intramuscularly or subcutaneously are 100 % bioavailable, since they are delivered directly into the bloodstream or body tissue.

The oral intake of a drug is usually associated with the largest variation in drug absorption. This route affects bioavailability, not only by the fractional uptake in the GI-tract, but also by the first-pass metabolism of the drug in the liver before reaching the systemic circulation (◘ fig. 4.33). The pregnancy-related reduced gastric acid output is paralleled by an overall higher mucus secretion, both effects combined, resulting in a less acid intra-gastric ambiance. Therefore, it is conceivable that this effect, together with the delayed gastric emptying, slower peristalsis in the GI tract and altered gut microbiome (Clarke et al. 2019) in pregnancy (Neuman and Koren 2017) affect drug absorption and with it, the therapeutic efficacy of most oral drugs. Meanwhile, the hemodynamic changes associated with the development of the hyperdynamic circulation (HDC) are unlikely to be relevant, as they do not include an appreciable change in the intestinal blood supply (detailed in ▶ Chap. 1).

Interestingly, reported data on bioavailability and therapeutic effect of most oral drugs, particularly those requiring repeated dosing, suggests that the overall effect of the pregnancy-related changes in GI function on bioavailability, is small (Koren and Pariente 2018). On the other hand, metabolization of drugs during their first passage across the liver parenchyma may reduce their bioavailability markedly. This effect applies e.g. to morphine, buprenorphine, propranolol, diazepam, and pethidine.

Importantly, nausea and vomiting in early pregnancy may also reduce drug availability for absorption after oral intake. Therefore, oral medications should be taken at a moment, when nausea is minimal. The raised circulating progesterone level tends to inhibit GI peristalsis, an effect that can be expected to enhance the development of nausea and vomiting.

4.7.2 Drug distribution

Drug distribution describes the reversible transfer of a drug between different locations after its entry into the systemic circulation. The volume of distribution (Vd) is a measure to describe the extent of dispersion of a systemic dose of medication throughout the body. It reflects a theoretical volume that an administered drug would occupy, if it were uniformly distributed at a concentration similar to that in plasma. The Vd is important to determine the loading dose of a drug needed to achieve a certain therapeutic level. Drugs that remain within the vascular bed have a Vd similar to the plasma volume, whereas soluble hydrophilic drugs, unbound to protein in the body, will have a Vd close to total body water (◘ fig. 4.34). Drugs that are highly bound to tissues, with a small proportion remaining in the intravascular space, will have a high Vd. By comparison, drugs that are highly bound to plasma proteins and/or have a large molecular weight will tend to concentrate intravascularly and will have a Vd close to 1. The Vd of a drug is useful in estimating the dose required to achieve a given plasma level. Drug distribution is influenced by factors, such as tissue perfusion, tissue binding, lipid solubility, and plasma protein binding.

During pregnancy, plasma volume expands by more than 40 % in concert with a rise in total body water, most of it occupying the extracellular compartment (◘ tab. 4.4). This adaptation dilutes hydrophilic drugs, leading to lower plasma levels, including that

4

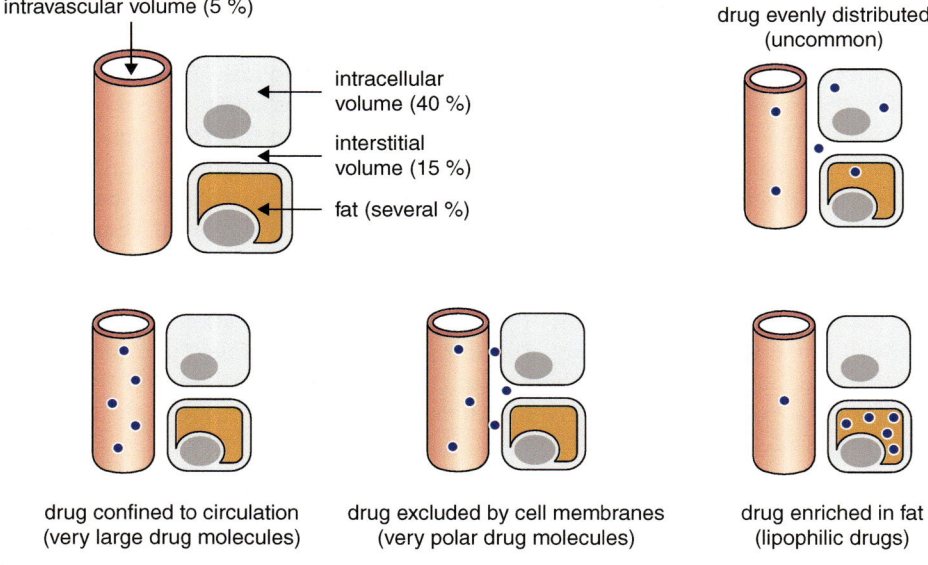

intravascular volume (5 %)

intracellular volume (40 %)

interstitial volume (15 %)

fat (several %)

drug evenly distributed (uncommon)

drug confined to circulation (very large drug molecules)

drug excluded by cell membranes (very polar drug molecules)

drug enriched in fat (lipophilic drugs)

◘ **Figure 4.34**   Volume of distribution (Vd) of a drug is defined as total number of drug molecules in the body (total dosage) divided by the plasma level. Very large drug molecules (e.g. proteins, polysaccharides) remain within the intravascular compartment (Vd = 1). If a large fraction of a drug accumulates in tissue, the Vd becomes large. This implies to lipophilic drugs that may have a Vd, that is many times larger than the actual total body volume

◘ **Table 4.4**   Pregnancy-induced changes (%) in the maternal body composition that affect pharmacokinetics during pregnancy (*adopted from* Ward and Varner 2019)

trimester of pregnancy	first	second	third
body weight	+6	+16	+23
total fat mass	+11	+16	+32
total body water	+11	+27	+41
plasma volume	+7	+42	+50
red blood cell volume	+4	+20	+28
hematocrit	−3	−8	−14
albumin	ns	−14	−28

of albumin. Albumin is the predominant protein in human plasma, with levels mostly declining after the first trimester, reaching a nadir in the third trimester. The fraction of albumin-bound drugs decreases with the fall in plasma albumin level resulting in higher levels of free circulating drug (for drugs that have limited clearance). This effect enables a higher tissue distribution and may be clinically relevant for certain drugs, particularly in advanced pregnancy. In general, small-molecular-weight and lipophilic drugs readily cross the placenta. The fetus and amniotic fluid may act as additional compartments, enabling drug accumulation reflected in a higher Vd of certain drugs.

4.7.3 **Drug metabolization**

Drug metabolization involves the chemical modification of a drug by specialized enzymatic systems. Some drugs, administered as inactive pro-drugs, need to be metabolized to be converted to their active form. However, metabolization of most drugs reduces their activity. The metabolic enzyme activity in different organs varies widely, depending on ethnicity, gender, age and enzyme polymorphisms, and is also a major source of variation in drug pharmacokinetics and response. The most frequently used drugs are metabolized in two phases. Phase I reactions involve oxidation, reduction, and hydrolysis and are mostly carried out in the liver by the cytochrome P450 (CYP) family of enzymes (Ward and Varner 2019). Phase II reactions involve conjugation by actions of uridine 5'-diphosphate glucuronosyltransferases [UGTs]. In most cases, these reactions follow phase I reactions and serve to facilitate excretion into urine or bile. Pregnancy may alter the activity of both phase I and phase II enzymes.

4.7.4 **Clearance**

Clearance is an important pharmacokinetic aspect of a drug. It is the (hypothetical) volume of plasma, cleared of the drug per unit time. Systemic clearance is the body's overall ability to eliminate a drug. Pregnancy can alter a drug's elimination (half-life), e.g. by altering its Vd or its clearance. The hepatic clearance of a drug is defined as the fraction of drug removed from blood by the liver (extraction ratio, ER) and depends on hepatic blood flow, uptake by hepatocytes and enzyme metabolic capacity. For drugs with a high liver ER (e.g. morphine and propranolol), the overall hepatic elimination is only limited by the hepatic blood flow. In contrast, hepatic clearance of drugs with a low ER (e.g. diazepam, caffeine) is limited by the intrinsic metabolic capacity of hepatocytes and the free plasma fraction of the drug.

4.7.5 **Drug elimination**

Renal drug excretion depends on glomerular filtration rate (GFR), tubular secretion, and reabsorption. Pregnancy induces a 50–60 % rise in GFR that lasts from early pregnancy until near term. If a drug is solely excreted by glomerular filtration, its renal clearance in pregnancy will increase as a function of GFR. Some drugs (e.g. cefazolin) display increased renal elimination during pregnancy. However, differences in renal tubular transport (secretion or reabsorption) and poorly elucidated pregnancy-induced changes in renal tubular transporters may have a major effect on renal drug clearance (Yacovino and Aleksunes 2012). For drugs with a narrow therapeutic window, a pregnancy-induced rise in clearance may lead to sub-therapeutic levels and deteriorating disease control. Conversely, to avoid increased toxicity, drug doses may need to be adjusted in the postpartum period, when pregnancy-induced changes in metabolic enzyme activity resolve.

4.7.6 Drug transporters

Drug transporters are widely expressed in many maternal organs and also in the placenta. These compounds regulate drug absorption, excretion and often the extent of drug entry into target organs. For example, drug transporters in hepatic sinusoids determine drug uptake into hepatocytes, where drugs may undergo biotransformation. Transporters in the biliary ductal system regulate secretion into the bile. In this context, the enterohepatic circulation is relevant. It refers to the transfer of bile acids, bilirubin, drugs and other liver products to the bile, to be deposited into the small intestines. In the enterohepatic circulation, certain products are hydrolyzed in the small intestine by bacterial flora, which may result in the liberation of liver-induced binding of a (lipophilic) drug, enabling its reabsorption. This process prolongs the action of a drug e.g. of digoxin, morphine and thyroxin through reabsorption by the enterocyte and return to the liver, as illustrated in ◘ fig. 4.35.

The enterohepatic circulation is an important phenomenon in the field of toxicology as many lipophilic xenobiotics undergo this process, that may also prolong their hepatotoxic properties. Renal transporters play an important role in regulating tubular secretion and reabsorption of water, solutes and drugs. For instance, renal transporters in the renal proximal tubules, are key in regulating the tubular secretion and reabsorption of drug molecules. These transporters are increasingly recognized as targets for clinically significant drug-drug interactions as elaborated elsewhere (Yin and Wang 2016).

Fetal development not only depends upon the transplacental exchange of nutrients, O_2 and metabolic waste products, but also upon the synthesis of hormones, peptides and steroids. The placenta separates the maternal and fetal circulations and with it, protects the fetus from xenobiotics in the maternal blood. It has been shown that – to some degree – nearly all drugs, administered during pregnancy, will reach the fetal circulation by passive diffusion. In the syncytiotrophoblast, a number of transporters have been identified on both the fetal and maternal side, that actively transfer drugs to the fetus.

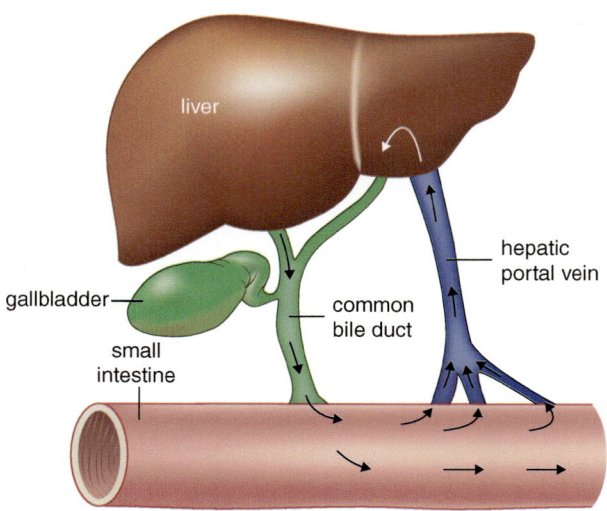

◘ **Figure 4.35**   The enterohepatic circulation, enabling hydrolysis of various hepatic products dissolved in the bile of the small intestines by bacteria in the local microbiome

Little is known about the regulation of the expression of placental drug transporters and how their activity varies with advancing pregnancy. Placental steroids, but also placental dysfunction modulate their expression. Changes in drug metabolism may alter drug dosage in pregnancy. For drugs with a narrow therapeutic window, increased clearance during pregnancy can lead to sub-therapeutic levels and worsening disease control. On the other hand, to avoid increased toxicity, drug doses may need to be adjusted in the postpartum period, when pregnancy-related metabolic enzyme activity changes resolve. In pregnancy, a more thorough approach would be to monitor free drug concentrations and adjust drug dosing to maintain the unbound concentration within its therapeutic range.

References

Abood A, Vestergaard P. Pregnancy outcome in women with primary hyperparathyroidism. Eur J Endocrinol. 2014;171:69–76.

Adam K. Pregnancy in women with cardiovascular diseases. Methodist Debakey Cardiovasc J. 2017;13:209–15.

Agrawal S, Agrawal S, Arnason T, Saini S, Belghiti J. Management hepatocellular adenoma: recent advances. Clin Gastroenterol Hepatol. 2015;13:1221–30.

Ahluwalia M, Hoag JB, Hadeh A, Ferrin M, Hadjiliadis D. Cystic fibrosis and pregnancy in the modern era: a case control study. Journal of Cystic Fibrosis. 2014;13:69–73.

Ahmad A, Ahmed A, Patrizio P. Cystic fibrosis and fertility. Curr Opin Obstet Gynecol. 2013;25:167–72.

Ala A, Walker AP, Keyoumars A, Dooley JS, Schilsky ML. Wilson's disease. Lancet. 2007;369:397–408.

Alexander EK, Pearce EN, Brent GA, et al. 2017 guidelines of the American thyroid association for the diagnosis and management of thyroid disease during pregnancy and the postpartum. Thyroid. 2017;27:315–89.

Alvarado-Mora MV, Locarnini S, Rizzetto M, Ribello-Pinho JR. An update on HDV: virology, pathogenesis and treatment. Antivir Ther. 2013;18:541–8.

Anand G, Beuschlein F. Management of endocrine disease: fertility, pregnancy and lactation in women with adrenal insufficiency. Eur J Endocrinol. 2018;178:R45–53.

Anderson LB, et al. Risk factors for developing post-traumatic stress disorder following childbirth: a systematic review. Acta Obstet Gynecol Scand. 2012;91:1261–72.

Ayers S, et al. The aetiology of post-traumatic stress following childbirth: a meta-analysis and theoretical framework. Psychol Med. 2016;46:1121–34.

Azulay CE, Pariente G, Shoham-Vardi I, Kessous R, Sergienko R, Sheiner E. Maternal anemia during pregnancy and subsequent risk of cardiovascular disease. J Matern Fetal Neonatal Med. 2015;28:1762–5.

Babenko O, et al. Stress-induced perinatal and transgenerational epigenetic programming of brain development and mental health. Neurosci Biobehav Rev. 2015;48:70–91.

Becker M et al. Depression during pregnancy and postpartum. Curr Psychiatry Rep. 2016;18:32 (9 pages).

Bennedsen BE. Adverse pregnancy outcome in schizophrenic women: occurrence and risk factors. Schizophr Res. 1998;33:1–26.

Bilezikian JP, Bandiera L, Khan A, Cusano NE. Hyperparathyroidism. Lancet. 2018;391:168–78.

Bioulac-Sage P, Sempoux C, Balabaud C. Hepatocellular adenomas: morphology and genomics. Gastroenterol Clin N Am. 2017;46:253–72.

Boafor TK, Olayemi E, Galadanci N, Hayfron-Benjamin C, Dei-Adomakoh Y, Segbefia C, Kassim AA, et al. Pregnancy outcomes in women with sickle-cell disease in low- and high-income countries: a systematic review and meta-analysis. BJOG. 2016;123:691–8.

Boga C, Ozdogu H. Pregnancy and sickle cell disease; a review of the current literature. Crit Rev Oncol Hematol. 2016;98:364–74.

Bolukbas FF, Bolukbas C, Horoz M, Ince AT, et al. Risk factors associated with gallstone and biliary sludge formation during pregnancy. J Gastroenterol Hepatol. 2006;21:1150–3.

Bonham CA, Patterson KC, Strek ME. Asthma and outcomes and management during pregnancy. Chest. 2018;153:515–27.

Breymann C. Iron deficiency anemia in pregnancy. Semin Hematol. 2015;52:339–47.

4

Brito V, Niederman MS. Pneumonia complicating pregnancy. Crit Chest Med. 2011;32:121–32.

Brummelte S, Galea LAM. Postpartum depression: etiology, treatment and consequences for maternal care. Horm Behav. 2016;77:153–66.

Calina D, Docea AO, Golokhvast KS, Sifakis S, Tsatsakis A, Makrigiannakis A. Management of endocrinopathies in pregnancy: a review of current evidence. Int J Environ Res Public Health. 2019;16(5). pii: E781. ► https://doi.org/10.3390/ijerph16050781.

Cappellini MD, Fiorelli G. Glucose-6-phosphate dehydrogenase deficiency. Lancet. 2008;371:64–74.

Carlberg KT, Singer ST, Vichinski EP. Fertility and pregnancy in women with transfusion-dependent thalassemia. Hematol Oncol Clin N Am. 2017;32:297–315.

Chaker L, Bianco AC, Jonklaas J, Peeters RP. Hypothyroidism. Lancet. 2017;390:1550–62.

Chen H, et al. Impaired CFDR-dependent amplification of FSH-stimulated estrogen production in cystic fibrosis and PCOS. J Clin Endocrinol Metab. 2012;97:923–32.

Chiossi G, Palomba S, Costantine MM, Falbo AI, Harirah HM, Saade GR, La Sala GB. Reference intervals for hemoglobin and hematocrit in a low-risk pregnancy cohort: implications of racial differences. J Matern Fetal Neonatal Med. 2019;32:2897–904.

Cho GJ, Kim YB, Kim SM, Hong HR, et al. Hepatitis A infection during pregnancy in Korea: hepatitis A infection on pregnant women. Obstet Gynecol Sci. 2013;56:368–74.

Choden T, Mandaliya R, Charabaty A, Mattar MC. Monitoring inflammatory bowel disease during pregnancy: current literature and future challenges. World J Gastrointest Pharmacol Ther. 2018;9:1–7.

Chowdhury AH, Lobo DN. Gallstones. Surgery. 2011;29:610–7.

Chrisoulidou A, Boudina M, Karavitaki N, et al. Pituitary disorders in pregnancy. Hormones. 2015;14: 70–80.

Christensen RD, Lambert DK, Henry E, et al. Unexplained extreme hyperbilirubinemia among neonates in a multihospital healthcare system. Blood Cells Mol Dis. 2013;50:105–9.

Chung AY, Duke MC. Acute biliary disease. Surg Clin N Am. 2018;98:877–94.

Cirino NH, Knapp JM. Perinatal posttraumatic stress disorder: a review of risk factors, diagnosis and treatment. Obstet Gynecol Surv. 2019;74:369–76.

Clark SM, Dutta E, Hankins GDV. The outpatient management and special considerations of nausea and vomiting in pregnancy. Semin Perinatol. 2014;38:496–502.

Clarke G, et al. Gut reactions: breaking down xenobiotic-microbiome interactions. Pharmacol Rev. 2019;71:198–224.

Cobey FC, Salem RR. A review of liver masses in pregnancy and a proposed algorithm for their diagnosis and management. Am J Surg. 2004;187:181–91.

Date RS, Kaushal M, Ramesh A. A review of the management of gallstone disease and its complications in pregnancy. Am J Surg. 2008;196:599–698.

De Bari O, Wang TY, Liu M, Paik CN, Portincasa P, Wang DQH. Cholesterol cholelithiasis in pregnant women: pathogenesis, prevention and treatment. Ann Hepatol. 2014;13:728–45.

De Franca Neto AH, Ramos do Amorim MM, Nobrega BM. Acute appendicitis in pregnancy: Literature review. Rev Assoc Med Bras. 2015;61:170–7.

De Genna NM, et al. Pregnancies, abortions, and births among women with and without borderline personality disorder. Womens Health Issues. 2012;22–4:e371–7.

De Leo S, Lee SY, Braverman LE. Hyperthyroidism. Lancet. 2016;388:906–18.

DeLoughery TG. Iron deficiency anemia. Med Clin N Am. 2017;101:319–32.

Den Hollander WJ, Schalekamp-Timmermans S, Holster IL, et al. Helicobacter pylori colonization and pregnancies complicated by preeclampsia, spontaneous prematurity, and small for gestational age birth. Helicobacter. 2017;22. ► https://doi.org/10.1111/hel.12364.

Dennis AT, Solnordal CB. Acute pulmonary edema in pregnant women (review). Anaesthesia. 2012;67:646–59.

Dhupar R, Smaldone GM, Hamad GG. Is there a benefit of delaying cholecystectomy for symptomatic gallbladder disease during pregnancy? Surg Endosc. 2010;2010(24):108–12.

Di Renzo GC, Spano F, Giardina I, Brillo E, Clerici E, Roura L. Iron deficiency anemia in pregnancy. Review. Woman's Health. 2015;11:891–900.

Diri H, Karaca Z, Tanriverdi F. Sheehan's syndrome: new insights into an old disease. Endocrine. 2016;51:22–31.

Dixon PH, Williamson C. The pathophysiology of intrahepatic cholestasis of pregnancy. Clin Res Hepatol Gastroenterol. 2016;40:141–53.

Drozdowski LA, Clandinin MT, Thomson ABR. Morphological, kinetic, membrane biochemical and genetic aspects of enteroplasticity. World J Gastroenterol. 2009;15:774–87.

Du X, Yuan Q, Yao Y, Li Z et al. Hypopituitarism and successful pregnancy. Int J Clin Exp Med. 2014;7:4660–5. eCollection 2014.

Dufernez F, Lachaux A, Chappius P, De Lumley L, Borst M, et al. Wilson disease in offspring of affected patients: report of four French families. Clin Res Hepatol Gastroenterol. 2013;37:240–5.

Dunkelberg JC, Berkley EMF, Thiel KW, Leslie KK. Hepatitis B and C in pregnancy: a review and recommendations for care. J Perinatol. 2014;34:882–91.

EASL Clinical Practice Guidelines: Wilson's disease. European association for study of liver. J Hepatol. 2012;56:671–85.

Edwards SM, Solveig A, Dunlop AL, Corwin EJ. The maternal gut microbiome during pregnancy. Am J Matern Child Nurs. 2017;42:310–7.

Ellegard EK. Pregnancy rhinitis. Immunol Allergy Clin N Am. 2006;26:119–35.

Evans CM, Simms LJ. Assessing inter-model continuity between the sections II and section III conceptualizations of borderline personality disorder in DSM-5. Personal Disord; Theory, Research and Treatment. 2018 May;8:290–6.

Eyden J, et al. A systematic review of the parenting and outcomes experienced by offspring of mothers with borderline personality pathology: potential mechanisms and clinical implications. Clin Psychol Rev. 2016;47:85–105.

Faa G et al. Review. Fetal programming of neuropsychiatric disorders. Birth Defects Research (part C). 2016;108:207–23.

Farrugia FA, Martikos G, Tzanetis P, et al. Pheochromocytoma, diagnosis and treatment: review of the literature. Endocr Regul. 2017;51:168–81.

Feghali M, et al. Pharmacokinetics of drugs in pregnancy. Semin Perinatol. 2015;39:512–9.

Fisher J, et al. Prevalence and determinants of common perinatal mental disorders in women in low- and middle-income countries: systematic review. Bull World Health Organ. 2012;90:139–49.

Fowden AL, Moore T. Maternal-fetal resource allocation: co-operation and conflict. Placenta. 2012;33:e11–5.

Frise CJ, Nelson-Piercy C. Peptic ulcer disease in pregnancy. J Obstet Gynecol. 2012;32:804.

Funder JW, Carey RM, Mantero F et al. The management of primary aldosteronism: case detection, diagnosis and treatment: an endocrine society clinical practice guideline. J Clin Endocrinol Metab. 2016;101:1889–916.

Gafni RI, Collins MT. Hypoparathyroidism. New Engl J Med. 2019;380:1738–47.

Galati SJ, Hopkins SM, Cheesman KC, et al. Primary aldosteronism: emerging trends. Trends Endocrinol Metabol. 2013;44:355–69.

Gaspersz MP, Klompenhouwer AJ, Broker MEE, et al. Growth of hepatocellular adenoma during pregnancy: a prospective study. J Hepatol. 2020;72:119–24.

Gelaye B, et al. Epidemiology of maternal depression, risk factors, and child outcomes in low-income and middle-income countries. Lancet Psychiatry. 2016;3:973–82.

Gentile S. Untreated depression during pregnancy short- and long-term effects in offspring. A systematic review. Neurosci. 2017;342:154–66.

Giles W, Murphy V. Asthma in pregnancy: a review. Obstet Med. 2013;6:58–63.

Glover V, et al. Prenatal maternal stress, fetal programming and mechanisms underlying later psychopathology – a global perspective. Dev Psychopathol. 2018;30:843–54.

Goodnight WH, Soper DE. Pneumonia in pregnancy. Crit Care Med. 2005;33:S390–7.

Grande I, Berk M, Birmaher B, Vieta E. Bipolar disorder. Lancet. 2016;387:1561–72.

Grasemann H, Ratjen F. Early lung disease in cystic fibrosis. Lancet. 2015;1:148–57.

Harris EL, et al. Psychiatric admission during pregnancy in women with schizophrenia who attended a specialist antenatal clinic. J Psychosom Obstet Gynecol. 2019;40:211–6.

Harrison PJ, Geddes JR, Tunbridge EM. The emerging neurobiology of bipolar disorder. Trends Neurosci. 2018;41:18–30.

Hatch Q, Champagne BJ, Maykel JA, et al. Crohn's disease and pregnancy: the impact of perianal disease on delivery methods and complications. Dis Colon Rectum. 2014;57:174–8.

Higham CE, Johannsson G, Shalet SM. Hypopituitarism. Lancet. 2016;388:2403–15.

Howard J, Oteng-Ntim E. The obstetrical management of sickle cell disease. Best Pract Res Clin Obstet Gynaecol. 2012;26:25–36.

Howdeshell KL, Ornoy A. Depression and its treatment during pregnancy: overview and highlights; Editorial. Birth Defects Res. 2017;109:877–8.

Howes OD, et al. The roles of genes, stress, and dopamine in the development of schizophrenia. Review. Biol Psychiatr. 2017;81:9–20.

Husebye ES, Allolio B, Arlt W, et al. Consensus statement on the diagnosis, treatment and follow-up of patients with primary adrenal insufficiency. J Intern Med. 2014;275:104–15.

Ibiebele I, et al. Appendicectomy during pregnancy and the risk of preterm birth. A population data linkage study. Aust NZ J Obstet Gynaecol. 2019;59:45–53.

Iijima S. Impact of maternal pheochromocytoma on the fetus and neonate. Gynecol Endocrinol. 2019;35:280–5.

Jha S, et al. Burden of common mental disorders among pregnant women: a systematic review. Asian J Psychiatr. 2018;36:46–53.

Johansen SL, et al. Management of perinatal depression with non-drug interventions. Brit Med J. 2019;364:1322 (15 pages).

Joshi MN, Whitelaw BC, Carroll PV. Hypophysitis: diagnosis and treatment. Eur J Endocrinol. 2018;179:R151–63.

Jung J, Rahman M, Rahman S, Thet Swe K, et al. Effects of hemoglobin levels during pregnancy on adverse maternal and fetal outcome: a systematic review and meta-analysis. Ann NY Acad Sci. 2019 Mai 31. ► https://doi.org/10.111/nyas.14112.

Kamoun M, Mnif MF, Charfi N, et al. Adrenal diseases during pregnancy; pathophysiology, diagnosis and management strategies. Am J Med Sci. 2014;347:64–73.

Kassenbaum NJ, et al. Global, regional and national levels and causes of maternal mortality during 1990–2013: a systematic analysis for the global burden of disease study 2013. Lancet. 2014;384:980–1004.

Kave M, Parooie F, Salarzaei M. Pregnancy and appendicitis: a systematic review and meta-analysis on the clinical use of MRI in diagnosis of appendicitis in pregnant women. World J Emerg Surg. 2019;14. ► https://doi.org/10.1186/s13017-019-254-1.

Kavitt RT, Lipowska AM, Anyane-Yeboa A, Gralnek IM. Diagnosis and treatment of peptic ulcer disease. Am J Med. 2019;132:447–56.

Kendall T, et al. Guidelines: borderline and antisocial personality disorders: summary of NICE guidance. BMJ. 2009;338:293–5.

Khan SJ, et al. Bipolar disorder in pregnancy and postpartum: principles of management. Curr Psychiatr Rep. 2016;18:13 (11 pages).

Khan AA, Clarke B, Rejnmark L, et al. Hypoparathyroidism in pregnancy: review and evidence-based recommendations for management. Eur J Endocrinol. 2019;180:R37–44.

Klompenhouwer AJ, Bröker MEE, Thomeer MGJ, Gaspersz MP, De Man RA, IJzerman JNM. Retrospective study on timing of resection of hepatocellular adenoma. Br J Surg. 2017;104:1695–703.

Ko CW, Beresford SAA, Schulte SJ, Matsumoto AM, Lee SP. Incidence, natural history, and risk factors for biliairy sludge and stones during pregnancy. Hepatology. 2005;41:359–65.

Koren G, Pariente G. Pregnancy-associated changes in pharmacokinetics and their clinical implications. Pharm Res. 2018;35:61 (7 pages).

Korevaar TIM, Medici M, Visser TJ, et al. Thyroid disease in pregnancy: new insights in diagnosis and clinical management. Nat Rev Endocrinol. 2017;13:610–22.

Kostic AD, Xavier RJ, Gevers D. The microbiome in inflammatory bowel disease: current status and the future ahead. Gastroenterology. 2014;146:1489–99.

Kourtis AP, Read JS, Jamieson DJ. Pregnancy and infection. New Engl J Med. 2014;370:2211–8.

Kovacs CS. Maternal mineral and bone metabolism during pregnancy, lactation and post-weaning recovery. Physiol Rev. 2016;96:449–547.

Kuo K, Caughey AB. Contemporary outcomes of sickle cell disease in pregnancy. Am J Obst Gynecol. 2016;215(505):e1–5.

Lacroix A, Feelders RA, Stratakis CA, Nieman LK. Cushing's syndrome. Lancet. 2015;386:913–27.

Lanas A, Chan FKL. Peptic ulcer disease. Lancet. 2017;390:613–24.

Landau E, Amar L. Primary aldosteronism and pregnancy. Ann Endocrinol (Paris). 2016;77:148–60.

Lao TT. Obstetric care for women with thalassemia. Best Pract Res Clin Obstet Gynaecol. 2017;39:89–100.

Larsson A, Palm M, Hansson L-O, Axelsson O. Reference values for clinical chemistry tests during normal pregnancy. BJOG. 2008;115:874–81.

Lee R, Nair M. Diagnosis and treatment of herpes simplex I virus infection in pregnancy. Obstet Med. 2017;10:58–60.

Leere JS, Vestergaard P. Calcium metabolic disorders: primary hyperparathyroidism, pregnancy-induced osteoporosis and vitamin D deficiency in pregnancy. Endocrinol Metab Clin N Am. 2019;48:643–55.

Lega I, Maraschini A, D'Aloja P, et al. Maternal suicide in Italy. Arch Women's Mental Health. 2020;23:199–206.

Leichsenring F, et al. Borderline personality disorder. Lancet. 2011;377:74–84.

Li Ren et al. Probiotic Lactobacillus rhamnosus GC prevents progesterone metabolite epiallaopregnanolone sulfate-induced hepatic bile acid accumulation and liver injury. Biochem Biophys Res Commun. 2019;520:67–72.

Lindsay JR, Nieman LK. The hypothalamic-pituitary-adrenal axis in pregnancy: challenges in disease detection and treatment. Endocrine Reviews. 2005;26:775–99.

Lonser RR, Nieman L, Oldfield EH. Cushing's syndrome: pathobiology, diagnosis and management. J Neurosurg. 2017;126:404–17.

Lopez A, Cacoub P, MacDougall IC, Peyrin-Biroulet L. Iron deficiency anaemia. Lancet. 2016;387:907–16.

Lumbers ER, Pringle KG. Roles of the circulating renin-angiotensin-aldosterone system in human pregnancy. Am J Physiol Regul Integr Comp Physiol. 2014;306:R91–101.

Lunjani N, Satitsuksanoa P, Lukasik Z, et al. Recent developments and highlights in mechanisms of allergic diseases: Microbiome. Allergy. 2018;73:2314–27.

Luzzatto L, Aresi P. Favism and glucose-6-phosphate dehydrogenase deficiency. New Engl J Med. 2018;378:60–71.

Magawa S, Tanaka H, Furuhashi F, Maki S, et al. A literature review of herpes simplex virus hepatitis in pregnancy. J Matern Fetal Neonatal Med. 2020;33:1774–9.

Malik A, Khawaja A, Sheikh L. Wilson's disease in pregnancy: case series and review of literature. BMC Research notes. 2013;6:421.

Malinowski AK, Shehata N, D'Souza R, Kuo KHM, Ward R, Shah PS, Murphy K. Prophylactic transfusion for pregnant women with sickle cell disease: a systemic review and meta-analysis. Blood. 2015;126:2424–35.

Mangla K, et al. Maternal self-harm deaths: an unrecognized and preventable outcome. Am J Obstet Gynecol. 2019;221:295–303.

Manoharan M, Sinha P, Sibtain S. Adrenal disorders in pregnancy, labour and postpartum – an overview. J Obstet Gynecol. 2019 aug 30; 1–10. ▶ https://doi.org/10.1080/01443615.2019.1648395.

McArdle JR. Pregnancy in cystic fibrosis. Clin Chest Med. 2011;32:111–20.

McCormack AL, Rabie N, Whittemore B, Murphy T, Sitler C, Magann E. HSV hepatitis in pregnancy: a review of the literature. Obstet Gynecol Surv. 2019;74:93–8.

McMullin MF, Bento C, Rossi C, Rainey MG, Girodon F, Cario H. Outcomes of pregnancy in patients with congenital erythrocytosis. Br J Haematol. 2015;170:586–8.

McMullin MF. Congenital erythrocytosis. Int J Lab Hem. 2016;38(suppl. 1):59–65.

Merikangas KR, et al. Prevalence and correlates of bipolar spectrum disorder in the world mental health survey initiative. Arch Gen Psychiatry. 2011;68:241–51.

Mikolasevic I, Filipec-Kanizaj T, Jakopcic I, et al. Liver disease during pregnancy: a challenging clinical issue. Med Sci Monit. 2018;24:4080–90.

Miloudi N, Brahem M, Ben Abid S, Mzoughi H, Arfa N, Tahar Khalfallah M. Acute appendicitis in pregnancy: specific features of diagnosis and treatment. J Visc Surg. 2012;149:e275–9.

Mohsen W, Levy MT. Hepatitis A to E: what's new? Int Med J. 2017;47:380–9.

Molitch ME. Prolactinoma in pregnancy. Best Pract Res Clin Endocrinol Metab. 2011;25:885–96.

Morton A. Primary aldosteronism and pregnancy. Review. Pregnancy Hypertens. 2015;5:259–62.

Mullur R, Liu YY, Brent GA. Thyroid hormone regulation of metabolism. Physiol Rev. 2014;94:355–82.

Muñoz M, Peña-Rosas JP, Robinson S, Milman N, Holzgreve W, Breymann C, et al. Patient blood management in obstetrics: management of anaemia and haematinic deficiencies in pregnancy and the post-partum period: NATA consensus statement. Transfus Med. 2018;28:22–39.

Murphy VE, Gibson P, Talbot PI, et al. Severe asthma exacerbations during pregnancy. Obstet gynecol. 2005;106:1046–54.

Murphy VE, Jensen ME, Gibson PG. Asthma during pregnancy: exacerbations, management, and health outcome for mother and infant. Semin Respir Crit Care Med. 2017;38:160–73.

Namazy JA, Schatz M. Management of asthma during pregnancy: optimizing outcome and minimizing risk. Semin Respir Crit Care Med. 2018;39:29–35.

4

Nault JC, Paradis V, Cherqui D, Vilgrain V, Zucman-Rossi J. Molecular classification of hepatocellular adenoma in clinical practice. J Hepatol. 2017;67:1074–83.

Neuman H, Koren O. The pregnancy microbiome. Nestle Nutr Inst Workshop Ser. 2017;88:1–9.

Nillni YI, et al. Treatment of depression, anxiety and trauma-related disorders during the perinatal period: a systematic review. Clin Psychol Rev. 2018;66:136–48.

Norman J, Politz D, Politz L. Hyperparathyroidism during pregnancy and the effect of rising calcium on pregnancy loss: a call for earlier intervention. Clin Endocrinol. 2009;71:104–9.

Ohkusa T, Kiodo S. Intestinal microbiota and ulcerative colitis. J Infect Chemother. 2015;21:761–8.

Ornoy A, et al. Antidepressants, antipsychotics, and mood stabilizers in pregnancy: what do we know and how should we treat pregnant women with depression. Review. Birth Defects Res. 2017;109:933–56.

Oteng-Ntim E, Meeks D, Seed PT, Webster L, Howard J, Doyle P, Chappell LC. Adverse maternal and perinatal outcomes in pregnant women with sickle cell disease: systemic review and meta-analysis. Blood. 2015;125:3316–25.

Owen MJ, et al. Schizophrenia. Lancet. 2016;388:86–97.

Papi A, Brightling C, Pedersen SE, et al. Asthma. Lancet. 2018;391:783–800.

Pare-Miron V, et al. Effect of borderline personality disorder on obstetrical and neonatal outcomes. Womens Health Issues. 2016;26–2:190–5.

Parkes I, Schenker JG, Shufaro Y. Parathyroid and calcium metabolism disorders during pregnancy. Gynecol Endocrinol. 2013;29:515–9.

Pastore PA, Loomis DM, Sauret J. Appendicitis in pregnancy. J Am Board Fam Med. 2006;19:621–6.

Patel EM, Swami GK, Heine P, Kuller JA, James AH, Grotegut CA. Medical and obstetric complications among women with cystic fibrosis. Am J Obstet Gynecol. 2015;212:98e1–9.

Pearce EN. Thyroid disorders during pregnancy. Best Pract Res Clin Obstet Gynecol. 2015;29:700–6.

Petrakos G, Andriopoulos P, Tsironi M. Pregnancy in women with thalassemia: challenges and solutions. Int J Women's Health. 2016;8:441–51.

Pfeiffenberger J, Beinhardt S, Gotthardt DN, Haag N, Freissmuth C, et al. Pregnancy in Wilson's disease: management and outcome. Hepatology. 2018;67:1261–9.

Phillips J, et al. The six most essential questions in psychiatric diagnosis: a pluralogue part 2: issues of conservatism and pragmatism in psychiatric diagnosis. Philos Ethics Humanit Med. 2012;7:8(16 pages).

Picano E, Pelikka PA. Ultrasound of extravascular lung water; a new standard for pulmonary congestion. Eur Heart J. 2016;37:2097–104.

Piel FB, Steinberg MH, Rees DC. Sickle cell disease. New Engl J Med. 2017;376:1561–73.

Portincasa P, Moschetta A, Palasciano G. Cholesterol gallstone disease. Lancet. 2006;368:230–9.

Rac MWF, Sheffield JS. Prevention and management of viral hepatitis in pregnancy. Obstet Gynecol Clin N Am. 2014;41:573–92.

Rac H, Gould AP, Eiland LS, et al. Common bacterial and viral infections: review of management in the pregnant patient. Ann Pharmacother. 2018 Dec 17;1060028018817935. (Epub ahead of print).

Rainey WE, Rehman KS, Carr BR. Fetal and maternal adrenals in human pregnancy. Obstet Gynecol Clin N Am. 2004;31:817–35.

Rebouissou S, Bioulac-Sage P, Zucman-Rossi J. Molecular pathogenesis of focal nodular hyperplasia and hepatocellular adenoma. J Hepatol. 2008;48:163–70.

Rees DC, Williams TN, Gladwin MT. Sickle-cell disease. Lancet. 2010;376:2018–31.

Rigg J, Gilbertson E, Barrett HL, et al. Primary hyperparathyroidism in pregnancy: maternofetal outcomes at a quaternary referral obstetric hospital, 2000-through 2015. J Clin Endocrinol Metab. 2019;2019(104):721–9.

Rogler G, Biederman L, Scharl M. New Insights into the pathophysiology of inflammatory bowel disease: microbiota, epigenetics and common signaling pathways. Swiss Med Wk. 2018;148:w14599.

Rogliani P, Ora J, Puxeddu E, Cazzola M. Airway obstruction: is it asthma or is it COPD? Int J Chron Obstruct Pulmon Disease. 2016;11:3007–13.

Rusner M, et al. Bipolar disorder in pregnancy and childbirth: a systematic review of outcomes. BMC Pregnancy and Childbirth. 2016;16:331 (18 pages).

Savajols E, Burguet A, Grimaldi M, Godoy F, Sagot P, Semama DS. Maternal haemoglobin and short-term neonatal outcome in preterm neonates. Plos One. 2014;9(2):e89530.

Schlüter DK, Griffiths R, Adam A, et al. Impact of cystic fibrosis on birthweight: a population-based study of children in Denmark and Wales. Thorax. 2018 July 19;1–8.

Schneider HJ, Aimaretti G, Kreitschmann-Andermahr I, et al. Hypopituitarism. Lancet. 2007;369:1461–70.

Scholl TO, Reilly T. Anemia, iron and pregnancy outcome. Review. J Nutr. 2000;130:443S–7S.

Serati M, et al. Perinatal major depression biomarkers: a systematic review. J Affect Disord. 2016;193:391–404.

Shao Z, Al-Tibi M, Wakim-Fleming J. Update on viral hepatitis in pregnancy. Cleve Clin J Med. 2017;84:202–6.

Sharma V, et al. Childbirth and prevention of bipolar disorder: an opportunity for change. Lancet Psychiatry. 2019;6:786–92.

Sheffield JS, Cunningham FG. Community-acquired pneumonia in pregnancy. Obstet Gynecol. 2009;114:915–22.

Shulman LP, Elias S. Cystic fibrosis. Clin Perinatol. 2001;28:383–93.

Silasi M, Cardenas I, Racicot K, Kwon JY, Also P, Mor G. Viral infections during pregnancy. Am J Reprod Immunol. 2015;73:199–213.

Sinesi A, et al. Anxiety scales used in pregnancy: a systematic review. BJ Psych Open. 2019;5:e5 (13 pages).

Smoller JW. Disorders and borders: psychiatric genetics and nosology. Am J Med Genet B Neuropsychiatr Genet. 2013;162B:559–78.

Srour SA, Devesa SS, Morton LM, Check DP, Curtis RE, Linet MS, Dores GM. Incidence and patient survival of myeloproliferative neoplasms and myelodysplastic/myeloproliferative neoplasms in the United States 2001–2012. Br J Haematol. 2016;174:382–96.

Sternlieb I. Wilson's disease and pregnancy. Hepatology. 2000;31:531–2.

Stilo SA, Murray RM. Non-genetic factors in schizophrenia. Curr Psychiatr Rep. 2019;21:100 (10 pages).

Stowasser M, Gordon RD. The renaissance of primary aldosteronism: what has it taught us? Heart Lung Circ. 2013;22:412–20.

Susser LC, et al. Selective serotonin reuptake inhibitors for depression in pregnancy. Am J Obstet Gynecol. 2016;215:722–30.

Taguchi N, Oda S, Kobayashi T, Naoe H, et al. Advanced parametric imaging for evaluation of Crohn's disease using dual-energy computed tomography enterography. Radiol Case Rep. 2018;13:709–13.

Tahel AT, Weatherall DJ, Cappellini MD. Thalassaemia. Lancet. 2018;391:155–67.

Tandon R, et al. Definition and description of schizophrenia in the DSM-5. Schizophr Res. 2013;150:3–10.

Tase A, Kamarizan MFA, Swarnkar K. Appendicitis in pregnancy: difficulties in diagnosis and management. Guidance for the emergency general surgeon: a systematic review. Int J Surg Open. 2017;6:5–11.

Taylor SM, Parobek CM, Fairhurst FM. Haemoglobinopathies and the clinical epidemiology of malaria: a systemic review and meta-analysis. Lancet Infect Dis. 2012;12:457–68.

Ten S, New M, McLaren N. Addison's disease: clinical review 130. J Clin Endocrinol Metab. 2001;86:2909–22.

Teodorescu A, et al. Dilemma of treating schizophrenia during pregnancy: a case series and a review of the literature. BMC Psychiatry. 2017;17:311 (4 pages).

Terrault NA, Bzowei NH, Chang KM, Hwang JP, Jonas MM, Murad MH. AASLD guidelines for treatment of chronic hepatitis B. Hepatology. 2016; 261–83.

Thomeer MG, Broker M, Verheij J, Doukas M, Terkivatan T, Bijdevaate D, De Man RA, Moelker A, IJzermans JN. Hepatocellular adenoma: when and how to treat? Update of current evidence. Therap Adv Gastroenterol. 2016;9:898–912.

Thorsness KR, et al. Perinatal anxiety: approach to diagnosis and management in the obstetric setting. Am J Obstet Gynecol. 2018;219:326–45.

Torres A, Niederman MS, Chastre J, et al. International ERS/ESICM/ESCMID/ALAT guidelines for the management of hospital-acquired pneumonia and ventilator-associated pneumonia. Eur Respir J. 2017a;50:1700582.

Torres J, Mehandru S, Colombel JF, Peyrin-Biroulet L. Crohn's disease. Lancet. 2017b;389:1741–55.

Ungaro R, Mehandru S, Allen PB, Peyrin-Biroulet L, Colombel JF. Ulcerative colitis. Lancet. 2017;389:1756–70.

Van de Mheen L, Smits SM, Terpstra WE et al. Haemolytic anaemia after nitrofurantoin treatment in a pregnant woman with G6PD deficiency. BMJ Case Rep. 2014. ▶ https://doi.org/10.136/brc-2013-010087.

Van der Weerd K, Van Noord C, Loeve M, et al. Pheochromocytoma in pregnancy: case series and review of literature. Eur J Endocrinol. 2017;177:R49–58.

Van der Woude CJ, Ardizzone S, Bengtson MB, Fiorino G, Fraser G, Katsanos K, Kolacek S, Juillerat P, Mulders AG, Pedersen N, Selinger C, Sebastian S, Sturm A, Zelinkova Z, Magro F. The second European evidenced-based consensus on reproduction and pregnancy in inflammatory bowel disease. J Crohns Colitis. 2015;9:107–24.

Vanders RL, Murphy VE. Maternal complications and the management of asthma in pregnancy. Womens Health. 2015;11:183–91.

Varlamov EV, McCartney S, Fleseriu M. Functioning pituitary adenomas- current treatment options and emerging medical therapies. Eur Endocrinol. 2019;15:30–40.

Venerito M, Vasapolli R, Rokkas T, Delchier J-C, Malfertheiner P. Helicobacter pylori, gastric cancer and other gastrointestinal malignancies. Helicobacter. 2017;22(Suppl. 1):e12413.

Vijay A, Elaffandi A, Khalaf A. Hepatocellular adenoma: an update. World J Hepatol. 2015;7:2603–9.

Ward RM, Varner MW. Principles of pharmacokinetics in the pregnant woman and fetus. Clin Perinatol. 2019;46:383–98.

Ware RE, De Montalembert M, Tshilolo L, Abboud MR. Sickle cell disease. Lancet. 2017;390:311–23.

Williams KE, Koleva H. Identification and treatment of peripartum anxiety disorders. Obstet Gynecol Clin. 2018;45:469–81.

Yacovino LL, Aleksunes LM. Endocrine and metabolic regulation of renal drug transporters. J Biochem Mol Toxicol. 2012;26:407–21.

Yin J, Wang J. Renal drug transporters and their significance in drug-drug interactions. Acta Pharm Sin B. 2016;6:363–73.

Yurdaydin C. Recent advances in managing hepatitis D. F1000Res. 2017;6:1596 (10 pages).

Zivot A, Lipton JM, Narla A, Blanc L. Erythropoiesis: insights in pathophysiology and treatments in 2017. Mol Med. 2018;24:11. ► https://doi.org/10.1186/s10020-018-0011-z.

Prevention & early detection of common pregnancy disorders

Abstract

The previous chapters provided an overview of the normal maternal adaptation to pregnancy. This information was then used as a reference to discuss the pathophysiology of common pregnancy disorders in seemingly healthy women and women with a preexistent chronic disorder. This final chapter summarizes the options to early identify in these two subgroups those women that are really at high risk to develop (one of) these complications, followed by a description of the options to prevent these complications to develop or at least, to minimize their clinical impact in case they do develop anyway.

5

Highlights

1. Educating women prior to conception is the best way to prevent common pregnancy disorders. Knowledge and information helps differentiate between common pregnancy discomforts and early signs of what could be a serious complication. It is most effective if the woman's own care provider communicates this guidance in a personal setting. During a prepregnancy consultation, the care provider should also inform/motivate his/her client on the importance of a healthy lifestyle. Such a consultation is likely to raise (1) a woman's self-confidence and positiveness in her relation with her care provider and (2) the chance she will alert her care provider more quickly when a relevant complication emerges;

2. Pregnant women at increased risk of a placental syndrome (PS) benefit from having the one-step FIGO-endorsed risk assessment between 11 and 14 weeks. This test identifies over 90 % of women that will develop an early-onset PS (< 34th week) and allows the timely use of low-dose aspirin prophylaxis, which has been shown to reduce the risk of developing early-onset PS by over 60 %.

3. The multifactorial risk profile of spontaneous preterm birth (sp-PTB) makes its early detection more complex. This may explain why two-thirds of sp-PTB cases occur unexpectedly and in the absence of a clear risk factor. Currently, it is only effective to offer screening to women at high risk of sp-PTB, because of a previous sp-PTB. Only these women benefit from screening in midpregnancy by measuring cervical length and serum fetal fibronectin levels, and if positive, to institute secondary prevention by cervical cerclage and intramuscular progesterone injections. Women at risk of sp-PTB for other reasons should follow primary prevention that consists of lifestyle and behavioral changes.

4. Gestational diabetes mostly affects women with modifiable risk factors already present before pregnancy. Therefore, it is most effective to offer preconceptional screening to all women at-risk because of advanced age, high BMI, demographic/ethnicity features and personal/family history. This screening consultation should include the measurement of fasting glucose and a glucose tolerance test, supplemented by realistic, personalized lifestyle and behavioral advices.

5.1 **General**

Discomforts often observed in uneventful pregnancy are usually mild and transient, but occasionally severe and even hampering normal functioning. Most of these annoyances are benign side-effects of the adaptations evolving in the various organ systems of the maternal body. In some cases, certain complaints may signal the presence of a subclinical disorder, associated with an increased risk, either to develop certain pregnancy complications or to aggravate the preexistent disorder. For instance, gallstone disease and gastrointestinal reflux disease are more likely to become symptomatic during pregnancy due to the slower peristalsis in the biliary and GI tracts, respectively. The same applies to the metabolic syndrome that predisposes to the development of gestational diabetes in the second half of pregnancy, and a preexistent thrombophilic condition (e.g. protein-S deficiency) that predisposes to thromboembolic events in pregnancy. On the other hand, new complaints developing in pregnancy, such as e.g. headache, are more complex. If a preexistent or 'primary' headache had been diagnosed before pregnancy as 'migraine', the complaint often tends to improve in advanced pregnancy, presumably because of the disappearance of cyclic fluctuations in steroid levels (Negro et al. 2017). However, migraine is also associated with a higher risk of developing a hypertensive disorder in pregnancy (Aukes et al. 2019). It follows that every 'new-onset' headache in pregnancy, but also a change in the clinical presentation of a primary headache requires thorough diagnostic work-up to avoid a delay in identifying the underlying cause and the potential negative impact of delayed clinical management (Negro et al. 2017). These inferences apply to all other primary complaints that develop in pregnancy, even when these complaints may initially mimic pregnancy-related effects.

In the seventies and eighties of the last century, various screening tests have been introduced to identify women at risk of developing common pregnancy complications – most frequently – with emphasis on identifying women at increased risk of developing early-onset preeclampsia (PE). Initially, screening consisted of recognizing these women based on unfavorable demographic features (such as poor socio-economic factors, older age) and/or on an unhealthy lifestyle or health issues (such as issues in their medical history, BMI > 30 kg.m^2, harmful nutrition/eating habits, sedentary lifestyle, smoking, low physical fitness). Such a selection procedure may seem clinically useful as it enables offering these women closer surveillance from early pregnancy onwards. However, a downside of this policy was a low sensitivity, giving rise to a high rate of 'by-catch' – the subgroup of 'false-positives' – prone to be subjected to unnecessary anxiety and medicalization. In this context, it is relevant to emphasize that the validity of a screening test depends on the following features: (1) Efficiency in case-finding (sensitivity, specificity and positive predictive value); (2) Whether health benefit of *early* detection exceeds that of later clinical detection; (3) Potential harm associated with the test procedure, and (4) Whether health benefits from testing outweigh screening costs. Ideally, these aspects should be determined by randomized controlled trials.

In the last decades, a wide range of new, more sensitive screening methods have been developed by adding biomarkers to demographic features and medical history. Recently, these procedures have been reviewed. Among the many reported tests that have been developed for the early detection of women at risk for early-onset PE, one was endorsed by the International Federation of Gynecology and Obstetrics (FIGO). This particular test consists of a one-step strategy carried out between 11 and 14 weeks of pregnancy (Poon et al. 2019). The logistics of the test and some background information is provided in the ■ figs. 5.1 and 5.2. The resulting estimate for risk combines the maternal risk profile based on demography plus medical/obstetrical history with the measurement of mean arterial pressure (MAP) and the biomarkers, serum placental growth factor (PLGF) and uterine artery pulsatility index (UAPI). The algorithm to calculate the risk predicted > 90 % of the cases of early-onset PE and 54 % of all PE cases, respectively, using a 10 % fixed false-positives rate (Akolekar et al. 2013). Among the many reported tests over the last 2 decades, this particular screening test was the only one, that was also externally validated in a large double-blind follow-up study (Rolnik et al. 2017). In that study, patients with a positive test outcome were randomized into a control – and a study group, using a placebo or 150 mg aspirin prophylaxis daily, respectively, from the day of screening until the 36th week of pregnancy. The rate of early-onset PE in the study group was more than 60 % lower than that in the control group.

5

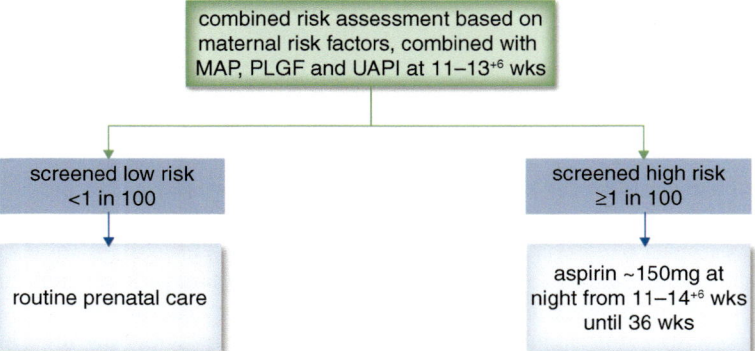

□ Figure 5.1   Logistics of the one-step, FIGO-endorsed risk assessment between 11 and 14 weeks to identify women destined to develop early-onset preeclampsia and her their eligibility for aspirin prophylaxis. *Abbreviations*: MAP, mean arterial pressure; PLGF, placental growth factor; UAPI uterine artery pulsatility index (*adopted from* Rolnik et al. 2017 and Poon et al. 2019)

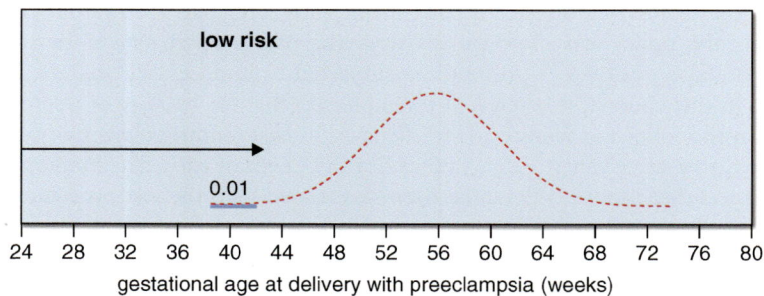

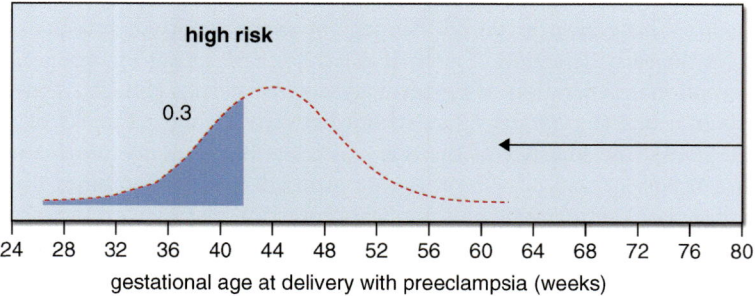

□ Figure 5.2   Gestational age (GA) distribution at the time of birth of women delivering because of preeclampsia (PE) in a low-risk (top) and high-risk (bottom) population. Using a competing risk model focusing on a high-risk population, the number of identified patients in the target range of GA (< 34 weeks) increases, since the entire at-risk population is 'pushed' to an earlier GA by combining demographic & medical history data with two biomarkers (dark area in bottom graph), thus increasing sensitivity of the test (*adopted from* Wright et al. 2015)

The usefulness of a screening test is reflected in the relationship between true-positives (sensitivity) and false-positive rate (1-specificity), known as a 'receiver operating characteristic' (ROC). The accuracy of the test is reflected in the area under the ROC curve (AUC). An AUC of 0.50 indicates that the test accuracy is no better than chance. Meanwhile, an AUC of over 0.90 indicates very good diagnostic accuracy. The reported AUC for detecting PE with onset before 32 weeks in the validation study mentioned above, was 0.896 (Tan et al. 2018). It follows that the FIGO-endorsed risk assessment was both accurate and clinically useful, as it identified almost 90 % of the women at high-risk of developing early-onset PE. Moreover, the identified at-risk women were found to have benefited from aspirin prophylaxis, resulting in more than 60 % fewer women developing early-onset PE, presumably due to the aspirin prophylaxis. Compared to no screening, this screening test has important health benefits, is associated with lower costs, and also shields test-negative women from anxiety and redundant diagnostic procedures.

Yet, the risk assessment did not really *prevent* early-onset PE. First, the observed values of both biomarkers in the test show that subnormal placental blood supply (high UAPI) and placental dysfunction (low PLGF) were already detectable by 11–14 weeks pregnancy in women destined to develop early-onset PE. Thus, the risk assessment did not predict early-onset PE, but rather identified women with *subclinical* early-onset PE. Therefore, aspirin did not prevent, but tempered the progression of subclinical early-onset PE. Secondly, around 10 % of the women that developed early-onset PE had a negative test outcome, a rather low figure. However, not only these false-negative women, but also an additional 36 % test-negative, at-risk women, developed PE anyway, but only after the 34th week (Akolekar et al. 2013; Tan et al. 2018). Even though, the clinical impact of PE developing after the 34th week is usually milder than that of early-onset PE, the later-onset PE that had developed in almost half (46 %) of test-negative at-risk women may also have a serious clinical impact on mother as well as the infant. This emphasizes that breaking down at-risk patients into subgroups of 'test-positives' and 'test-negatives', as if these subgroups are mutually exclusive, has various undesirable effects, even though the actual test result is accurate. These effects relate to the a priori selection of only at-risk women to be tested. This aspect does not devaluate the FIGO-endorsed risk-assessment. However, these unexplored and underreported shortcomings should not be ignored in the global appraisal of the test's possibilities and limitations and therefore, should also be taken into account in clinical decision making.

Meanwhile, the clinical urge to develop better risk assessments to prevent common pregnancy disorders does have to overcome the restraint caused by our still limited insight into the onset of many common pregnancy complications. As a matter of fact, prevention of the 3 most common pregnancy complications, placental syndromes, preterm birth and gestational diabetes (GDM), is most effective by the earliest possible detection of their onset. For any risk assessment intended to identify women that deviate from normality already in the first trimester, one should keep in mind that embryo implantation initiates a unique, and intimate interaction between embryo and decidua that still largely unfolds beyond our current scientific horizon.

The maternal adaptation to pregnancy consists of three components. (1) Accepting the semi-allograft infant as a temporal host, (2) Providing the infant with the means to grow and mature in line with its genetic potential, and (3) at term, providing the infant a safe exit from the uterine cavity to the outer world. These key features require adaptive changes in the maternal immune function, the presence of a uterus capable of accommodating and nourishing the infant throughout pregnancy and at term, providing the means and conditions for a safe delivery. Last but not least, the transition to maternity also includes the physical and mental preparation of the pregnant woman. These events result in the maternal adaptive changes listed in ▪ tab. 5.1.

Our understanding of the events that evolve in the window of embryo implantation is still incomplete. Yet, promising targets for the earliest possible detection of a placental syndrome are events involved in either the development of immunotolerance or the initial events that accompany the institution of the hemodynamic and metabolic adaptations.

▪ Table 5.1 Pregnancy-induced physiologic changes along with some common collateral effects.

trigger	intended effect	adaptive response	effects	risks
1. crosstalk of dNKs with decidual stroma cells and EVTs	suppression local innate immune function	acceptance semi-allograph (embryo)	mild systemic inflammatory response	higher vulnerability for viral infections (?)
2. relaxin, along with progesterone and other placental vasodilators; initially raised, later on, reduced insulin sensitivity	vascular relaxation	total peripheral vascular resistance ↓	hyperdynamic circulation→ renal hyperfiltration & a-v shunting ↑	relative hypovolemia; risk of orthostasis ↑ → excessive RAAS activity
	SMCR surrounding central and art. baroreceptors	downwards reset setpoints of arterial BP and osmolality	sodium and water retention; Expansion ECV	orthostatic edema ↑
	securing fetal supply of O_2 and metabolic substrates	hyperphagia, preferential glucose availability for fetus (low-threshold IR)	stimulation of production clotting factors	risk of developing obesity, gestational DM, and thrombosis
	central nervous system	downwards resetting CO_2-setpoint in respiratory center	respiratory vital and minute volume ↑	restless legs, insomnia, fatigue, neuropathy's (carpal tunnel syndr.) ↑
3. relaxin, ↓ P/E ratio, placenta & membranes aging	preparation birth canal	laxity of all joints and ligaments ↑	hyperflexible joints	pelvic/girdle pain, backache/ imbalance ↑

Abbreviations: EVTs, extra-villous trophoblasts; RAAS, renin-angiotensin-aldosterone system; a-v, arteriovenous; SMCR, smooth muscle cell relaxation; BP, blood pressure; ECV, extracellular volume; P/E ratio, progesterone/estrogen ratio; IR, insulin resistance; DM, diabetes mellitus

5.2 Placental syndromes (PS)

Theoretically, an attractive target to avert the development of a *placental syndrome* is an event that closely relates to embryo implantation, such as the preparational response of the innate immune system at the implantation site. Based on our current insights in the physiology of embryo implantation, plausible targets for elucidating its disruption and the events evolving in the early phases of placentation are listed in ◘ tab. 5.2.

The development of *maternal immunotolerance* towards the embryo begins 2–3 days before embryo implantation, when natural killer (NK) cells in the maternal blood accumulate in the decidua (dNK), where endometrial stromal cells induce their maturation and with it, alter their phenotype (Leno-Duran et al. 2014). This maturation of dNK cells accelerates with the blastocyst implantation into the maternal decidua. Then, mature dNK cells begin to release specific cytokines, growth factors and angiogenic factors that finetune decidual remodeling and optimise local conditions for blastocyst implantation and invasion. An important development is the binding of dNK cells to HLA-G on extravillous trophoblast cells (EVTs) using their inhibitory receptor KIR2DL4 (◘ fig. 5.3). This link abolishes the dNKs' cytotoxicity, thus inducing immunotolerance of EVTs as detailed previously (Leno-Duran et al. 2014; Ferreira et al. 2017; Ander et al. 2019).

◘ **Table 5.2** Attractive targets for a screening program intended to identify in the first-trimester, women at increased risk of developing a placental syndrome

adaptation to be evaluated	measurements between 8 and 10 weeks	what does result tell you?	what remains obscure?
immunotolerance	*at implantation site*: number & expression patterns of dNK cells and EVTs, and % dNK-cells bound to EVT. *peripheral blood*: BSE; leucocytosis	local degree of immune tolerance; development of a mild *physiologic* systemic leukocytosis	yes/no higher vulnerability for certain viral infections
hyperdynamic circulation	*serum levels* of urea, creat, Hct and osmol (expected ↓), PV (expected ↑) 24-h urine creat/albumin	evolution/degree of HD-circulation, hemodilution and renal hyperfiltration	how to determine adequacy of *relative* hypovolemia?
	CO (HR, SV) (expected ↑), 24-h-*BP monitoring*; beat-to-beat variation (expected ↑)	basal CO and sympathetic response resembling that to standard exercise	is the rise in CV sympathetic activity normal or excessive?
anabolic metabolism	leptin, *serum levels* of pre-prandial glucose & insulin	degree & evolution anabolic metabolism	is degree of developing anabolism 'normal'?

Abbreviations: dNKs, decidual natural killer cells; EVTs, extravillous trophoblast cells; BSE, blood cell sedimentation rate; Hct, hematocrit; creat, creatinine; osmol, osmolality; PV, plasma volume; HR, heart rate, SV, stroke volume; HD, hyperdynamic; RQ, respiratory quotient

5

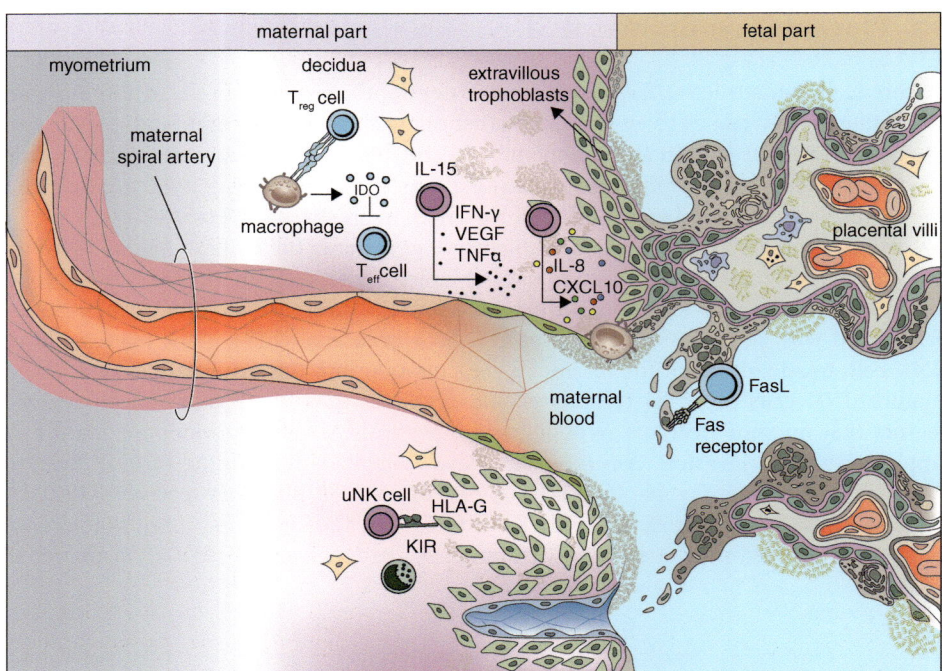

◘ Figure 5.3 Regulation of maternal immunotolerance towards the conceptus. The decidua basalis contains an abundance of uNKs, that mature in the decidua in response to uterine IL-15. By releasing a wide range of cytokines (e.g. IFN-γ, VEGF, TNF-α, IL-8) and chemokines (e.g. CXCL10), mature uNKs promote decidual remodeling, blastocyst implantation and EVTs' decidual invasion. uNKs also bind to HLA-G, expressed by EVTs, which protects them against uNK-mediated cytotoxicity. Finally, the enzyme IDO, released by decidual macrophages prevents T-cell activation, thus further limiting local cytotoxicity. *Abbreviations*: uNKs, uterine natural killer cells; IL, interleukin; EVTs, extravillous trophoblast cells; HLA-G, human leukocyte antigen G; IDO, indoleamine-2,3-dioxygenase; KIR, killer cell inhibitory receptor. FasL, ligand of the Fas protein, which is involved in apoptosis, the process of physiologic programmed cell death (*adopted from* Ander et al. 2019)

Adequate maternal immunotolerance is pivotal for a successful pregnancy and requires the proper regulation, not only of the number of dNK cells that accumulate in the decidua basalis at the time of implantation, but also of their functions. Verification of normal immunotolerance in a clinical setting requires insight into the expression patterns of both dNKs and EVTs during blastocyst implantation. At present, it is illusive to get access to this information as it may require sampling of these decidual cells by biopsy, which represents an invasive procedure imposed to the relatively small implantation site. Most likely, this disturbs local physiology, presumably resulting in a spontaneous miscarriage.

In the 8 to 10 weeks after embryo implantation, the mother develops a *hyperdynamic circulation (HDC)*. This implies that her total peripheral vascular resistance (TPVR) gradually falls, accompanied by a circa 30–40 % compensatory rise in cardiac output (CO) without appreciable rise in basal metabolic rate (Spaanderman et al. 2000a). The fall in TPVR results from a pregnancy-induced relaxation of vascular smooth muscle cells (VSMCs) (Duvekot et al. 1995) primarily triggered by the luteal hormone relaxin

(Conrad 2011) as detailed in ▶ chap. 1. The rise in CO appears to be a safeguard to avert a fall in arterial pressure and cerebral blood flow in response to the fall in TPVR. Therefore, it is not surprising that most of the generated extra CO is metabolically redundant and directed to the kidneys and arteriovenous (a-v) shunts in the systemic vascular bed. The HDC that develops in pregnancy, induces eccentric cardiac remodeling (shown in ▶ chap. 1 ◘ fig. 1.12), closely resembling the one observed in endurance-trained athletes (Weiner and Baggish 2012; De Haas et al. 2017). Eccentric cardiac remodeling enables the ejection of a larger stroke volume, thus increasing cardiac efficiency.

An essential aspect in the pregnancy-induced HDC development is a transient state of cardiovascular underfill, that triggers both volume retention and a rise in cardiovascular sympathetic activity. This, in turn, leads to concomitant increases in cardiac preload, inotropy and chronotropy to boost CO (which compensates for the fall in cardiac afterload). If the underfill state of the vascular bed lasts for an extended period, backup adjustments will emerge to replace the increased cardiovascular sympathetic tone. The most important cardiac adaptive response in this respect is the pregnancy-induced cardiac remodeling depicted in ▶ chap. 1, ◘ fig. 1.12, that improves cardiac efficiency by enabling prolonged ejection of a larger stroke volume without requiring the support of a concomitantly raised cardiovascular sympathetic tone. It is unclear, why HDC and resulting ECR already develop in the first half of pregnancy, when maternal metabolic demands are only marginally increased (De Haas et al. 2017). Presumably, early cardiac remodeling secures the timely preparation of the maternal heart for the approximate 40 % extra cardiac work required in the second half of pregnancy. This averts the need for a rise in cardiovascular sympathetic tone during a period of pregnancy, when such a compensation would compromise the uteroplacental blood flow. Indirect support for this idea comes from the observation that failure to develop HDC and eccentric cardiac remodeling early in pregnancy predisposes a woman to a placental syndrome in advanced pregnancy (Aardenburg et al. 2006).

If embryo implantation fails because of defective immunotolerance, luteal insufficiency or a genetic defect of the embryo, the trigger for the development of HDC will be absent as well (Donaghay and Lessey 2007). However, when both embryo implantation and the related trigger for the development of a HDC are normal, the vasodilator response to relaxin may also be subnormal or absent, because of defective end-organ responsiveness resulting from reduced arterial compliance. This may apply to women with essential hypertension (Spaanderman et al. 2000b).

In a normal pregnancy, the first signs of the developing HDC are already discernible one week after embryo implantation (Davison and Lindheimer 1989). It is plausible that subnormal HDC development contributes to the defective embryo implantation and early placentation in women developing a placental syndrome later on in pregnancy. As a matter of fact, excessive hypovolemia in this critical period may induce such a strong rise in cardiovascular sympathetic tone that it also raises uteroplacental vascular resistance, and with it, compromises early placental development. Therefore, a more beneficial risk assessment than the FIGO-endorsed test for these women may be to *determine the quality of the HDC development* between the 8th and 12th pregnancy weeks. The test result will already be available several weeks earlier than the FIGO-endorsed test, enabling both an earlier start of aspirin prophylaxis, and the option to explore, whether additional prophylaxis e.g. tempering of the excessive sympathetic cardiovascular tone, enhances the effect of aspirin.

Preventing a *placental syndrome* is best served by discerning the increased risk for this complication as early as possible. Therefore, a first medical consultation should be planned 3 to 6 months before an intended conception and may be offered to (1) all healthy nulliparous women, but at least to nulliparous women, who are at increased risk, because of obesity, obvious signs of an unhealthy lifestyle, poor stress coping, or a family history of placental syndromes; (2) women with a history of early-onset placental syndrome, and (3) women affected by one of the preexistent medical disorders discussed in ► chap. 3 and 4. During this pre-pregnancy risk assessment all relevant details of a woman's own medical history and that of her family, along with her lifestyle, socioeconomic condition nutritional state and eating habits should be recorded, followed by a general physical exam and finally the exams listed in ◘ tab. 5.3. The embryo is most vulnerable to epigenetic programming in the first-trimester of pregnancy. Therefore, this particular consultation should also be used to inform the woman about the importance of these aspects and discuss with her the options to optimize her lifestyle (Cuneo 2017; Oostingh et al. 2019) and eating habits, as delineated elsewhere (Jones et al. 2017; Baker et al. 2018; Reijnders et al. 2019). In the third subgroup mentioned above, the prepregnant medical evaluation should be followed by the woman's visit to the specialist that performs the regular check-ups of her medical disorder. During this appointment, the woman should be informed about the possible effects of pregnancy on her medical disorder, the impact of pregnancy on her current medication, and the possible necessity to replace these drugs by pregnancy-friendly alternatives.

The pre-pregnancy medical check-up will be extra useful, when its outcome can be utilized as a reference for the results obtained from a follow-up medical exam at the end of the first trimester of pregnancy as detailed in ◘ tab. 5.3. Such a comparison provides the best possible insight into magnitude and quality of a woman's HDC development in pregnancy (Spaanderman et al. 2001).

◘ **Table 5.3**   Content of a prepregnant and first-trimester medical check-up of risk profile in the three subgroups as detailed in the text.

systems to be evaluated	measurements before, and again between 8 and 12 weeks pregnancy	what does result mean?
baseline renal/volume functions and their response to pregnancy	serum levels of creatinine, hematocrit, osmolality, C-reactive protein (CRP), & erythrocyte sedimentation rate (ESR); In a 24-h urine collection: creatinine and albumin	degree of hypo-osmolality (dilution), basal creatinine clearance (GFR), pregnancy-induced rise GFR, and that in albuminuria
cardiovascular function & sympathetic activity	24-hrs blood pressure (BP) & heart rate (HR) recording; BP/HR sitting & standing; ECG and cardiac output (CO) measurement	hyperdynamic response (HR/CO), degree of orthostasis and of the rise in CV sympathetic activity
uterine BF velocity	pulsatility index (PI) in the uterine artery	risk fetal growth restriction
anabolic metabolism	leptin, pre-prandial glucose and insulin	extent of developing anabolism

Pregnancy puts extra strain upon the cardiovascular, renal and metabolic functions. It follows that the focus of both the prepregnant and first-trimester medical check-ups is first, to identify subclinical abnormalities in the circulatory, renal, and metabolic functions in the non-pregnant state, and second, to explore whether these issues affect the adaptive response to pregnancy in these three systems. ◻ Table 5.3 lists the measurements that should be included in both sets of medical tests, along with the information that will be provided by the test results.

Feasibility, efficiency and cost/effectiveness of the strategy proposed above is currently evaluated in a properly powered, prospective study. It follows that the most effective, evidence-based preventive procedure with respect to a placental syndrome for the time being, is the FIGO-endorsed test between 11 and 14 weeks pregnancy as discussed earlier in this chapter. One may argue, whether it is ethical to deny the aspirin prophylaxis to the test-negatives within the pre-selected at-risk group, as the associated risk of adverse side effects is very low.

5.3 Preterm birth (PTB)

PTB is the leading cause of neonatal mortality and morbidity worldwide, accounting for about 75 % of perinatal deaths and more than half of long-term infant morbidities. Unfortunately, almost all known intrinsic and extrinsic factors potentially involved in causing spontaneous preterm birth unrelated to placental dysfunction (sp-PTB) are only traceable after midpregnancy (Talati et al. 2017). It follows that currently, no suitable *early* target is available, that causally relates to sp-PTB.

Both pathophysiology and clinical presentation of PTB is complex, because PTB is a multifactorial complication with at least the following six factors contributing to its pathogenesis: (1) Mechanical properties of the uterus (distensibility) and the cervix (to remain closed), (2) Pregnancy-induced endocrine environment suppressing myometrial activity until near-term, (3) Size and growth rate of the intrauterine content (fetus, placenta and amniotic fluid), (4) Aging of placenta and membranes (eventually triggering an inflammatory response), (5) Signature of primarily the cervicovaginal microbiota, and (6) Possible presence of genetic variants in the innate immune function that predispose to a pathologic inflammatory response (Strauss III et al. 2018).

The risk of sp-PTB is also influenced by external factors, such as socioeconomical background, chronic diseases, nutritional state, ethnicity, smoking and experienced psychological stress (Voltolini et al. 2013). The 6 features listed above, are both gestational age-dependent and mutually interrelated. Early identification of women destined to have their pregnancy ending in a sp-PTB is further complicated by the fact that the mechanism that results into irreversible sp-PTB eventually merges into the deregulation of the immune system and an exaggerated inflammatory response. This may explain, why two-thirds of sp-PTB cases occur unexpectedly and in the absence of a clear risk factor (Vogel et al. 2018). The overlap of sp-PTB with normal term birth complicates the search for a consistent, cost-effective, first-trimester screening test to identify low-risk patients doomed to develop sp-PTB. The screening test at present, only offered to women at high risk of sp-PTB because of a previous sp-PTB, consists of measuring cervical length and/or serum fetal fibronectin levels in midpregnancy. However, the accuracy in predicting sp-PTB in *low-risk* nulliparous, singleton pregnancies using these two predictors is low (Esplin et al. 2017; Bloom and Leveno 2017).

■ **Table 5.4**   Preterm birth risk factors reported in odds ratio (OR) and relative risk (RR) (*adopted from* Wade et al. 2020)

	risk factor	impact on PTB
1.	multiple pregnancy	OR ≅ 6–10
2.	prior preterm birth	OR ≅ 5–6
3.	short cervix (< 20 mm)	RR ≅ 3–6
4.	genital infections	OR ≅ 2–8
5.	tobacco use (> 20 sig/d)	OR ≅ 1.5
6.	pyelonephritis	OR ≅ 1.3
7.	inter-pregnancy Interval (< 6 m)	OR > 1.2

Recent studies suggest that the signature of the cervicovaginal microbiota and vaginal β-defensin-2 levels in at-risk women has the potential to identify women at risk for sp-PTB earlier (Elovitz et al. 2019). This line of research is likely to result in the development of a screening test based on detecting specific microbial signatures in maternal blood in midpregnancy (Subramaniam et al. 2020). For the time being, the only method to early identify women at risk of sp-PTB is combining demography with features of the medical and obstetrical history (■ tab. 5.4), unfortunately, a risk assessment with modest sensitivity (Wade et al. 2020).

Since an accurate screening test for sp-PTB in early pregnancy is lacking, many women at increased risk of sp-PTB due to either demographic features or medical/family history, could be offered some preventive measures, which should be non-invasive and without relevant side effects (because of the likelihood of instituting these measures to a relatively large subgroup of 'false-positive' women). Therefore, it is not surprising that *primary preventive measures for sp-PTB* in general consist of lifestyle and behavioral changes, such as exercise, better eating habits and the use of nutritional supplements, preferably supported by nutritional education (Matei et al. 2019). Also, screening for lower genital tract infections reduces the risk of sp-PTB (Medley et al. 2018; Matei et al. 2019). Prolongation of pregnancy observed in women on low-dose aspirin prophylaxis to prevent early-onset PE, may be a welcome side-effect of the improved placental function in most of these women. In the *secondary* prevention of sp-PTB, intravaginal progesterone supplementation and cerclage in women with a short cervix have been found effective (Matei et al. 2019). The evidence is rather limited for interventions, such as intramuscular progesterone injections in multiple pregnancies, cervical pessary in singleton pregnancies with a short cervix and treatment of periodontal disease (Medley et al. 2018).

5.4 Gestational diabetes (GDM)

GDM is the most common metabolic disorder affecting up to 7 % of pregnancies worldwide (Donovan et al. 2019). A pregnancy complicated by GDM is not only associated with a high rate of maternal complications during pregnancy (such as preterm birth, placental syndromes) and labor (such as assisted vaginal delivery, cesarean delivery for dystocia or fetal distress). The metabolic abnormalities in GDM may also induce epigenetic programming in the fetus, excessive fetal growth and various neonatal complications, such as respiratory distress syndrome, cardiomyopathy and hypoglycemia. As GDM mostly affects women with modifiable risk factors already present before pregnancy, it is most effective to aim for *preconceptional screening of women at-risk for GDM* based on age, BMI, demography, ethnicity and personal/family history, as elaborated elsewhere (Donovan et al. 2019). This strategy identifies women at risk for GDM fairly accurately, creating the possibility to offer them a program for assisted and targeted lifestyle changes, known to reduce the risk of developing GDM. First-trimester screening for GDM has been discussed in ▶ chap. 2 and included in ◘ tab. 5.3.

The pregnancy-related changes in the *maternal metabolism* develop in two phases as discussed in ▶ chap. 1 and illustrated in ◘ fig. 1.18. In the first half of pregnancy the maternal energy stores are expanded in response to various hormonal changes. Meanwhile, the second half of pregnancy is dominated by the mobilization of these energy stores to meet the progressive growth of energy demands, not only of the conceptus, but also of the (then increased) maternal basal metabolism. To this end, the early-pregnancy maternal endocrine environment induces an increase in appetite and with it, hyperphagia, and a higher insulin sensitivity to support the build-up of fat and glycogen stores (Augustine et al. 2008). In the second half of pregnancy, this effect is reversed as reflected in the low-threshold insulin resistance (as detailed in ▶ chap. 1) and leptin resistance (Ladyman et al. 2010) (▶ chap. 1, ◘ fig. 1.18). With respect to screening tests in the first trimester, it is important to take into account the anabolic state of the metabolism. The identification of at-risk women for GDM may benefit most of preconceptional screening, enabling pre-pregnancy preventive measures (Donovan et al. 2019).

Screening of at-risk women for GDM in the first-trimester and the subsequent clinical management of women at increased risk for GDM, has been discussed in ▶ chap. 2.

Chapters 3 and 4 focused on course and outcome of pregnancy in women with a preexistent chronic disorder. Most of these disorders are managed by prescription drugs. Therefore, we supplemented ▶ chap. 4 with a section on the effect of pregnancy on pharmacokinetics and the consequences for the management of pregnant women with a preexistent disorder that require ongoing medical treatment during pregnancy. Yet, the clinical management of these patients during pregnancy is beyond the scope of this book and therefore, the interested reader is referred to review articles and guidelines that discuss this management in more detail, including the possible necessity to switch to alternative medication.

In summary, the inferences presented in this chapter indicate that first-trimester *screening for placental syndromes* in at-risk women by the so-called one-step FIGO-endorsed risk assessment is both medically beneficial and cost-effective. Possible improvement may emerge from current studies designed to determine the predictive potential of magnitude and quality of the HDC development in the first trimester of pregnancy. Such an HDC-test may identify women responding abnormally to the endogenous HDC-trigger, along with those with limited renal reserves. *Early screening for sp-PTB* in a low-risk population is currently not feasible by evidenced-based tests, although developments are in progress to identify at-risk women by a test based on detecting specific microbial signatures in maternal blood in midpregnancy (Subramaniam et al. 2020). *Screening for GDM* would benefit most of the pre-pregnant evaluation of insulin resistance and insulin reserves, followed by a program of supervised lifestyle and nutritional adjustments as detailed in ▶ chap. 2 and reported recently (Baker et al. 2018; Van Dijk et al. 2019). If a woman at-risk for GDM presents for the first time in pregnancy, the pre-pregnant check-up can be performed in the first trimester of pregnancy.

All risk assessments mentioned above are only feasible, if quality, capacity and organization level of the maternal care system are adequate. To this end, care provision requires subdivision into levels of medical complexity, that is to say, basic, specialty, sub-specialty and regional perinatal care, as detailed elsewhere (ACOG 2019).

In pregnancy, a unique transient physiologic condition develops with two genetically different individuals closely interacting with one another. It secures the vital preservation of the species. To this end, the reproductive function has been strengthened during the course of evolution. Yet, particularly its complexity in key adaptations in the maternal immune, cardiovascular and metabolic functionality to host the infant in the maternal body, to enable it to grow and mature according to its genetic potential, implies that some women will not be able to meet these preconditions. If maladaptation in one of these functions can be detected early on by a screening test, both the mother and infant will benefit from the timely institution of targeted preventive measures to at least delay the onset, or minimize the severity of the suspected complication. Besides, women identified as being at risk for a certain pregnancy complication (and therefore, advised to participate in a special prevention program), will likely gain a motivational boost to both follow the clinical advice and alert their health care provider on a timely basis, when early signs of that specific complication develop.

References

Aardenburg R, et al. A low plasma volume in formerly preeclamptic women predisposes to the recurrence of hypertensive complications in the next pregnancy. J Soc Gynecol Invest. 2006;13:598–603.

ACOG. Levels of maternal care. Obstetric Care Consensus No. 9 American College of Obstetricians and Gynecologists. Obstet Gynecol. 2019;134:e41–55.

Akolekar R, et al. Competing risk model in early screening for preeclampsia by biophysical and biochemical markers. Fetal Diagn Ther. 2013;33:8–15.

Ander SE, et al. Immune responses at the maternal-fetal interface. (review) Sci Immunol. 2019;4:10.

Augustine RA, et al. From feeding one to feeding many: hormone-induced changes in bodyweight homeostasis during pregnancy. J Physiol. 2008;586:387–97.

Aukes AM, Yurtsever FN, Boutin A, et al. Associations between migraine and adverse pregnancy outcomes: systematic review and meta-analysis. Obstet Gynecol Survey. 2019;74:738–48.

Baker M, et al. Intervention strategies to improve nutrition and health behaviours before conception. Lancet. 2018;391:1853–64.

Bloom SL, Leveno KJ. Unproven technologies in maternal-fetal medicine and the high cost of US health care. JAMA. 2017;317:1025–6 (editorial).

Conrad KP. Maternal vasodilation in pregnancy: the emerging role of relaxin. Am J Physiol Regul Integr Comp Physiol. 2011;301:R267–75.

Cuneo J. Women's Health. Pregnancy and conception. Prim Care Clin Office Pract. 2017;44:369–76.

Davison LM, Lindheimer MD. Volume homeostasis and osmoregulation in human pregnancy. Balliere's Clin Endocrinol Metab. 1989;3:451–72.

De Haas S et al. Cardiac remodeling in normotensive pregnancy and in pregnancy complicated by hypertension: systematic review and meta-analysis. Ultrasound Obstet Gynecol. 2017;50:683–96è.

Donaghay M, Lessey BA. Uterine receptivity: alterations associated with benign gynecologic disease. Semin Reprod Med. 2007;25:461–75.

Donovan BM, et al. Development and validation of a clinical model for preconception and early-pregnancy risk prediction of gestational diabetes mellitus in nulliparous women. PLoS-ONE. 2019;14(4):e215173.

Duvekot JJ, et al. Maternal volume homeostasis in early pregnancy in relation to fetal growth restriction. Obstet Gynecol. 1995;85:361–7.

Elovitz MA, et al. Cervicovaginal microbiota and local immune response modulate the risk of spontaneous preterm delivery. Nature Comm. 2019;10(1305):8 pages.

Esplin MS, et al. Predictive accuracy of serial transvaginal cervical lengths and quantitative vaginal fetal fibronectin levels for spontaneous preterm birth among nulliparous women. JAMA. 2017;317:1047–56.

Ferreira LMR et al. HLA-G: at the interface of maternal-fetal tolerance. (review). Trends Immunol. 2017;38:272–86.

Jones C, et al. Fetal programming and eating disorder risk. J Theor Biol. 2017;428:26–33.

Ladyman SR, et al. Hormone interactions regulating energy balance during pregnancy. J Neuroendocrinol. 2010;22:805–17.

Leno-Durán E, et al. Liaison between natural killer cells and dendritic cells in human gestation. Cell Mol Immunol. 2014;11:449–55.

Matei A, et al. Primary and secondary prevention of preterm birth: a review of systematic reviews and ongoing randomized controlled trials. Eur J Obstet Gynecol Reprod Biol. 2019;236:224–39.

Medley N et al. Interventions during pregnancy to prevent preterm birth: an overview of Cochrane systematic reviews. Cochrane Database Syst Rev. 2018;11:CD012505.

Oostingh EC, Hall J, Koster MPH, et al. The impact of maternal lifestyle factors on preconceptional outcomes: a systemic review of observational studies. Reprod Biomed Online. 2019;38:77–94.

Poon LC, et al. The International Federation of Gynecology and Obstetrics (FIGO) initiative on pre-eclampsia: A pragmatic guide for first-trimester screening and prevention. Int J Gynecol Obstet. 2019;145(suppl. 1):1–33.

Negro A et al. Headache and pregnancy: a systematic review. J Headache Pain. 2017;18(106):20.

Reijnders IF, Mulders AGMGJ, Van der Windt M et al. The impact of maternal lifestyle on clinical features and biomarkers of placental development and function: a systematic review. Hum Reprod Update. 2019;25:72–94.

Rolnik DL, et al. Aspirin versus placebo in pregnancies at high risk for preterm preeclampsia. New Engl J Med. 2017;377:613–22.

Spaanderman MEA, et al. Cardiac output increases independently of basal metabolic rate in early human pregnancy. Am J Physiol Heart Circ Physiol. 2000a;278:H1585–8.

Spaanderman MEA, et al. Latent hemodynamic abnormalities in symptom-free women with a history of preeclampsia. Am J Obstet Gynecol. 2000b;182:101–7.

Spaanderman MEA, et al. Preeclampsia and maladaptation to pregnancy: A role for atrial natriuretic peptide? Kidney Int. 2001;60:1397–406.

Strauss JF III, et al. Spontaneous preterm birth: advances towards discovery of genetic predisposition. Am J Obstet Gynecol. 2018;218(292–314):e2.

Subramaniam A, et al. Midtrimester microbial DNA variations in maternal serum of women who experience spontaneous preterm birth. J Matern Fetal Neonatal Med. 2020;33:367–559.

Talati AN, et al. Pathophysiology of preterm labor with intact membranes. Semin Perinatol. 2017;41:420–6.

Tan MY, et al. Screening for pre-eclampsia by maternal factors and biomarkers. Ultrasound Obstet Gynecol. 2018;52:186–95.

Van Dijk MR, Koster MPH, Oostingh EC. A mobile app lifestyle intervention to improve healthy nutrition in women before and during early pregnancy: single-center randomized controlled trial. J Med Internet Res. 2020;22:e15773.

Vogel JP, et al. The global epidemiology of preterm birth. Best Bract Res Clin Obstet Gynecol. 2018;52:3–12.

Voltolini C et al. Understanding spontaneous preterm birth: from underlyng mechanisms to predictive and preventive interventions. Reprod Sci. 2013;20:1274–92 (Review).

Wade EE et al. The state of the science of preterm birth. Assessing contemporary screening and preventive strategies. J Perinat Neonat Nurs. 2020;34:113–24.

Weiner RB, Baggish AL. Exercise-induced cardiac remodeling. Prog Cardiovasc Dis. 2012;54:380–6.

Wright D, et al. Competing risk models in screening for preeclampsia by maternal characteristics and medical history. Am J Obstet Gynecol. 2015;213(62):e1–10.

Supplementary Information

Index – 269

Index

U

V

W

Z

Your free e-book on Mijn BSL

Every copy of this book is accompanied by a unique activation code that gives the owner free and unlimited access to the online version of the book, including online extras.

How do I obtain online access to the book on Mijn BSL?
Simply go to ►www.bsl.nl/activatie, follow the steps and enter the activation code below to access your online product.

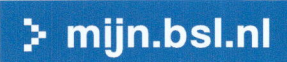

Your unique activation code:

XCKY-3TMA-V4F7-R89E

Have you already activated your code? Log in directly at ►www.mijnbsl.nl.

Need technical support?
Are you having problems logging in or are you experiencing other technical difficulties? Please contact onlineklantenservice@bsl.nl

Printed by Printforce, the Netherlands